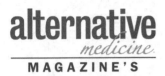

alternative *medicine*
MAGAZINE'S
Definitive Guide to Weight Loss

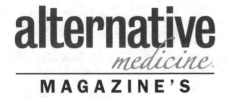

alternative *medicine.*
MAGAZINE'S

Definitive Guide to Weight Loss

10 Healthy Ways to
Permanently Shed Unwanted Pounds

SECOND EDITION

Ellen Kamhi, Ph.D., RN, HNC

CELESTIAL ARTS
Berkeley | Toronto

Many of the designations used by manufacturers and sellers to distinguish their products are claimed as trademarks. Where the publisher is aware of a trademark claim, such designations, in this book, have initial capital letters.

The information contained in this book is based on the experience and research of the author. It is not intended as a substitute for consulting with your physician or other health-care provider. Any attempt to diagnose and treat an illness should be done under the direction of a health-care professional. The publisher and author are not responsible for any adverse effects or consequences resulting from the use of any of the suggestions, preparations, or procedures discussed in this book.

Cartoons copyright ©2002 and 2003 by Randy Glasbergen, www.glasbergen.com.

Photograph of Swimming Dragon pose by T. K. Shih.

Photographs for the Super Seven Home Workout by Brad Kevelin.

"Six Myths About Stress" adapted from *The Stress Solution* by Lyle H. Miller, PhD, and Alma Dell Smith, PhD, available at www.apahelpcenter.org, thanks to the American Psychological Association.

Optimum Foods for Ayurvedic Body Types chart adapted from *The Ayurvedic Encyclopedia* by Swami Sada Shiva Tirtha, copyright 1998.

Key Healthy Recipes coutesy of Sprouts Farmers Market, www.sprouts.com.

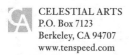

CELESTIAL ARTS
P.O. Box 7123
Berkeley, CA 94707
www.tenspeed.com

Distributed in Australia by Simon and Schuster Australia, in Canada by Ten Speed Press Canada, in New Zealand by Southern Publishers Group, in South Africa by Real Books, and in the United Kingdom and Europe by Publishers Group UK.

Cover design by Chloe Rawlins
Text design by Chris Hall

LIBRARY OF CONGRESS CATALOGING-IN-PUBLICATION DATA
Kamhi, Ellen.
     Alternative Medicine Magazine's definitive guide to weight loss : 10 healthy ways to permanently shed unwanted pounds / by Ellen Kamhi. — 2nd ed.
          p. cm.
     Summary: "This book uses alternative medicine methods to offer safe, simple ways to lose weight. It provides the tools to make better food choices, use supplements wisely, start exercising, resolve emotional issues, and correct the underlying imbalances that may be contributing to weight gain." — Provided by publisher.
     Includes bibliographical references and index.
     ISBN-13: 978-1-58761-259-6
     ISBN-10: 1-58761-259-3
     1. Weight loss — Popular works. 2. Nutrition — Popular works. 3. Alternative medicine — Popular works. I. Title.
     RM222.2.K25 2007
     613.2'5 — dc22   2006020000

First printing this edition 2007
1   2   3   4   5   —   11 10 09 08 07

Contents

About the Author

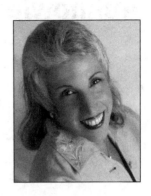

Ellen Kamhi, Ph.D., RN, HNC

Ellen Kamhi attended Rutgers and Cornell universities, sat on the Panel of Traditional Medicine at Columbia Presbyterian Medical School, and is a clinical instructor at Stony Brook Medical School. She was nominated for the March of Dimes Woman of Distinction in 2004 and received the J. G. Gallimore award for research in science. A respected authority in the field of natural healing, Dr. Kamhi is a professional member of the American Herbalist Guild (AHG), is nationally board certified as a holistic nurse (a-HNC), and works to bring together a body of modern and ancient practices and philosophies that use less invasive, less toxic, natural techniques to enhance wellness. Ellen Kamhi is the author of *Cycles of Life: Herbs and Energy Techniques for the Stages of a Woman's Life* and *The Natural Guide to Great Sex* and coauthor of *The Natural Medicine Chest* and *Arthritis: An Alternative Medicine Definitive Guide*, and appears daily on radio and television. She is quoted in mainstream magazines, including the *New York Post*, the *New York Times*, *Self*, *Latina*, and *Marie Claire*, and is on the editorial board of the peer review journal *Alternative Therapies in Health and Medicine*. Along with Dr. Eugene Zampieron, ND, Ellen is cofounder of Natural Alternatives Health Education and Multimedia, which sponsors international workshops on natural medicine. She also participates in the design and development of herbal and nutritional products for Nature's Answer, in Hauppauge, NY, and sees patients in private practice.

The Natural Nurse, www.naturalnurse.com

Acknowledgments

I am so happy to have this opportunity to share the diet, exercise, and lifestyle protocols that have helped keep me, my family, and my patients in tip-top shape, even as we move into advanced years. Writing a book is a time-consuming labor of love, and an effort that usually relies on the expertise and assistance of others. I would like to thank those who have shaped, inspired, influenced, motivated, and supported my efforts. To my parents, Julius, who still works full-time, and Sondra, who swims two miles a day, and my children, gourmet chef Brenda, personal trainer Titus, and naturopathic physician Ali, thank you for all your love and support. To my friends Dr. Michael and Lois Posner, who were occasionally successful at pulling me away from my work marathons, and for providing clinical insight used in this book. To Bill for his photography, and who shares so many of my interests, including herbs, healthy eating, and working out. To MyKey, who lightened my life with love and laughter during the writing of this manuscript. To all my wonderful teachers, especially Serafina Corsello, MD, whose intensity, fortitude, depth of knowledge, and wonderful healthy cooking is always a joy! To Nature's Answer, for providing me with the ongoing opportunity to be involved with the production of wholesome herbal and nutritional products. To my business partner and soul brother, Eugene Zampieron, for his ongoing, intense investigations into the highest level of knowledge about natural medicine. To G-D, the ultimate source of healing.

Important Information for the Reader

Your health and that of your loved ones is important. Treat this book as an educational tool that will enable you to better understand and assess your condition and treatment options and choose the best course of treatment when a health problem arises, as well as how to prevent health problems such as obesity from developing in the first place. It could save your life.

Remember that this book on weight management is different. It is not a diet book. Unlike the countless fad diets, alternative medicine recognizes that one size does not fit all. Fad diets don't work because they do not address the unique biochemistry of each individual, nor do they take into account the underlying imbalances that may have caused you to gain weight in the first place. Rather than simply emphasizing weight loss, this book will instead show you how to correct imbalances and reduce toxicity so that you will gradually return to a healthy weight. This book is about alternative approaches to health — approaches which may not be understood by mainstream physicians. We urge you to discuss the treatments described in this book with your doctor. We have been gratified to learn that many of our readers have found their physicians open to new ideas presented to them.

Use this book wisely. As many of the treatments described in this book are, by definition, alternative, they have not necessarily been investigated, approved, or endorsed by any government or regulatory agency. National, state, and local laws may vary regarding the use and application of many of the treatments discussed. Accordingly, this book should not be substituted for the advice and care of a physician or other licensed health-care professional. Pregnant women and people using prescription medications, in particular, are urged to consult a physician before commencing any therapy. Ultimately, you must take responsibility for your health and how you use the information in this book.

All of the factual information in this book has been drawn from the scientific literature. To protect privacy, all patient names have been changed. Branded products and services discussed in the book are evaluated solely on the independent and direct experience of the health-care practitioners quoted. Reference to them does not imply an endorsement nor a superiority over other branded products and services, which may provide similar or superior results.

A weight-loss program should be undertaken only under the supervision of a qualified health-care practitioner. Anyone with heart disease, atherosclerosis, diabetes, sleep apnea, osteoarthritis, gallstones, hypertension, or a family history of heart disease, or women who are pregnant or breast-feeding should consult with their doctor before embarking on a weight-loss program. Neither the publisher nor the author of this book take responsibility for any adverse effects experienced due to using any of the suggestions contained in this book.

Introduction: Dieting Is Not the Answer

Let's be clear about it from the start: Dieting is not the answer. Good health is the key to weight management. Ultimately, weight loss is less about dieting and more about regaining a state of health. This book outlines a healthy lifestyle plan that can literally extend your life and improve your overall quality of life while keeping you svelte, sexy, and energetic into your golden years. To achieve significant and permanent weight loss, you need to come up with a plan that incorporates healthier eating, exercise, stress reduction, and healing any underlying imbalances. This approach will help you feel and look better for a lifetime. I invite you to use this book as a guide to finding a personal plan that you can live with. And let's emphasize *you!*

By now, you may have been riding the fad diet merry-go-round for quite some time and might feel ready to jump off. You've followed one regimented diet after another, eaten the prescribed prepackaged or powdered foods, counted calories, given up flavor in favor of low fat, and gone to the support groups. And you may even have lost some weight, but only to see the pounds

IN THE INTRODUCTION

- We're Getting Fatter
- Serious Health Conditions Linked to Being Overweight
- What Causes Weight Gain?
- Are You Overweight?
- Why This Book Is Different
- How to Use This Book

Bingeing and the Low-Calorie Diet

The average individual will begin to lose weight when they eat fewer than 1,500 calories per day (SEE QUICK DEFINITION). However, low-calorie diets often go much lower than this amount, some to as low as 300 calories per day. Many people who try to bring their calorie intake down to this level develop overeating or bingeing behaviors, uncontrollably eating a large quantity of food in a short period of time.

Bingeing is not a sign of weakness or lack of willpower, but rather a response to the biochemical disruptions caused by a very low-calorie diet. Among the disruptions is reduced activity of the thyroid gland (SEE QUICK DEFINITION). When food intake is reduced, the thyroid responds by secreting fewer hormones, thus lowering metabolism (SEE QUICK DEFINITION) and conserving the body's energy resources. This slowing of metabolism works against the dieter's goal, as less body fat will be burned when metabolism slows. In time, the body will attempt to correct the imbalance and restore thyroid function, often by bingeing. Binge eating may also be a physiological response to an increase in plasma ghrelin levels, so severely restricting calories is clearly not the answer.

reappear after you went off the program. It is a sad fact that most people who lose weight through dieting end up gaining the pounds back—and then some. Many factors are responsible for this. Of course, returning to previous habits of poor eating and not exercising play an important role. Most people grow weary of the restrictions associated with extreme diets. Many health experts also question the long-term safety of fad diets. In addition, the hormone known as ghrelin, which regulates appetite, may hold the key to this ping-pong effect experienced by most dieters (see page 163). When people begin to lose weight due to dietary restriction, they often experience an increase in plasma ghrelin levels, which in turn increases appetite. This rise in ghrelin among dieters may represent the body's evolutionary response to restricting calories and may be part of the reason why people who lose weight through dieting often experience an increase in appetite.[1]

 A **calorie** is a measure of the energy-producing potential contained in food. In practical terms, the number of calories in a particular food tells you how much fuel you're getting from eating it.

We're Getting Fatter

The unmistakable fact is that Americans are getting fatter. We are growing more and more overweight even as we obsess about our appearance. The increased incidence in obesity in the United States is so severe that it has prompted establishment of federal clinical guidelines on the identification, evaluation, and treatment of overweight and obesity, developed by the combined efforts of the National Heart, Lung, and Blood Institute and the National Institute of Diabetes and Digestive and Kidney Diseases. The shocking truth is that 97 million adults in the United States are overweight or obese. In fact, the Department of Epidemiology and Public Health at the University of Miami School of Medicine concluded, "Obesity has emerged as one of the most important public health issues in the United States."[2]

Higher body weight isn't simply a matter of appearance or vanity, it's associated with increased mortality from all causes,[3] and from specific illnesses, including the following:

- High blood pressure
- Type 2 diabetes (SEE QUICK DEFINITION)
- Coronary heart disease
- Stroke
- Gallbladder disease
- Osteoarthritis
- Sleep disturbances
- Respiratory problems
- Endometrial, breast, prostate, and colon cancers

 QUICK DEFINITION The thyroid gland, one of the body's seven endocrine glands, is located in the throat area, and wraps around the windpipe right behind the Adam's apple. It is the body's metabolic thermostat, controlling body temperature, energy use, and, in children, the body's growth rate. The thyroid controls the rate at which organs function and the speed with which the body uses food. Hypothyroidism is a condition of low or underactive thyroid gland function that can produce one or more of as many as 47 symptoms, including fatigue, depression, lethargy, weakness, weight gain, and low body temperature. A resting body temperature below 97.8°F may indicate hypothyroidism.

Metabolism is the biological process by which energy is extracted from the foods consumed, producing carbon dioxide and water as by-products for elimination. There are two kinds of metabolism constantly underway in the cells: anabolic and catabolic. The anabolic function produces substances for cell growth and repair, while the catabolic function controls digestion, disassembling food into forms the body can use for energy.

The association between obesity and early death is so clearly defined that physicians reporting in the New England Journal of Medicine cite the following as potential causes for lowering overall life expectancy in the United States:

- Two-thirds of American adults are overweight or obese.
- As many as 30% of U.S. children are overweight.
- Childhood obesity has more than doubled within the past 25 years.

- Within the past 20 years, childhood diabetes has increased tenfold.[4]

In addition to health risks, societal costs of an overweight population include expenses for medical care and workers' compensation and millions of dollars in lost productivity, which continues to be a burden for everyone. Health-care costs related to obesity increased tenfold between 1987 and 2002, and there's no end in sight.[5]

Serious Health Conditions Linked to Being Overweight

Here's a roundup of just a few of the serious health conditions linked to being overweight:

Diabetes

The incidence of type 2 (adult-onset) diabetes has tripled in the last 40 years, and it continues to rise. A vast majority (80%) of those with adult-onset diabetes are overweight. Studies have found that losing weight helps diabetics control their disease with less reliance on medications. Losing weight also reduces the risk of developing diabetes in the first place.[6]

 Diabetes mellitus is a degenerative illness that centers around the hormone insulin and the pancreas. In type 1 diabetes, the pancreas is unable to manufacture insulin. This accounts for a very low percentage of people who have diabetes. In type 2 diabetes, the pancreas produces insulin, but the body's cells don't respond to it and can't absorb glucose from food. As blood glucose levels continue to rise, the pancreas releases more insulin to deal with the excess blood sugar. The result is both a state of low blood sugar and too much insulin (hyperinsulinism).

 For more on **diabetes**, see chapter 5, Strengthen Your Sugar Controls, pages 132–33.

Heart Disease

Obesity increases your chances of getting heart disease, independent of other risk factors.[7] One study concluded that obesity tripled the chances of developing hypertension in people between the ages of 20 and 75.[8] Another study, which followed over 100,000 women, found a direct link between weight gain and the likelihood of stroke, particularly strokes caused by blood clots; as more weight was gained, the risk of stroke increased.[9]

Cancer

Obesity is also an independent risk factor in the development of many different forms of cancer. Studies from around the world link obesity to a wide variety of cancers, including prostate, breast, endometrial, colon, stomach, and kidney, to name a few.[10]

Other Conditions

Obesity is a contributing factor in a number of other health problems, including osteoarthritis,[11] gallbladder disease, gout,[12] and cataracts.[13]

What Causes Weight Gain?

The cause of weight gain is pretty straightforward: you consume more calories from food than your body uses or burns off in its daily tasks. But whether or not a person becomes obese depends on a number of factors, including genetics, societal influences, psychological makeup, and degree of physical activity.

Many people blame being overweight on external situations, such as "It runs in my family" or "I have a thyroid condition." However, only about 1% of obesity is actually a medical condition. Here are some of the most common causes of these rare instances:

 For a complete discussion of the thyroid, see chapter 6, Overcome a Sluggish Thyroid, page 150. For more on stress and the adrenal glands, see chapter 4, Heal Your Emotional Appetite, page 101.

- Hypothyroidism: The thyroid gland does not produce enough thyroid hormone.

- Cushing's syndrome: The adrenal glands produce an excess amount of the hormone cortisol, which causes fat accumulation in the face, upper back, and abdomen.

- Pharmaceutical drugs: Antidepressants, steroid medications, drugs for high blood pressure, and seizure drugs may cause increased body weight.

Although genetics may be partially responsible for obesity that runs in families, a stronger association exits between excess weight gain and dietary and lifestyle habits learned in childhood, including the kinds of food families tend to eat (for example, high-fat or processed foods). Studies have shown that the environment created by parents, through their own eating and exercise habits, greatly influences their children's risk of being overweight. Overweight families tend to have diets that are higher in fat and junk food. In addition, these same families habitually watch more television and have other sedentary habits.[14]

The consumer culture of the United States influences Americans to eat more and consume the worst kinds of food — fast foods, processed foods, and high-fat foods — which offer the least nutrition and the most potential for adding body fat and decreasing overall wellness. Americans are eating too much, period. Overconsumption is rampant in the United States, and unfortunately is spreading to other areas of the world as fast-food chains go international. The movie *Super Size Me*, which follows the health of a man as he eats only McDonald's food for a month, focuses on the fast-food practice of offering supersize portions of high-fat foods.[15] Portions that are served in the United States are usually much larger than serving sizes listed on food charts. This is referred to as "portion distortion" by the National Institutes of Health. Here are a few examples: A couple of decades ago, most people drank an 8-ounce cup of coffee; with milk and sugar that's just 45 calories. Today's 16-ounce cup of mochaccino has a whopping 350 calories! The size of a piece of meat, such as a steak, that is listed on food charts is approximately 3 ounces, or about the size of a deck of cards. But the actual portion served usually ranges from 6 to 12 ounces — four times the size! The food industry is doing its part to keep us "living large," spending billions every year on advertising. Studies have shown that the promotion of high-calorie junk food contributes to the growing epidemic of childhood obesity.[16] Take the National Heart, Lung, and Blood Institute's Portion Distortion Quiz at http://hin.nhlbi.nih.gov/portion.

Psychological factors play a significant role in weight gain, as many people overeat in response to stress, anger, sadness, boredom, or other emotional factors unrelated to hunger or nutritional needs.[17] Foods affect moods by triggering the release of endorphins, the body's natural painkillers, and the brain chemical serotonin, a mood regulator. Unfortunately, comfort foods such as chocolate, carbohydrates, and sweets may temporarily elevate mood, but they also trigger cravings that lead to overeating. Because emotional eating is one of the main factors involved in obesity, recognizing and addressing psychological factors related to overeating is of utmost importance in achieving and maintaining a healthy weight. Understanding and controlling your emotional eating may take some effort. You'll need to learn to recognize addictive and self-sabotaging patterns, and if a self-help approach isn't sufficient, psychological counseling may be necessary.

Exercise is probably the most important strategy if you want to lose weight and keep it off. The amount of exercise you get on a regular basis will strongly affect your weight. Our lives in general are less physically active than those of previous generations, and most people aren't getting enough exercise to make up for it. Only one-quarter of U.S. adults are meeting minimum exercise requirements, and this has a massive negative effect on both weight and overall health.[18] Children in the United States regularly spend two to an astounding six hours per day watching television or sitting in front of a computer! This consistent inactivity is reflected in the unfolding tragedy of ever-increasing numbers of obese children.[19]

 For more on the role of **psychological factors in weight problems**, see chapter 4, Heal Your Emotional Appetite, page 97. For more on the **importance of exercise**, see chapter 2, Start Exercising, page 52.

Everybody is different. You probably know people who can eat anything they want without ever seeming to gain an ounce, while you have to watch everything you eat. That's because each of us has a different metabolism. Plus, metabolism changes as we age. Decreased hormone levels along with reduced activity leads to a slower metabolism, potentially causing weight gain. The way you put on the pounds and the ease or difficulty with which you lose them is unique to you.

Are You Overweight?

You probably know if you're overweight: your clothes may seem a little tight or your body may feel uncomfortable or bulky to you. A quick look in the mirror may confirm the extra pounds. However, an ideal weight for you should be based on how healthy you feel, not on how you or others think you should look. One of the easiest ways to get a general picture of where you are on the weight spectrum is to use the guidelines issued by the U.S. Department of Health and Human Services, which appear below. These general guidelines give normal weight ranges based on height and age.

When you've found your correct weight range, keep in mind your frame size (small, medium, or large) and gender when considering where you fall in a given range. Specifically, those with a smaller frame should be on the lower end of a given range, while those with a larger frame will be on the higher end. Men will generally fall on the higher end of their weight range because they tend to have higher muscle and bone mass, and women will be on the lower end of the range. Again, these are meant as general guidelines, not necessarily goals. Always bear in mind your unique physiology.

Optimum Weight Ranges		
Height	Weight (in pounds)	
	Ages 19 to 34	Ages 35 and up
5' 0"	97–128	108–138
5' 1"	101–132	111–143
5' 2"	104–137	115–148
5' 3"	107–141	119–152
5' 4"	111–146	122–157
5' 5"	114–150	126–162
5' 6"	118–155	130–167
5' 7"	121–160	134–172
5' 8"	125–164	138–178
5' 9"	129–169	142–183
5' 10"	132–174	146–188
5' 11"	136–179	152–194
6' 0"	140–184	155–199
6' 1"	144–189	159–205
6' 2"	148–195	164–210
6' 3"	152–200	168–216
6' 4"	156–205	173–222
6' 5"	160–211	177–228
6' 6"	164–216	182–234

Weight Ranges for Older Adults

Some physicians believe that a small amount of weight gain is normal as we get older because the metabolism slows and people tend to exercise less, but they don't necessarily consume fewer calories. Seniors who continue to exercise while also maintaining a healthy eating regimen don't necessarily put on extra pounds. The following chart gives acceptable weights for people over 50. The middle of the weight range for each age and height is considered the ideal weight.

Body Mass Index

Calculating your body mass index (BMI) is another way to determine if you are overweight, and it's a little more precise than the height–weight charts. BMI is the ratio of your weight to your height.

Optimum Weight Ranges for Older People		
Height	Weight (in pounds)	
	Ages 50–59	Ages 60 and up
5' 0"	114–142	123–152
5' 1"	118–148	127–157
5' 2"	122–153	131–163
5' 3"	126–158	135–168
5' 4"	130–163	140–173
5' 5"	134–168	144–179
5' 6"	138–174	148–184
5' 7"	143–179	153–190
5' 8"	147–184	158–196
5' 9"	151–190	162–201
5' 10"	156–195	167–207
5' 11"	160–201	172–213
6' 0"	165–207	177–219
6' 1"	169–213	182–225
6' 2"	174–219	187–232
6' 3"	179–225	192–238
6' 4"	184–231	197–244

I've provided a mathematical formula for those who would like to calculate their BMI, but you can skip to the reference chart below to figure out your BMI without having to do the math.

1. Multiply your weight in pounds by 704. For example, a person who weighs 160 pounds would multiply 160 by 704, which equals 112,640.

2. Convert your height to inches (for example, 5 foot 10 equals 70 inches), then multiply it by itself. In this example, 70 inches multiplied by 70 inches equals 4,900.

3. Divide the answer from step 1 by the answer in step 2: 112,640 divided by 4,900 equals 22.99. Round this to the nearest whole number to determine your BMI. So a person who's 5 foot 10 person and weighs 160 pounds has a BMI of 23.

The higher your BMI, the greater your health risk. Physicians generally consider a BMI between 18.5 and 24.9 to be acceptable. Those with a BMI from 25.0 to 29.9 are considered overweight and at a higher

BMI	19	20	21	22	23	24	25	26
Height (feet, inches)				Body Weight (pounds)				
4'10"	91	96	100	105	110	115	119	124
4'11"	94	99	104	109	114	119	124	128
5'0"	97	102	107	112	118	123	128	133
5'1"	100	106	111	116	122	127	132	137
5'2"	104	109	115	120	126	131	136	142
5'3"	107	113	118	124	130	135	141	146
5'4"	110	116	122	128	134	140	145	151
5'5"	114	120	126	132	138	144	150	156
5'6"	118	124	130	136	142	148	155	161
5'7"	121	127	134	140	146	153	159	166
5'8"	125	131	138	144	151	158	164	171
5'9"	128	135	142	149	155	162	169	176
5'10"	132	139	146	153	160	167	174	181
5'11"	136	143	150	157	165	172	179	186
6'0"	140	147	154	162	169	177	184	191
6'2"	144	151	159	166	174	182	189	197
6'3"	148	155	163	171	179	186	194	202
6'4"	152	160	168	176	184	192	200	208
	Healthy Weight						Overweight	

risk for weight-related diseases, and those with a BMI of 30 and higher are considered obese.[20]

BMI should not be used as a weight guide by pregnant women, body-builders or other competitive athletes, children, or the elderly (particularly those who are sedentary or frail), since it may overestimate body fat in athletes and others who have a muscular build, and it may underestimate body fat in older persons and those who have lost muscle mass.

No single table or measurement should be relied on solely to indicate a weight problem. Use them as a general guide. If they indicate a potential weight problem, it is best to check with your health-care professional for further evaluation.

27	28	29	30	31	32	33	34	35
Body Weight (pounds)								
129	134	138	143	148	153	158	162	167
133	138	143	148	153	158	163	168	173
138	143	148	153	158	163	168	174	179
143	148	153	158	164	169	174	180	185
147	153	158	164	169	175	180	186	191
152	158	163	169	175	180	186	191	197
157	163	169	174	180	186	192	197	204
162	168	174	180	186	192	198	204	210
167	173	179	186	192	198	204	210	216
172	178	185	191	198	204	211	217	223
177	184	190	197	203	210	216	223	230
182	189	196	203	209	216	223	230	236
188	195	202	209	216	222	229	236	243
193	200	208	215	222	229	236	243	250
199	206	213	221	228	235	242	250	258
204	212	219	227	235	242	250	257	265
210	218	225	233	241	249	256	264	272
216	224	232	240	248	256	264	272	279
Overweight			Obese					

Source: Adapted from *Clinical Guidelines on the Identification, Evaluation, and Treatment of Overweight and Obesity in Adults: The Evidence Report.* 1998. NIH/National Heart, Lung, and Blood Institute (NHLBI).

Are You an Apple or a Pear?

In addition to your BMI, it is important to determine where you carry your fat. People generally fall into one of two basic body shapes, apple or pear. Apple-shaped people tend to gain weight above the waist and in the abdominal area. The apple shape, more prevalent among men, indicates increased risk of developing health problems related to obesity. Pear-shaped people carry extra fat on their hips, thighs, and buttocks. More women follow this pattern of weight gain, which is associated with a lower risk of developing heart disease, diabetes, and other weight-related diseases.

To more precisely determine which body shape you have, calculate your waist-to-hip ratio:

1. Measure your waist at its narrowest point (just above the navel).

2. Measure your hips at their widest point (around your buttocks).

3. Divide your waist measurement by your hip measurement.

For example, a woman with a waist size of 35 inches and a hip size of 38 inches would have a waist-to-hip ratio of 0.92. If this number is higher than 1.0 for men or 0.8 for women, it indicates an apple body type and increased risk for weight-related health problems. Men with a waist circumference of more than 40 inches and women with waists larger than 36 inches are also at greater risk. In fact, studies indicate that waist circumference may be the best single indicator of cardiovascular risk factors.[21]

Body Fat or Body Lean?

All of these charts, measurements, and calculations are intended to help you determine if you have a weight problem. They are relatively easy ways of estimating your body fat based on your overall weight and standards for your height and age. However, there are a number of ways to more directly measure your body fat (as opposed to lean body tissue, such as muscle and bone), all of which are generally performed in a physician's office, health club, or weight-loss clinic. One method uses calipers to measure skin fold thickness at various points on the body. Another method, hydrostatic weighing, involves weighing a person repeatedly both in and out of water; since fat is lighter than water, this allows calculation of the proportion of fat to other tissues. A third way of determining body fat is through bioelectric impedance, in which a weak electric current is passed through the body. Because fat tissue is a poor conductor compared to lean body mass, the percentage of fat in the body can be estimated. Cost and convenience may be factors in whether you choose to use one of these methods.

How Do You Feel?

A final determinant of whether you have a weight problem is how you feel. Your level of health and vitality is an important measure of your ideal weight. So, answer a few questions about your overall state of health:

- Do you have plenty of energy, or would you like to have more?
- What health problems do you have?
- Does your weight hamper your movements or activities?
- Do you feel comfortable with your size?
- Are you victimized by eating behaviors, like compulsive over-eating, that leave you debilitated physically and emotionally?
- Would you like to feel better than you do?

Take an honest look at how excess weight may factor into your general state of health. Keep in mind that being overweight or obese can contribute to a variety of health problems, including heart disease, adult-onset diabetes, and cancer, among others.

If you have tried to lose weight before, consider what you did in the past that didn't work for you and start from a different place. Establish realistic, healthy goals for yourself and, as best as you can, be clear about the reasons why you are undertaking this process again and what you are willing to do to achieve success. You know yourself well, and what does and does not work for you. Give yourself the tools, knowledge, and support to reach your goal. Ultimately, you are the one who must decide if losing weight and making other lifestyle changes will improve your health.

Why This Book Is Different

This is not a diet book. Alternative medicine focuses on improving your overall health and fitness, which leads to healthy weight maintenance as an excellent secondary effect. This approach helps you lose weight and keep it off! It is essential to understand the factors that went into creating a weight problem in any given person, because obesity is never caused by one thing alone and no two people have exactly the same causal factors.

Alternative medicine employs a battery of diagnostic tools—physical examination, dietary assessment, emotional evaluation, and tests for immune, digestive, and detoxification function—to build an individualized picture of a person's condition. Skilled alternative practitioners take the time needed to investigate underlying imbalances that may contribute to weight gain, including an underactive thyroid, hormone imbalances, food allergies, yeast infections, and parasites. Alternative medicine not only respects differences between individuals, its also concentrates its diagnosis and treatment plan around this customized approach. Rather than giving you one more fad diet, we provide you with the tools you need to make better food choices, use supplements wisely, start an exercise program that works for you, deal with any emotional issues, and correct any underlying imbalances or toxicity that may be contributing to your weight gain.

How to Use This Book

Take this quiz to determine which part of the book you should begin to use first:

1. I am ready to deeply commit to my overall health and wellness. (Start with part I. After doing a serious detoxification protocol as outlined in chapter 1 for six months, most people will find themselves automatically at their ideal weight.)

2. I feel I am in control of my life. I am satisfied with how I look and feel. I just want to lose a few pounds. (Go directly to part III, Customize Your Weight-Loss Program.)

3. I know I am overweight, but I'm not ready to give up my lifestyle. It seems too overwhelming and difficult. (Start with part I, chapter 2. Start exercising as a first step.)

In this introduction, you've learned a bit about why dieting doesn't work, health problems associated with excess weight, and how to determine if you're at risk. You've also learned that the approaches in this book go beyond weight loss and appearance; what you learn here will support and improve your health and enhance your quality of life. You're probably highly motivated to get started, so let's begin.

Part I
Change Your Lifestyle

GLASBERGEN

"Eat less and exercise more? That's the
most ridiculous fad diet I've heard of yet!"

one

Detoxification

Detoxification is one of the first steps for anyone who is serious about losing weight permanently. To embark on this path indicates that you fully recognize that you are in control of your lifestyle habits, and that only you can change them. You are beyond searching for the quick fix and are truly ready to make a pro-active commitment to feel well and look great.

The body's detoxification systems need to be functioning optimally in order to break down fat and increase energy. In this chapter, you'll find an outline of a detoxification program that will help you clear your liver, kidneys, skin, and bowels—the main organs of detoxification. Many people find that following this program for one week two to three times per year eliminates symptoms of bloating, indigestion, allergies, sinus problems, and a host of other illnesses. An added bonus of detoxifying is natural weight control, along with increased energy, an elevated mental and emotional state, and a renewed sense of self-

IN THIS CHAPTER

- The Link between Toxins and Weight Gain
- Basic Detoxification Strategies
- The Jump-Start Detox
- Toxic Colon Leads to Weight Gain
- Diagnosing Toxicity
- Alternative Medicine Detoxification Therapies
- Success Story: Reversing Obesity through Detoxification
- Success Story: Colon Cleansing Reduces Excess Weight
- Success Story: Losing Weight through Lymphatic Cleansing

awareness and self-control. I'll refer back to this chapter on detoxification many times throughout the book, since it is actually the basic first step in any weight-loss program.

If you want to try a detox, but aren't sure you're ready for the serious commitment of a full detoxification, begin with "Jump-Start Detox," on page 7. Then, skip ahead to chapter 2, Start Exercising. You can return to the rest of chapter 1 as soon as you're ready

The Link between Toxins and Weight Gain

The body puts on extra pounds over time, a phenomenon linked to years of poor diet, not enough exercise, stress, reliance on medications, and many of the other factors discussed in this book. All of these poor lifestyle choices lead to an accumulation of various kinds of toxic waste products in the body. One particularly troublesome result of this is a breakdown in the ecology of the gastrointestinal tract, which leads to a variety of health problems ranging from obesity, fatigue, depression, and impaired immune function to chronic constipation, gas, acne, and lower back pain.

An unhealthy colon can also lead to food cravings and allergies. These conditions, along with a general malaise, contribute to self-destructive eating habits that translate into weight gain. Additionally, the accumulated debris in a toxic colon can actually add several pounds to a person's weight. And as the body's ability to process toxins becomes increasingly impaired, it creates more fat cells to store toxins. In this way, toxins can literally make you fat.

The vast majority of these complaints and symptoms can be alleviated by cleansing, healing, and supporting the intestinal system, where most digestion and absorption of nutrients occurs. Keeping this passageway clean and alive with healthy digestive microbes is vital to maintaining a healthy body weight. As you'll learn in this chapter, alternative medicine offers natural, gentle, and effective methods that can restore the intestinal environment and simultaneously facilitate weight loss.

In fact, permanent weight loss is one of the natural side effects of a detoxification protocol.

Why Detoxification Is More Crucial Now Than Ever

Detoxification has been widely recognized throughout history as a way to rest and heal the body. It's increasingly important these days, as our environment and food become increasingly saturated with pollutants and chemicals and the body's mechanisms for elimination of toxins can't keep up with the chemical deluge. All organs involved in detoxification, which include the intestines, liver, lymphatic system, kidneys, skin, connective tissue, and respiratory system, can become overloaded. The constant circulation of toxins in the body taxes the immune system (SEE QUICK DEFINITION), which must continually strive to destroy or eliminate them.

Basic Detoxification Strategies

Once you have decided that you are ready to embark on a healthy new lifestyle, which automatically leads to a healthy weight, there are basic strategies you can use to enhance your success and speed the process along. Detoxification is chief among these, but a detoxification program should be tailored to a person's specific condition, including disease state, toxic burden, and the functional capacity of their major organs of detoxification: the intestines, liver, and lymphatic system, among others. People who are obese are often too toxic or too deficient in functional capacity to attempt to aggressively and rapidly rid the body of toxins. It is best to work with a knowledgeable health-care practitioner who can guide you through the stages of the detoxification process. The process must progress at a rate that your body can handle without causing greater injury.

 The **immune system** guards the body against foreign, disease-producing substances. Its "workers" are various white blood cells including 1 trillion lymphocytes and 100 million trillion antibodies. Lymphocytes are found in high numbers in the lymph nodes, bone marrow, spleen, and thymus gland.

During detoxification, many people experience a healing crisis, a brief worsening of symptoms immediately followed by significant improvement. Although the healing crisis is uncomfortable, it usually indicates that toxins are being effectively removed from the body. However, a health-care professional should be alerted when symptoms worsen during detoxification to avoid complications or injury. You can support your body during this process and minimize any healing crisis by increasing your consumption of antioxidants in fruits, vegetables, and supplements prior to beginning a detoxification program.

Before getting started on a detoxification program, it's also important to make fundamental changes to your diet and lifestyle so that you don't introduce more toxins for your body to process. Here are some basic steps you can take to reduce your toxic load:

Use only organically raised foods: This is a crucial general guideline when making food choices. Eat foods that are certified as having been grown organically. They will be free of the contaminants, synthetic pesticides and herbicides, hormones, preservatives, dyes, artificial colorings, and antibiotics found in conventionally raised foods. Many health food stores offer organic produce and meat, as do some farmers' markets and even some conventional grocery stores.

Get the poisons off your vegetables: Since the U.S. Food and Drug Administration tests only about 1% of produce for pesticide residues, cleaning your food is the only way to ensure that you aren't eating agricultural poisons. Even organic foods may have residues of potentially harmful substances. There are several natural products now on the market for washing fruits and vegetables. They remove many toxins and help prevent food-borne illnesses, too.

Maintain a household free of toxic chemicals: Remove chemical contaminants and toxic household cleansers from your home, or at least limit your exposure to them. Instead, use natural cleaning products, such as distilled white vinegar, baking soda, borax, lemon juice, citrus cleaners (not petroleum-based), castile soaps, and environmentally safe commercial products. These products are available in many health food stores or by mail order; increasingly, they're even available in standard supermarkets.

Breathe clean air: Since the average American spends most of their time indoors, indoor air quality is crucial. Unfortunately, indoor air ranks near the top of the list of polluted environments. Toxic substances such as pollens, dust mites, mold spores, tobacco smoke residues, benzene, chloroform, chemical gases, and formaldehyde are now commonly found in tightly sealed indoor environments. Whenever possible, open windows in your house, even if for only part of the day. In nature, a thunderstorm can clean up stagnant air in a local environment by way of ionization and ozone release. Commercial air filters are available that produce ions and low levels of ozone (O_3), creating air that's refreshed as after a thunderstorm. Common houseplants can also be used as filters to remove pollution from indoor air, an idea that first came out of NASA space research in the 1970s. Scientists discovered that not only do plants recycle oxygen, they remove air pollutants too.[1] Common plants that are especially effective include English ivy, spider plants, peace lily, snake plant, pothos, philodendrons, palms, mums, and ferns.

Filter your household water: Tap water is a major source of toxic chemicals, which the liver is required to process. A practical and economical solution is to get countertop water filters for your home and office; they are more cost-effective than commercially purified and bottled water. Filtration through reverse osmosis is another option. These systems force water through a microporous membrane under pressure. They are most effective against inorganic pollutants like nitrates, and metals like lead. Deionization resins are also used to accomplish this purpose.

The Jump-Start Detox

If you've only just begun to implement the suggestions above, it's too soon for you to use the more thorough detoxification therapies described later in this chapter. However, you can begin to get a taste for detoxification by following the simple program outlined below.

Preparing for Detoxification

Prepare for detoxification by gathering all the herbs and foods you'll need beforehand so you can relax and enjoy the process. Read through this section to get an overview before you begin, so that you'll know what you need and what to expect. Cook a full pot of Detoxifying Vegetable Soup. You can eat all you want of this soup throughout the day. It is high in minerals and helps to stave

Any detoxification effort should always be planned and carried out under professional supervision. Alcoholics, diabetics, people with eating disorders, those recovering from substance abuse, and people who are underweight, morbidly obese, or physically weak, as well as those who have an underactive thyroid or hypoglycemic condition, are urged not to detoxify without consulting a licensed health-care professional.

off food cravings. It also contains a lot of sulfur-containing vegetables, which helps to support the liver in its detoxification process.

■ Detoxifying Vegetable Soup

When preparing this Natural Nurse recipe, it is best to use only organic ingredients. Also, don't use aluminum cookware; stainless steel or glass is much better. Aluminum can leach into food from aluminum cookware and aluminum foil. This metal has been found in the brains of people who suffer from Alzheimer's. Nori, a type of sea vegetable, is available in natural foods stores, Asian markets, and sometimes in the Asian foods section of other grocery stores.

1 onion
1 cabbage
2 cloves garlic
2 carrots
2 stalks celery
1 bunch parsley
5 leaves of kale
2 sheets nori
4 pieces of okra
1 cup brown rice
Bragg's Liquid Aminos to taste
2 quarts of water

Combine all of the ingredients and simmer for 1½ hours.

Freshly prepared vegetable and fruit juices are immensely nutritious and can play an important role in detoxification. Use organic vegetables and fruits for juicing whenever possible. The juice is most nutritious and healing when consumed right away, but you can also freeze fresh juices for future use. If you do store fresh juices in the refrigerator, pour them in an airtight glass container, and fill it to the brim; the less oxygen in the container, the fresher the juice remains. Here's the juice blend I recommend to support detoxification:

■ Rainbow Feather Veggie Juice

Drink at least 8 ounces of this Natural Nurse juice per day to support detoxification. You can also substitute a high-quality "green food" drink powder from the health food store.

½ beet root
3 to 5 beet greens
1 cucumber
½-inch slice ginger
1 to 3 carrots
2 stalks celery
½ bulb fennel
1 bunch parsley and/or cilantro
2- to 4-inch piece burdock and/or yellow dock root
1 lemon, juiced

1 tablespoon spirulina, chlorella, or any of the organic "green
food" combinations available in health food stores

Juice the beet, greens, cucumber, ginger, carrots, celery, fennel, parsley, and burdock in a juicer. Add the lemon juice and spirulina and
dilute by 50% with filtered or purified water.

Mini Fasting

There are many methods of detoxification. Most employ some degree
of fasting to allow the digestive system to eliminate toxins that have
accumulated over time. Fasting does not involve starvation. Try a mini
fast, along with herbs to cleanse the bowels, reduce constipation, support the liver, and increase flow of lymph fluid. For three days, eat as
much of the Detoxifying Vegetable Soup as you like, and drink as much
water and herbal tea as you want. Also drink green vegetable juices and
"green food" supplements mixed in water, up to four glasses per day.
Any two fruits can be included as snacks but are optional. You can continue for up to seven days if you like.

When you end your mini fast, don't eat any fried, processed, or sugar-
laden foods for at least another two days. This will give your bowels
and liver a rest. Avoiding these foods altogether is the best choice for
permanent weight loss. If you feel emotionally threatened by the idea of
permanently giving up these kinds of foods, allow yourself one "cheat"
day a week until you're content to follow a healthy eating regime all
the time.

Colon Detox

If you experience constipation during detoxification, try the herb cascara sagrada along with ¼ teaspoon psyllium seeds in 8 ounces of water
two times per day (see "Colon-Cleansing Supplement Programs," page
35). You may find it helpful to do an enema on any day that you fail to
have a bowel movement during detoxification. See "Enemas," page 35,
for more information.

Liver Detox

The liver is an important organ of detoxification. It acts just like a pool
filter, removing impurities from the blood. When it becomes overburdened by the accumulation of too many toxins, it can no longer break
down fat efficiently, which is necessary for weight loss. Herbs can aid
the liver in this process, especially dandelion, burdock, fo-ti, licorice
root, and milk thistle.

Lymph System Detox

The lymphatic system (SEE QUICK DEFINITION) plays an extremely important role in removing waste products from the body and aids in weight loss by filtering out toxins that are released by fat cells as they break down. Detoxification makes the lymph fluid less viscous (thick), allowing it to flow more easily throughout all body tissues and reducing the pressure on the lymph nodes. Please note, however, that during the detoxification process the lymph nodes may temporarily become tender because the body is eliminating a lot of waste during this process. You can stimulate circulation of lymph fluid using several techniques. Exercise is helpful, and jumping on a mini trampoline is the most effective form of exercise for this purpose. Massage and dry skin brushing can also help (see "Dry Skin Brushing," page 46). Herbs can also be used to support the lymph system; cleavers, red clover, and nettles are especially effective.

 The **lymphatic system** consists of lymph fluid and the structures (vessels, ducts, and nodes) involved in transporting it from tissues to the bloodstream. Lymph fluid occupies the space between the body's cells and contains plasma proteins, foreign particles, and cellular wastes. Lymph nodes are clusters of immune tissue that work as filters, or "inspection stations," for detecting and removing foreign and potentially harmful substances in the lymph fluid. While the body has hundreds of lymph nodes (more than 500), they are mostly clustered in the neck, armpits, chest, groin, and abdomen. The lymphatic system is the body's master drain, collecting and filtering the lymph fluid and conveying waste products and cellular debris to the bloodstream, ultimately allowing them to be cleared from the body.

 For more on **exercise and the lymphatic system,** see chapter 2, Start Exercising, pages 62–63.

Castor Oil Pack

Applied externally to any area of the body, a castor oil pack can be one of the most helpful therapies available, relieving spasms, pain, and discomfort. It increases circulation to the area, softens tissues, and can actually pull toxins out through the skin. Adding thuja oil (red cedar) or lavender oil increases the effectiveness of a castor oil pack. (For complete instructions, see "Castor Oil Pack Instructions," page 40.)

Following the procedures outlined in the "Jump-Start Detox" will do much to put you on the road to better health and a slimmer body, but ideally you'd take detoxification to the next level with the therapies described in the rest of this chapter. If you're not yet ready for a serious detox, skip ahead to chapter 2 and return to the rest of chapter 1 when you're ready. If you are ready, or even if you just want more detailed information reducing your exposure to toxins, testing your toxin levels, and what's involved with detoxifying specific organs, read on. Following the detoxification programs outlined later in this chapter will be immensely beneficial to your overall health, and help you achieve a healthy weight as part of the process.

Toxic Load

An analogy may help exemplify the negative cumulative effects of undischarged toxicity: Our organs of detoxification accumulate toxins like a barrel collecting rainwater. If the amount of toxins being absorbed exceeds the amount of toxins eliminated, the barrel eventually overflows. Once that happens, toxic substances circulate throughout the system, progressively damaging organs and tissues and creating numerous acute or chronic problems, much as the overflowing rainwater may damage the foundation of a house. This can lead to allergies, immune system breakdown, chronic degenerative conditions, and obesity.

Our bodies are designed to handle a certain level of toxins, but stress, environmental pollution, and poor dietary choices can overtax the system. Biopsies of fat samples taken from patients found over 300 foreign chemicals, concentrated most notably in the brain, the nervous system, and breast milk.[2] Another study discovered 167 pollutants in the blood and urine of people tested, including an average of 56 carcinogens in each person.[3] No matter how healthy our diet and lifestyle, we are all exposed to toxins on a daily basis—not just from the environment but also from within. Even normal metabolic processes can produce toxins that are harmful if out of balance.

Toxins in the Environment

Toxins emanate from a variety of noxious sources, mixing together in our bodies to form a chemical cocktail of industrial by-products, pesticides, herbicides, household contaminants, and biological contaminants. In addition, processed or genetically altered foods, alcohol, tap water (which usually contains heavy metals), and other chemicals, such as newspaper ink, add to this potentially dangerous mixture.

Office workers are exposed to toxic air that's continuously recycled throughout sealed buildings.[4] Considering that most people in industrialized nations spend more than 90% of their time indoors, indoor pollutants can cause chronic exposure to toxic substances. In many cases, ventilation systems are poorly designed and inadequate.[5] The combined

Environmental estrogens are foreign compounds and/or chemical toxins that mimic the effects of estrogen in the body. Environmental estrogens, also called xenobiotics or xenoestrogens, are present primarily in man-made chemicals ("greenhouse gases," herbicides, and pesticides such as DDT) and industrial by-products (from manufacture of plastics and paper, as well as from the incineration of hazardous wastes).

The **endocrine glands**, including the testicles, ovaries, pancreas, adrenals, thyroid, parathyroid, and pituitary, are central to the regulation and normalization of all the body's complex, interconnected systems, from metabolism and heat production to spermatogenesis and uterine preparations for pregnancy.

influence of electromagnetic pollution and toxic fumes produced by construction materials can result in seemingly inexplicable illnesses that affect neurological and biochemical processes. Sick building syndrome (SBS) refers to a host of symptoms produced by low-grade toxic environmental conditions in living or office spaces. SBS symptoms include headaches, memory loss, fatigue, infections, irritability, impaired balance, and respiratory, eye, and skin diseases.[6] All of these suppress the immune system, rendering those afflicted susceptible to chronic illness.

Another huge problem is xenobiotics, or environmental estrogens (SEE QUICK DEFINITION). These chemicals have been linked to hormone dysregulation, which leads to weight gain.[7] Each year, an estimated 1,000 new synthetic chemicals of this variety enter the world market, swelling the planetary total to well over 100,000—a figure that seems bound to continue to rise rapidly. All of these are completely foreign and potentially harmful to the human body, especially to the function of the digestive system and endocrine glands (SEE QUICK DEFINITION). Evidence is accumulating that these chemicals, even at very low concentrations and exposures, cause "hormone havoc"—autoimmune diseases, clinical depression, reproductive system disorders, and obesity—among other problems.

Toxins enter the body through breathing, by swallowing, or via the skin's pores. (Those same pores, of course, also facilitate the elimination of toxic chemicals.) In the United States, tap water commonly contains chlorine, aluminum, pesticides, lead, copper, and other toxic substances.[8] Approximately 70% of the toxins from tap water enter the body through the skin; the remaining 30% enter via ingestion.

Conventional dental amalgams or "silver" fillings are actually made of tin, copper, silver, nickel, zinc, and the toxic metal mercury. These fillings disintegrate over time and have been shown in some instances to release toxic metals into the body. Mercury toxicity affects bones, joints, the central nervous system, and the brain.[9] Symptoms of mercury toxicity include joint aches and pains, as well as immune dysfunction. Mercury and other toxic metals increase free radicals, which attack cell membranes.

Copper, which is toxic at high levels, is a particular problem in tap water when copper pipes are used for plumbing. High copper intake has been found to interfere with the formation of healthy fats, increase free radical damage, and interfere with kidney function, all of which can have a negative impact on maintaining a healthy weight.[10] People who drink unfiltered water, as well as welders, metal and construction workers, plumbers, and auto mechanics, can be exposed to potentially toxic levels of copper. Other sources include birth control pills, intrauterine devices, and many fungicides and pesticides—all of which contain copper as a main ingredient.

Chemicals found in dry-cleaning fluids (trichloroethylene), paint solvents (toluene), municipal water supplies (phenol and chlorine), carpets and flooring (formaldehyde), and some imported produce (DDT pesticide residues) are also potentially harmful. Studies have proven that these chemicals can interfere with proper nerve and muscle function, cause skeletal and muscular changes, and interfere with reproductive function.[11] Often only a very small dose of these toxic agents is required to produce injurious effects, especially in hypersensitive individuals.

Inner Toxins

Environmental toxins are only one layer of the toxic load that our bodies must process. Endotoxins—toxins produced within the body—are also potentially dangerous if not efficiently eliminated. Endotoxins include uric and lactic acid, homocysteine, nitric oxide, intestinal toxins, and cellular debris from dead microorganisms. These normal by-products of metabolic processes are typically broken down by the liver and excreted from the body. But in someone with a compromised immune system, they tend to accumulate in the blood, where they burden the detoxification pathways or initiate an allergic reaction. The immune system views these substances as a threat and sends

 QUICK DEFINITION An **antibody** is a protein molecule made from amino acids by white blood cells in the lymph tissue and set in motion against a specific foreign protein, or antigen, by the immune system. Antibodies, also referred to as immunoglobulins, may be found in the blood, lymph, saliva, and gastrointestinal and urinary tracts, usually within three days after the first encounter with an antigen. The antibody binds tightly with the antigen as a preliminary step in removing it from the system or destroying it.

antibodies (SEE QUICK DEFINITION) to bind with the substance (termed an antigen), forming structures known as circulating immune complexes. If too many immune complexes accumulate, the kidneys can't excrete enough of them via the urine, in which case they are stored in soft tissues, triggering inflammation, water retention, and weight gain.

For example, arginine and ornithine (important amino acids) enter the body as part of a normal diet, but if they are not digested properly, they undergo unfavorable chemical changes. Ornithine is converted by bowel bacteria into a toxic substance called putrescine, which in turn degrades into polyamines, such as spermadine, spermine, and cadaverine (literally meaning "the essence of dead cadavers"). These chemicals cause many allergic-type symptoms as well as fatigue, emotional stress, and weight gain.

Toxic Colon Leads to Weight Gain

At birth, the inner lining of the intestines is pink, clean, and supple. Over time, however, a combination of poor diet, stress, and exposure to environmental toxins can cause the intestines to become swollen, stagnant, and caked with debris. The accumulated material can often contribute several pounds to the weight of the colon.

False Linings

Intestinal mucus makes the stool gummy, causing it to stick to the intestine walls, build up, and eventually harden into plaque. This "false lining" reduces the diameter of the intestinal passageway, leaving only a narrow opening through which waste can travel. As this lining thickens, it becomes increasingly difficult to regularly empty the bowel, and the lining can block absorption of essential nutrients. In addition, "unfriendly" microorganisms overgrow, replacing "friendly" bacteria, such as *Lactobacillus acidophilus* (see "Friendly and Unfriendly Bacteria," page 15). When this happens, the contents of the intestines putrefy and harmful chemicals are generated, which can cause inflammation, bloating, and numerous health problems, including weight gain.

Toxins that build up in the colon can pass through the intestinal wall and accumulate in the lymphatic system—the network of vessels and nodes that drain the body of toxic substances. When the flow of toxins from the colon becomes too heavy, circulation of the lymph fluid becomes blocked and toxins back up throughout the body, further compromising the immune system.

Toxins Tack On the Pounds

Unhealthy or compromised intestinal function has a major impact on weight. Although the weight of the accumulated fecal matter can contribute somewhat to being overweight, it is the effects of this accumulated matter that causes the greater problem. People with a toxic colon do not absorb nutrients from food efficiently. This can trigger a false hunger reaction that drives them to overeat. Furthermore, toxic by-products from the colon drain the body of energy, lower metabolism, and overburden other organs of detoxification, such as the liver and kidneys. Let's take a look at some of the factors that can contribute to the formation of mucoid plaque, disturb the balance of intestinal microflora, and cause the development of toxic bowel syndrome and obesity:

Friendly and Unfriendly Bacteria

The estimated 100 trillion bacteria that live in the human intestines do so in a delicate balance. Certain bacteria, such as *Lactobacillus acidophilus* and *Bifidobacterium bifidum*, are "friendly" bacteria that support numerous vital physiological processes. They help ensure that bowel movements are regular and frequent, and they also oppose the overgrowth of yeasts and parasites. Other bacteria, such as staphylococcus and clostridium, are also present but are considered "unfriendly" because they produce a variety of toxic substances. A healthy proportion of microorganisms in the colon is 85% friendly bacteria to no more than 15% unfriendly bacteria. Unfortunately, in most people the proportions are the exact opposite. A number of factors can throw off the balance of intestinal flora, including stress, the use of antibiotics and other drugs, and processed foods.

- Acid diet: Acid-forming foods, such as sugars, processed grains, eggs, and meat, contribute to the formation of intestinal plaque. Overeating also causes too much acid.

- Processed foods and refined carbohydrates: Foods made from bleached white flour, such as white bread, pastas, pastries, and cakes, are almost totally devoid of fiber. Because most of the nutrients have also been lost during processing, they tend to deprive the body of vitamins, minerals, enzymes, and other wholesome nutrients. Instead, they form a nonnutritive gooey mass in the intestines and disrupt the normal function of digestive enzymes that normally break down food. One of the most important keys to weight loss is to eliminate these foods and replace them with foods high in fiber and nutrients, such as dark-green leafy vegetables.

- Stress and tension: Stress causes the release of excess acid in the intestines as well as constriction of the walls of the bowel and sphincter muscles, hindering the passage of fecal material.

- Food allergies: The intestines often produce mucus in response to food allergies, leading to constipation, cramps, bloating, diarrhea, and other bowel symptoms.

- Parasites and candida: Digestive problems can also arise due to infestation of the colon by parasites or candida. Parasites commonly enter the body through contaminated food or water supplies (both domestic and from foreign travel), and induce a wide variety of reactions, including swelling of joints, asthma, arthritis, heightened allergies, menstrual disorders, prolonged bowel disorders, and weight loss or weight gain.

- Antibiotics: Antibiotics are prescribed by physicians to kill the harmful bacteria causing an infection. Unfortunately, because these drugs don't distinguish between unfriendly and friendly microbes, they cause a massive die-off of friendly bacteria. (Steroids and birth control pills can have a similar effect.) When friendly bacteria are not replaced through diet or supplements, unfriendly bacteria quickly lay claim to the intestines, often causing a yeast overgrowth.

For more on **food allergies,** see chapter 7, Break Food Allergies and Addictions, page 165.

Diagnosing Toxicity

In addition to weight gain, many common symptoms are caused by toxicity, such as headaches, bloating, gas, fatigue, depression, lower back pain, sallow complexion, dark circles under the eyes, tender abdomen, abnormal body odor, and bad breath. Constipation is usually present. Conventional physicians often consider one bowel movement a week to be normal, but in natural medicine the goal is to have one to three bowel movements a day. Any less indicates that the stool is being retained in the body, which allows for the reabsorption of potentially toxic waste materials.

In addition to studying symptoms and lifestyle patterns, natural healthcare practitioners use the following diagnostic tests to assess the level of toxins that may be affecting a person's health. These tests are usually not available through conventional physicians, who are not trained in the importance of toxins in overall health, as well as in weight management. (See Resources for laboratories that perform these tests.)

Comprehensive digestive stool analysis: This test assesses digestive inadequacies that can contribute to a variety of health issues, including obesity. The panel consists of a group of nearly two dozen tests performed on a stool sample. The tests reveal how well food is digested, how efficiently nutrients are absorbed, the proportions of friendly versus unfriendly bacteria in the intestine, whether or not the diet contains adequate fiber, the degree of fat absorption, the status of digestive enzymes, and the presence of the yeastlike fungus candida. All of these factors can contribute to digestive imbalance and difficulty losing weight. This test must be ordered by a health-care practitioner.

Functional liver detoxification profile: A liver that is unable to adequately detoxify the body's store of toxins and waste products may contribute significantly to obesity. Excess free radicals and by-products of incomplete metabolism resulting from poor detoxification can interfere with the movement of substances across cell membranes and damage to the cells' "energy factories," the mitochondria (SEE QUICK DEFINITION). The functional liver detoxification profile helps assess the liver's ability to convert potentially dangerous toxins into harmless substances that can then be eliminated by the body. This conversion process occurs in two major chemical reactions referred to as phase I and phase II. The detoxification profile determines the presence of enzymes needed to start the conversion process and the rate at which phase I and phase II detoxification are operating.

 Mitochondria are organelles present in every cell of the body. They have a highly organized internal structure with many internal membranes. Enzymes responsible for converting proteins, carbohydrates, and fats into energy are located on these membranes.

Oxidative stress profile: This test assesses the degree of free radical damage in the body and measures the body's levels of glutathione, an amino acid complex central to detoxification. It involves a urine analysis done by diagnostic laboratories.

Testing transit time: In the early 1900s, most people in the United States had a brief intestinal transit time; it normally took 15 to 20 hours from the time food entered the mouth until it was excreted as feces. Today, many people have a seriously delayed transit time. It may take as long as 50 to 70 hours for food to make the journey from the mouth to excretion. This allows the stool to putrefy, harmful microorganisms to flourish, and toxins to be reabsorbed by tissues and lymph vessels, triggering water retention and weight gain. Begin a transit time test by eating a test food that's likely to be identifiable in your stool, such as corn kernels, sesame or sunflower seeds, or beets Note the time that you ingest the test food. Then, watch for the material to appear in your stool — specifically, whole undigested kernels or seeds or a marked red color from the beets. The time between eating the test food and the appearance in your stool is your transit time.

Urine analysis: Alternative health-care professionals rely on urine analysis to assess a patient's digestive function and enzyme status. The person's total urine output is collected over a 24-hour period to determine concentrations of various substances in the urine. The urine analysis provides information on digestion and assimilation along with an analysis of nutritional deficiencies, kidney function, levels of bowel toxicity, and pH. Conventional doctors can order a urine test to assess all the parameters listed below. For a urine analysis that measures levels of nutrients and enzymes, the Loomis Urinalysis technique is used. The following specific values are measured in urine analysis:

- Volume: Total urine output, either excessive (polyuria) or minimal (oliguria), in relation to the specific gravity (see below). This indicates how well the kidneys are functioning.
- Indican (Obermeyer test): Indican, which comes from putrefying proteins in the large intestine, is extremely toxic and may cause inflammation, among other symptoms. Indican levels in the urine indicate the degree of toxicity, putrefaction, gas, and fermentation in the intestines. The higher the level, the greater the intestinal toxicity.
- Calcium phosphate: In this measure of the status of carbohydrate digestion, a reading of 0.5 is normal.
- pH: This value indicates how acidic or alkaline the urine is on a scale of 0 to 14, with urine pH usually ranging from 4.5 to 8.0 and with 7.0 being neutral.
- Chloride: Chloride levels reflect salt residues in the urine and give information on salt intake and assimilation.
- Specific gravity (SP): In this measure of the weight of total dissolved substances in the urine against an equal amount of water,

a normal reading of 1.020 means that the urine is 20% heavier than water. Specific gravity shows the general water content (hydration) of the body. Values typically range from 1.005 to 1.030; a high reading indicates concentrations of dissolved substances and possible kidney stress. Low levels may indicate that the body is maintaining too much fluid.

- Total sediment analysis: This indicates the amount of dissolved organic and mineral substances remaining in the urine after digestion; an optimal total reading for the three sediment categories is 0.5. The three sediment categories are calcium phosphate, uric acid, and calcium oxalate. Calcium phosphate indicates the status of carbohydrate digestion. Uric acid is a by-product of the breakdown of purines (a kind of protein), mostly excreted by the kidneys; a high reading of uric acid may indicate gout. Calcium oxalate indicates the status of fat digestion; a reading of 0 signifies optimum fat digestion.

- Vitamin C: Levels of vitamin C indicate body reserves of this key nutrient; a reading of 1 is high, 2 to 5 is normal, and 6 to 10 is deficient.

Hair trace mineral analysis: This test measures the levels of critical minerals and toxic metals in the body's tissues. The minerals present in the hair cell during its formation are locked within the hair structure. Both minerals and toxic metals exist in higher concentration in the hair than in the blood, making them easier to measure through hair analysis. Hair analysis provides an average reading that indicates levels over a several-month period; it gives a larger picture of the body's metabolic changes over time. A 1-gram sample of hair is cut and sent to the laboratory by the health-care practitioner. (The hair cannot be dyed, permed, bleached, or treated, but pubic hair can be substituted.) The laboratory burns the hair, then views and quantifies the elements present by means of atomic spectroscopy. The U.S. Environmental Protection Agency states that hair analysis is an accurate, inexpensive screening tool for heavy metal toxicity.

ToxMet Screen: This test is an inexpensive but detailed analysis of the levels of specific heavy metals in the body based on a urine sample. Levels of four highly toxic metals — arsenic, cadmium, lead, and mercury — are tested, as well as ten potentially toxic elements, including aluminum, bismuth, boron, nickel, and strontium. Finally, information is gathered on the levels of 14 essential metals and minerals, such as copper, calcium, chromium, molybdenum, selenium, and vanadium. When test results exceed limits believed to be safe, the report indicates a high concentration.

EDTA lead versenate 24-hour urine collection test: This test must be administered by a physician. EDTA (ethylenediaminetetraacetic acid), a chemical that binds with heavy metals and pulls them out of the body, is administered intravenously. The patient's urine is then collected over a 24-hour period and analyzed by a laboratory for proportions of heavy metals present in the urine.

Iridology: A useful alternative medicine technique for assessing the state of the colon, lymphatic system, and other internal organs is iridology, in which the iris (the colored portion of the eye) is studied. Iridologists have mapped the entire body on the iris, and iridology looks for small markings such, as black spots, speckles, tiny yellow clumps, or white circles on its surface to detect disease in various organs and systems. When the colon is toxic, a ringed formation will appear on the iris.

Tongue analysis: In traditional Chinese medicine (SEE QUICK DEFINITION), the tongue is used to diagnose a host of internal conditions. To do a tongue analysis, do not eat any food after 5 p.m. on the day before you will do the diagnosis; also do not include any meat in your last meal. Upon arising the next morning, immediately look at your tongue. A coating on the tongue may indicate a clogged colon; the thicker the coating, the more severe the problem. For an in-depth tongue analysis, consult with a health-care practitioner trained in traditional Chinese medicine.

Traditional Chinese medicine (TCM) which originated over 5,000 years ago, is a comprehensive system of medical practice that heals the body according to the principles of nature and balance. A TCM physician considers the flow of vital life force energy (qi) in a patient through close examination of the person's pulse, tongue, body odor, voice tone and strength, and general demeanor, among other elements. Underlying imbalances and disharmony in the body are described in terminology analogous to the natural world (heat, cold, dryness, dampness, or wind).

Darkfield microscopy: Darkfield microscopy is a way of studying living whole blood cells under a specially adapted microscope that projects a dynamic image of the blood, magnified 1,400 times, onto a video screen. The skilled practitioner can detect early signs of illness in the form of abnormalities in the blood known to produce disease. Relevant technical features in the blood include color, blood components, and the size of certain immune cells. The amount of time the blood cell stays viable indicates the overall health of the individual. Darkfield microscopy reveals distortions of red blood cells (which indicate nutritional status), possible undesirable bacterial or fungal life forms, and blood ecology patterns indicative of health or illness. In cases of lymph stagnation, the blood cells will appear to be coagulating or sticking together excessively, which makes the blood viscous. This may indicate an overburdened lymph system, which makes it more difficult to lose weight.

Electrodermal screening: Electrodermal screening (EDS) is a form of computerized information gathering based on physics, not chemistry. A blunt, noninvasive electric probe is placed at specific points on the patient's hands, face, or feet corresponding to acupuncture points at the beginning or end of energy meridians. Minute electrical discharges from these points provide information about the condition of the body's organs and systems, useful for the physician in evaluation and developing a treatment plan. The trained EDS practitioner conducts an "interview" with the patient's organs and tissues, gathering information about the status of those systems and their energy pathways. In EDS, specific points can be used to detect impaired functioning or blockage of the body's detoxification systems.

See Resources for information about laboratories that offer these diagnostic tests.

Alternative Medicine Detoxification Therapies

Detoxification strategies can help reverse the accumulation of toxins that otherwise promote the destruction of body tissues and contribute to other degenerative conditions. You can choose from several different methods of detoxification, including fasting, drinking fresh juices, and following specific diets. Related therapies for detoxification include colon- and bowel-cleansing treatments, bodywork, lymphatic drainage, aromatherapy, and nutritional and herbal support to bolster

 For more on the role of **psychological factors in weight problems,** see chapter 4, Heal Your Emotional Appetite, page 97.

the organs of detoxification. Any program of detoxification must also address the mind to foster positive thoughts and feelings. The mind-body connection must not be overlooked during weight loss.

The first step in most detoxification protocols is a general body cleanse, utilizing such methods as eating nutrient-specific diets, fasting, and consuming fresh juices. These methods are the cornerstone of detoxification therapy and are critical for successful and permanent weight loss. Avoiding solid foods and ingesting only liquids or teas allows the body to focus on cleansing, breaking down circulating toxins. Fasting improves energy levels, reduces allergies and acne, aids in weight loss, and sharpens mental acuity.

After accomplishing this general cleansing, you can implement treatments that focus on the main detoxification organs in the body: the colon, liver, and lymphatic system, along with the kidneys, skin, and lungs. All of these must be cleansed of accumulated toxins and waste matter before the body can easily and efficiently break down fat and build healthy muscle. You'll find information and therapies about detoxifying each of these organs later in this chapter.

Fasting

Each cell needs a constant supply of nourishment in the form of oxygen, proteins, glucose, amino acids, fatty acids, vitamins, minerals, and trace elements. Equally important to the cells is waste removal. Metabolic wastes must be carried away from the cells by the lymphatic system, the "garbage disposal" of the cells. When nutritional deficiencies, sluggish metabolism, a stagnant lymphatic system, and environmental and internal toxins have choked the cells, fasting is a necessity. Water fasting is done by consuming only filtered water and/or herbal teas, with zero caloric intake. This type of fasting causes a rapid release of toxins from the body, where they have been buried in the fat for long periods of time. This kind of fast is not recommended for beginners! Incorporating vegetable or fruit juices and "green foods" into a fasting regime is less aggressive than a water-only fast and is better tolerated by most people with borderline hypoglycemia (low blood sugar— SEE QUICK DEFINITION).

Preparation for Fasting

Fasting traditionally starts at the beginning of a new season (typically autumn or spring), but it can be undertaken at any point during the year. Because it's such a powerful therapy for detoxification, you need to begin releasing some toxins before you fast; the detox tea described below will help with this. You also need to boost your nutritional reserves by eating nutritious foods and using the supplements below. Also consider incorporating more fresh juices and "green foods" into your diet before fasting (see "Juicing," pages 29–30 and "Green Foods," page 30). **You should drink the tea and take the supplements for a full month before beginning the fast.** In the meanwhile, you'll probably want to continue reading this chapter so that you'll fully understand the detoxification process. You may also want to read ahead and start incorporating some of the suggestions in upcoming chapters, particularly in regard to moderate exercise, a healthier diet, and a healthier emotional relationship to food and eating.

 Hypoglycemia, or low blood sugar (glucose), is a condition often associated with diabetes. Glucose is the primary source of fuel for the brain. In healthy people, the release of insulin acts to keep blood sugar levels fairly constant. When the pancreas produces too much insulin, however, blood glucose levels drop suddenly. Symptoms of hypoglycemia include anxiety, weakness, and sweating.

Detox Tea

Mix together equal parts of dandelion, burdock, red clover, and peppermint. Use 1 tablespoon of this blend per cup of tea. To prepare, bring filtered water to a boil, then pour it over the tea blend. Allow the blend to steep for 5 minutes, then pour the tea through a strainer. Drink six or more cups of the tea daily for one month prior to a fasting period, and continue to drink it while fasting.

Supplements: The following supplements will both boost your nutritional reserves and support your body's mechanisms of detoxification. For one month prior to starting a fast, take the following supplements:

- Multivitamin-multimineral without copper: two to three tablets with each meal
- Multiple antioxidant: two to three tablets with each meal
- Lipotropic factors to support detoxification, such as black radish root, beet leaf, and ox bile extract: three tablets, two times a day
- Bioflavonoids (liquid form preferred): 1 tablespoon per day
  You should also continue taking these supplements while fasting.

Diet to Prepare for Fasting

For one week before you begin the fast, eliminate refined, canned, and processed foods, hydrogenated oils and rancid fats, alcohol, caffeine, refined sugars, most animal products, and any foods that cause food allergies and toxic reactions. Additional foods to avoid include yeast, wheat and other high-gluten grains, cow's milk and dairy products, refined or concentrated natural sugars (even fruit juices), corn, and nightshade vegetables (tomatoes, peppers, eggplant, and potatoes). Organic vegetables and fruits should be incorporated into the diet daily. Also incorporate into your daily diet two glasses of Rainbow Feather Veggie Juice (pages 8–9) and six or more cups of the detox tea described above.

Mucus-Cleansing Diet

You might also consider boosting the effectiveness of your fast by following a mucus-cleansing diet for three to five days before you start fasting. Mucus is created by the body to trap toxins or disease-causing organisms circulating in the sinus cavity and gastrointestinal tract. An overabundance of mucus causes stagnation of all body systems. The mucus-cleansing diet consists of foods and beverages that help thin and dislodge mucus.

An excellent combination to start with is the Lemonade Special (based on a fasting protocol developed by Stanley Burroughs in the 1970s). Lemons help loosen mucus and cleanse the liver. (Those with candida infections should use the herbal sweetener, stevia, rather than honey.) Here's the recipe and the procedure for using the lemonade:

1. Place the freshly squeezed juice of an organic lemon into a 1-quart glass jar.

2. Fill the jar with filtered water.

3. Add 1 teaspoon of raw honey (or substitute 2–3 drops of the naturally sweet herb stevia).

4. Add a pinch of ground cayenne pepper (or a little fresh grated horseradish).

5. Make an 8- to 12-ounce glass in the morning and continue to drink it throughout the day. Take a few gulps at least once per hour. If you finish the first 8- to 12-ounces, prepare another batch. You should finish two to four full glasses of the combination per day.

Drink water throughout the day, as well. It's also a good idea to drink an herbal tea consisting of equal portions of peppermint, spearmint, fenugreek, eucalyptus, ginger, and licorice. These herbs have mucus-removing properties. Use 1 tablespoon of this blend per cup of tea. To prepare, bring filtered water to a boil, then pour it over the tea blend. Allow the blend to steep for 5 minutes, then pour the tea through a strainer. Drink 5 to 6 cups per day of this tea combination, and/or the mucous cleansing tea.

You can also enjoy either the Detoxifying Vegetable Soup (pages 7–8) or a potassium-rich broth throughout the day. To prepare the broth, simmer about 1 cup each of chopped celery, carrots, beets, onions, parsley, kale, and parsnips and 4 cloves of garlic in 2 quarts of filtered water for 45 minutes. Use only organically grown produce. You can add sea salt or Bragg Liquid Aminos (containing soybeans and filtered water) to enhance the flavor. Strain the broth and store it in the refrigerator, consuming it within a day or two.

Steamed carrots, mustard greens, onions, and garlic should be eaten throughout the day as an accompaniment. You can top these vegetables with grated horseradish (fresh, not pickled).

15-Day Fast

It's best to ease into this fast over a three-day period. The fast itself lasts for five days, after which you should take a full week to slowly reintroduce healthy foods back into your diet.

Day 1: Eliminate beans and whole grains. Eat only fruits, vegetables (raw or cooked), tofu, nuts, seeds, and juices. Always dilute juices by 50% to 75% with purified water. Drink at least eight glasses of water daily. Drink the detox tea described above, using stevia to sweeten it if you wish. Take the nutritional supplements discussed above for the duration of the fast.

Day 2: Consume only fruit and raw or steamed vegetables. Eliminate tofu, nuts, and seeds. Limit portions to decrease the capacity of your stomach.

Day 3: Eat only raw vegetables and fruits and chew them thoroughly.

Days 4 through 8: Eliminate all solid foods. Drink unlimited quantities of warm herbal tea throughout the day. Consume liberal quantities of water, which will dilute your body fluids and flush your lymphatic, circulatory, and urinary systems; your urine must stay diluted to avoid damaging your kidneys. During these five days, take the following supplements to support your organs of detoxification and minimize any temporary worsening of symptoms (healing crisis):

- Milk thistle (80% standardized silymrin): 450 mg, three times a day
- Artichoke root (5% standardized cynarin): 300 mg, three times a day
- SAMe (S-adenosylmethionine): 500 mg, twice daily
- NAC (N-acetylcysteine): 500 mg, twice daily
- Glutathione: 150 mg, twice daily
- L-glutamine (an amino acid that supports regeneration of the gastrointestinal barrier and is particularly useful during a fast): 4 grams daily

 When calories are restricted, toxins embedded in fatty tissues are liberated and can be flushed out of the body. Releasing too many toxins at once can overwhelm the organs of detoxification, so care must be taken to decide how rapidly to mobilize the pollutants in the body. It is imperative to consult with a health-care practitioner before starting any detoxification therapy.

 For more on the role of **food allergies and weight gain**, see chapter 7, Break Food Allergies and Addictions, page 165.

Day 9: Take a full week to ease into your healthy diet again. On the first day of eating solids, consume only one light meal of steamed or baked vegetables such as squash, sweet potatoes, or carrots. Eat only one type of vegetable; don't mix them. With your meal, take one to three capsules of digestive enzymes or bromelain (an enzyme from pineapples) to help support your digestive system, which has now been inactive for an extended time.

Day 10: Now you may supplement your diet with more varieties of cooked foods and a raw salad (with a dressing of flaxseed oil, lemon juice, and sea salt). Look for reactions to foods as you reintroduce them into your diet. Work with a health-care practitioner to determine the extent of any hidden food allergies and sensitivities

Days 11 through 13: Reintroduce into your diet easily digested proteins. Organic tofu and whole grains such as brown rice, millet, quinoa, amaranth, and buckwheat are good choices. Avoid foods with a high gluten content, such as wheat, spelt, rye, barley, and oats.

Days 14 through 15: Now you can begin following a normal healthy diet. At this point, you have successfully completed the fast.

Activity during a Fast

During a fast, it's important to get enough rest and to conserve your energy. Vigorous exercise is discouraged because it increases your physiological need for glucose (SEE QUICK DEFINITION), which will come from fat, or from muscle protein if you push yourself too hard. Light aerobic exercise, such as walking or swimming, is fine, and stretching, yoga, and tai chi are encouraged. Stress, whether physical or psychological, hampers your healing and even promotes abnormal levels of toxins in the blood by producing stress hormones and free radicals. Focus on reducing any negative emotions through creative endeavors, such as meditating or writing in a journal. Good strategies to deal with potential food obsessions or excessive hunger during fasting are light exercise, sleep, or avoidance of situations where food is prominent. Avoid being around food as much as possible, and have someone else prepare meals for the family if this is one of your responsibilities. Many people find that food cravings abate after the first couple of days of fasting. If possible, take time off from your job or normal routine during the fast.

 Glucose, a type of sugar, is the main fuel used by the brain. After a meal is eaten, the pancreas produces insulin to enable sugars to be metabolized. If you are eating a lot of carbohydrates, your body will become accustomed to producing a lot of insulin and, over time, you may experience insulin resistance. The result is that your body may store the carbohydrates as fat rather than making them available as fuel that can be burned off by your body.

Shorter Fasts

In this modern world, it isn't always practical to do a 15-day fast. Fortunately, some shorter fasts are also quite effective. If you'd like to detox but don't have the time available for a longer fast, try one of the fasts described below.

Two-day fast: For two days, drink 2 to 3 eight ounce glasses of Rainbow Feather Veggie Juice daily (pages 8–9), along with 4 to 5 cups of the Detox Tea (page 23), and two whey-, rice-, or soy-based protein powder shakes a day. Select a protein powder that has very few ingredients. They vary greatly; read the label and take special note of the section titled "other ingredients."

Three- to five-day fast: Follow the guidelines for the two-day fast, adding an organic vegetable soup prepared with the following ingredients: 1 cabbage, 4 leaves of kale, 2 carrots, 1 onion, 2 cloves garlic, 1 bunch of parsley, and 2 stalks of celery. Cut the vegetables into bite-size pieces and place them in a soup pot with 1 gallon of filtered water. Simmer for 1 hour, then add Bragg Liquid Aminos (available in most health food stores) to taste. You may eat a bowl of this soup as many times a day as you choose.

Three- to five-day mono diet: For those who find it difficult to complete a liquid fast, try eating only one type of nonallergenic food for several days. It's best to consult with your health-care professional when deciding what food to eat on a mono diet. Good choices include pears, brown rice, apples, squash, or carrots (if hypoglycemia is not a problem). If using a fruit or vegetable, it can be prepared raw, boiled, steamed, or baked. You should drink at least 2 quarts of filtered water and/or herbal tea daily during the mono diet. Three to five days is a typical duration for a mono diet; when you're ready to end the diet, slowly reintroduce healthy foods.

Skin and Bowel Detoxification while Fasting

About one-third of all body impurities are eliminated through the skin, commonly referred to as the "third kidney." During a fast, your sweat and sebaceous secretions will contain higher concentrations of fat-soluble pollutants, heavy metals, and salts. Shower or bathe three times per day during a fast to avoid reabsorbing these toxins. Adding Epsom salts, baking soda, sea salt hydrogen peroxide, ginger root, bentonite clay, and/or burdock root to the bath will help remove toxins more quickly. Taking showers or baths in which the temperature of the water alternates between hot and cold aids in detoxification and flushes the lymphatic system. You can also encourage drainage of lymphatic fluid through your skin by using a loofah sponge or soft brush on dry skin.

Fat-soluble toxins present in your body, made up primarily of bile formed by the liver, will be flushed out through the stool during a fast.

The stool of an individual fasting typically contains more toxins than normal. For this reason, it's important to avoid constipation and to encourage elimination through colonics, enemas, and herbal support.

Experiences during a Fast

Many people report a spectrum of feelings as they proceed through a fast. Most experience physiological and psychological withdrawal effects during the first three days or, in some cases, for longer periods. The more prepared your body is, the fewer and less intense the side effects, which may include transient headaches, fluctuations in energy level, hypoglycemia, bad breath, increased body odor, constipation, nausea, rectal mucus discharge, acne, and a temporary aggravation of many conditions. Serious side effects are very rare, especially among people who follow the prefasting program outlined above, and usually only occur when people who should be under medical supervision undertake long fasts. More severe side effects can include fainting or dizziness, dangerously low blood pressure, cardiac arrhythmias, severe vomiting or diarrhea, kidney problems, and gout. As emphasized, it's important to consult with a practitioner who's knowledgeable about fasting before you undertake this vital aspect of detoxification.

Support Therapies for Fasting

Specific nutrients, particularly the "green foods" and fresh juices, can help support the body nutritionally during an intensive fast. They're also useful for promoting cleansing and weight loss on a daily basis.

Juicing

Many people attempt to fast on juice. While juice fasts have positive benefits, the carbohydrates in the juice decrease the rate of toxin removal. Fresh juices can, however, prepare your body for fasting, and they're so healthful that they should become a part of your daily diet. Fresh juices are a simple way to obtain the 8 to 10 daily servings of fruits and vegetables recommended by the National Cancer Society, National Cancer Institute, and the American Heart Association. Due to their high concentration of vitamins, minerals, natural sugars, intact enzymes, and phytonutrients (plant compounds with health-protecting qualities), they're particularly helpful in repairing damaged tissues. They are also easily digested, and their nutrients can be quickly utilized by the body. Here are some tips on juicing:

- Use only organic, nonirradiated fruits and vegetables.

- If organic produce isn't available, wash off pesticide residues using fruit and vegetable washes.

- Always peel away the skins of citrus fruits before juicing (except lemons and limes), but retain as much of the white layer between the peel and fruit as possible, because it's rich in vitamin C and bioflavonoids (SEE QUICK DEFINITION).

- Remove pits, stones, and hard seeds from fruits such as cherries, plums, and mangoes.

- Juice the stems and leaves of most produce, such as beets, grapes, and apples, but remove the greens of carrots and rhubarb.

- Fruits with a low water content, such as papayas, mangoes, avocados, and bananas, won't juice well, but they can be prepared in a blender as smoothies.

- Juiced watermelon with the rind helps cleanse the kidneys.

- Cherries and all berries are especially high in bioflavonoids.

- Okra and cabbage contain the amino acid glutamine, which helps repair the intestinal lining. (When the intestinal lining loses integrity, it allows inflammation-provoking substances to enter the bloodstream and body tissues.)

- Pineapple and papaya contain natural plant enzymes that aid in digestion and nutrient absorption. Add a little ginger to pineapple juice for extra enzyme power and to soothe any gastrointestinal irritation.

 QUICK DEFINITION

A **bioflavonoid** is a pigment within plants and fruits that acts as an antioxidant to protect the body against damage from free radicals and excess oxygen. In the body, bioflavonoids enhance the beneficial activities of vitamin C, and they are often included in vitamin C supplements. Originally called vitamin P, these vitamin C "helper" substances include citrin, hesperidin, catechin, rutin, and quercetin. When taken with vitamin C, bioflavonoids increase the absorption of vitamin C in the liver, kidneys, and adrenal glands. As antioxidants, they also protect vitamin C from destruction by free radicals.

"Green Foods"

Commonly referred to as "green" foods, blue-green algae, chlorella, spirulina, wheatgrass, and barley grass act as powerful antioxidants, support the liver, and aid in detoxification. See chapter 9, page 229 for more information about green foods.

Physical Therapies for General Detoxification

Chiropractic adjustments can help to move toxins out of the system. Peristalsis, the wavelike contractions that move material through the colon, occurs as a result of nerve impulses that originate in the spinal nerves. The stimulation of the proper function of these nerves can be improved by removing stress that may occur due to misalignment of the spine. Chiropractic adjustments can help normalize the action of the ileo-cecal valve, the valve that separates the small intestine from the large intestine. If this valve goes into spasms and shuts too tightly, material remains in the small intestine longer than it should, extending transit time. Chiropractic adjustments also remove subluxations (misalignments of the vertebrae), which can interfere with many of the normal metabolic reactions in the body.

Massage can also be beneficial by helping to relax the abdominal muscles and encourage normal peristalsis, thus aiding in prevention of the buildup of fecal material. Since stress is also a factor in toxicity, massage's natural tranquilizing effect can help by restoring calm and soothing the digestive tract. In addition, it directly helps to improve circulation of blood and lymph fluids, which supports the body's natural detoxification processes, as well as the breakdown of fat.

Reflexology is based on the idea that there are reflex areas in the hands and feet that correspond to every part of the body, including the organs and glands. By applying gentle but precise pressure to these reflex points, reflexologists can release blockages that inhibit energy flow and cause pain and disease. Stimulating certain reflex points in the feet has a positive effect on internal organs. This helps to improve the function of the organs of detoxification, and supports weight loss by helping the body get rid of toxins more effectively.

Success Story: Reversing Obesity through Detoxification

Michelle, 50, had a host of debilitating symptoms, including obesity, gum disease, food allergies, recurring depression, and severe gastrointestinal dysfunction (chronic diarrhea and diverticulitis, an inflammation of the intestinal lining). Although she was only 5 foot 3, Michelle weighed 220 pounds and had never exercised in her life. She had tried numerous popular diet plans, but none had worked. Her weight had become such a problem that she couldn't even see her own knees.

She knew that her diet was very poor. She had consumed an average of 16 to 18 diet colas every day since her student years, when she needed the quick caffeine boost the sodas provided. As a self-described "soda-holic," Michelle kept two cases of sodas in her car, just in case she needed a boost while on the road. She primarily ate out, and she never cooked any whole foods. When she did eat vegetables (which was seldom), they were frozen or canned.

Finally, in desperation, Michelle visited a nutritionist who specialized in detoxification. He explained to Michelle that if a person is in a state of ill health and gastrointestinal dysfunction, they cannot rush into a detoxification program. In people who are chronically ill and whose systems are deeply imbalanced, the body lacks the energy and proper organ function to manage the complex processes of detoxifying. Such people must prepare for detoxification slowly by going through a process of changes over time, and in Michelle's case, she had to wean herself off diet sodas for five months before she was ready or able to drop the "addiction."

To prepare Michelle for detoxification, the nutritionist slowly introduced supplements that would help her immune and digestive systems, specifically vitamin C, garlic, pancreatic enzymes, hydrochloric acid (the stomach's primary digestive "juice"), and flaxseed oil. Michelle began to eat more fresh vegetables and fish. After five months of preparation, Michelle was still unable to handle detoxification. A lifetime of poor eating habits and 15 years of steady intake of diet soda had seriously imbalanced intestinal bacteria, impairing Michelle's digestion. The nutritionist added probiotics acidophilus and bifidus along with whey protein to promote the growth of beneficial microflora and aloe vera juice to improve her intestinal health. Michelle also used a very high-quality vegetarian protein powder as a meal replacement once per day.

After another six months, Michelle really started to notice a change in her body. Her clothes were beginning to feel loose, and her energy level was much better. This gave her the motivation she needed to finally give up her sodas, and that was a great psychological victory for her. Her bowel movements were much improved, indicating healthier functioning of her intestines.

Michelle was finally ready to begin the full detoxification regimen. This consisted of a two-week intensive phase in which she primarily ate foods that produced no allergic reactions or excessive mucus, avoiding foods such as dairy products, white flour, wheat, corn, and sugar. The core of this two-week phase was a high-protein rice concentrate powder, with beneficial omega-3 essential fatty acids (SEE QUICK DEFINITION), herbal tea, and vegetable juices.

This kind of detox protocol helps the liver, the body's chief organ of detoxification, rid the body of toxins and accumulated waste matter. It also supports the other organs of detoxification, the kidneys, bladder, intestines, skin, lungs, and lymphatic system, and even the mind. As toxins are flushed out, many people report feeling uplifted in their thoughts and mood. However, during the process of clearing toxins there may be moments of mental agitation, irritation, and sudden mood shifts, as well as headaches and muscle pains, but these negative reactions are temporary, usually lasting only one or two days at most. To offset and hopefully prevent these common detox symptoms, Michelle took antioxidants, herbs, vitamins (C and E), fatty acids, and minerals.

Michelle didn't experience any problems during the two-week detoxification program because her system had been prepared for over a year to handle it. After the fast, Michelle commented, "This process did not happen overnight. It's been a gradual lifestyle adjustment. I feel as if somebody has taken a vacuum cleaner through my insides and cleaned them out. My taste buds suddenly feel alive again for the first time in years. And I actually crave healthy foods, such as broccoli and okra. I don't miss drinking soda at all!"

> **QUICK DEFINITION**
> **Essential fatty acids** (EFAs) are unsaturated fats required in the diet. Omega-3 and omega-6 fatty acids are the two principal types. Omega-3 fatty acids are found in flaxseed, canola, pumpkin, walnut, and soy oils. Fish oils, especially from salmon, cod, and mackerel, also contain important omega-3 fatty acids. Omega-6 fatty acids are found in most plant and vegetable oils, including safflower, corn, peanut, and sesame, as well as evening primrose, black currant, and borage.

Since her initial fast five years ago, Michelle has repeated the process for one week every six months and has clearly developed a permanent commitment to her health. She feels better than ever, having dropped 60 pounds and four dress sizes, and she's grown leaner in terms of body fat. Her food choices are primarily fresh vegetables, some fruits, fish, chicken, eggs, and a limited amount of grains. Reversing a lifetime of indolence, Michelle also began a regular exercise program by taking a daily lunchtime walk. In fact, this year Michelle walked the 26-mile Los Angeles Marathon, and next year she intends to run it!

The following treatments focus on the main detoxification organs in the body, the colon, liver and lymphatic system, along with the kidneys, skin and lungs. All of these must be cleansed of accumulated toxins and waste matter before the body can easily and efficiently break down fat and build healthy muscle.

Colon Cleansing

Normal colon function yields two to three bowel movements per day, following meals. The average American eliminates less than once per day, which means that most people are actually constipated. With constipation, the stool is hard and dry. Hardened fecal stones (fecoliths) get caught in the folds of the colon, contributing to toxic buildup. In traditional cultures, where 5 to 10 times more unprocessed fiber is eaten than in the standard American diet, the stool is typically larger and softer, and elimination occurs more frequently. There is a corresponding lower incidence of colon cancer and other gastrointestinal diseases in these cultures.

Colon cleansing is commonly recommended by natural health practitioners as a remedy to this situation, and as an effective method of detoxification. Enemas and colonic irrigations, in which water or some other fluid is used to flush out the lower portion of the colon, can help restore intestinal health.[12] Certain supplement programs are also helpful.

Colon Hydrotherapy

Colon hydrotherapy involves the gentle infusion of warm, filtered water into the colon. Although it can be slightly uncomfortable for some people, colon hydrotherapy is unsurpassed in its ability to detoxify the colon, correct disordered intestinal bacteria (dysbiosis), and treat intestinal permeability (leaky gut syndrome). It also tones the muscles of the colon and stimulates peristalsis (the wavelike contractions of the intestines), which propels food through the digestive tract and prevents the buildup of destructive wastes.

 Pregnant women and people with severe heart disease, appendicitis, aneurysm, gastrointestinal hemorrhage, severe hemorrhoids, colon cancer, intestinal wall herniation, severe colitis, and intestinal blockages should not undergo colon hydrotherapy.

Colonic hydrotherapy, or a colonic, begins with the insertion of a small rectal tube (speculum) into the patient by the therapist, nurse, or physician. Water, which may be oxygenated or enhanced with the addition of food-grade hydrogen peroxide, ozone, botanical antimicrobials, nutritional supplements, or friendly intestinal flora (probiotics), is gently infused into and out of the intestines. The temperature, water pressure, and flow are continuously monitored throughout the treatment. The colonic machine is self-sanitizing, featuring a built-in check valve that prevents wastewater from returning and contaminating the water source. All instruments used in the treatment are sterile and disposable, eliminating any possible contamination of the patient.

The water pressure used during the colonic treatment is a safe and gentle 5 pounds per square inch. The treatment usually lasts about an hour, which includes time for evacuating the bowels after the treatment. A series of 8 to 12 colonic treatments is often prescribed, depending on the person's diagnosis. The medications or therapeutic substances infused during the treatments are changed often so as to expose disease-causing microorganisms in the colon to the widest spectrum of disease fighters, guaranteeing maximum eradication. Many people report an instant weight loss immediately following a colonic. It is not unusual to drop 5 to 7 pounds of old fecal matter by the end of a 45-minute treatment. In addition, the abdomen becomes much more flat. This helps with weight-loss motivation, as well.

Enemas

An enema involves injecting water into the colon via a small plastic tube inserted into the rectum. The tube is attached to an enema bag, which is basically just a compressible sack, and generally about 1 cup to 1 quart of warm water is used. The water flushes out the lower portion of the colon. Enema bags can be purchased in any drug store. They are actually the same as douche bags, and are sold with different attachments to be used to either purpose. Enemas can easily be done at home. Adding medicinal herbs or the friendly bacteria *Lactobacillus acidophilus* makes an enema even more effective. Enemas help purge both the colon and liver of accumulated toxins, dead cells, and waste products.

Colon-Cleansing Supplement Programs

Begin a colon-cleansing supplement program by combining ½ teaspoon psyllium seed powder, 1 teaspoon vitamin C powder, and 8 ounces of water, drinking it immediately after mixing the ingredients and following it with another 8 ounces of water or herb tea. Do this once daily. After two days, begin taking a combination of herbs such as barberry, wormwood, and cascara sagrada, which help to destroy unfriendly bacteria and stimulate elimination through the colon. Also, begin a regimen of supplementation to help rebuild a healthy intestinal lining, including L-glutamine, plantain, slippery elm, ginkgo, and skullcap. Continue taking the herbs and supplements daily for a month, then reduce to one or two times per week.

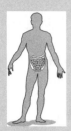

The Origins of Colon Hydrotherapy

Accounts of bowel cleansing date back to ancient Egypt. The Ebers Papyrus, an ancient Egyptian manuscript on health and spirituality, contains hieroglyphs that depict the use of gourds and rushes as a rudimentary enema bag to infuse liquids into the colon through the anus. The Essene Gospel of Peace contains a translation from the ancient Hebrew Dead Sea Scrolls that describes the use of goatskins and reeds to perform an enema as both a medical and spiritual cleanser.[13] About eight decades ago, natural health-care pioneer John Harvey Kellogg, MD, of Battle Creek, Michigan, used colon therapy to avoid surgery in a majority of patients afflicted with gastrointestinal diseases.[14] The popularity of colon therapy reached its zenith in the 1920s and 1930s. At that time, colonic irrigation machines were a common sight in hospitals and physicians' offices. Although interest declined with the advent of pharmaceutical and surgical treatments, colon therapy is once again gaining in popularity and is now commonly used by alternative medicine practitioners.

Increased interest in colon health has led to a surge in the number of over-the-counter colon-cleansing products. Most of these products utilize supplements containing a combination of herbs, nutrients, enzymes, and toxin absorbers designed to help remove the mucoid plaque lining in the colon and enhance digestion and absorption of nutrients. Many of these supplements include ingredients that also cleanse the liver, gallbladder, and lymphatic system. If they're quality products, their labels and included information will also recommend a diet of organic whole foods high in natural fiber and dark-green leafy vegetables.

Success Story: Colon Cleansing Reduces Excess Weight

"My weight crept up on me so slowly that I hardly noticed what was happening," says Betty, 32, who was 5 foot 1 and weighed 140 pounds. Betty tried commercial diet drinks and succeeded in losing a few pounds; however, she soon gained it all back and then some. She also began to feel increasingly run-down, and sadly, when she tried to have a baby, suffered a miscarriage.

Betty finally decided to see a holistic nutritionist, whose exam revealed that her problems were related to a buildup of fecal material in her colon (the end portion of the large intestine). The nutritionist recommended that Betty undergo a colon cleanse. "At first, the idea seemed a little weird to me and I was scared," Betty remarked. She didn't think she had a problem with her colon, as she wasn't troubled by either constipation or diarrhea. Nevertheless, she decided to give the cleanse a try.

"I went on a brief, supervised juice and water fast and took herbal cleansing formulas in the morning and before bed," she said. Betty was taught how to do enemas at home and also visited a colon therapist for a series of colonic irrigations, a treatment that involves flushing out the entire colon with warm, filtered water. Soon after the treatment, Betty began to see results. "Thick black and dark brown matter literally poured out of my body," she reports. "I couldn't believe all that stuff was inside me, and I can't tell you how much better I felt once it was gone."

After the fast and colonic irrigations, the nutritionist recommended herbs and a cleansing diet that helped to flush Betty's liver and gallbladder. Combined, all of these treatments restored Betty's vitality. "I don't worry about dieting now," she said. "My body has more muscle and less fat, too. I weigh around 100 pounds, and I've stayed at that weight for the past four years."

Liver Detoxification Therapies

The liver, located beneath the right lower part of the rib cage, is the largest organ in the body and one of the most complicated, rivaled only by the brain. The liver collects and removes foreign particles and chemicals from the blood and detoxifies these poisons through three systems: the Kupffer cells; phase I and phase II biotransformation systems, involving over 75 enzymes; and production of bile. Each system feeds into the others, and all three must be operating at full efficiency for proper detoxification.

Approximately 3 pints of blood are filtered by the liver each minute. The Kupffer cells are stationary white blood cells that engulf foreign matter in the blood before it passes through the rest of the liver. When the liver is damaged, toxic, congested, or sluggish, the Kupffer cells become overburdened and the filtration system breaks down, allowing increased levels of antigens, foreign proteins, bowel microorganisms, and dietary waste products to pass through the liver and enter the general circulatory system. Inflammatory agents called cytokines are also released, contributing to the development of inflammation and obesity. Bile, a yellowish brown, orange, or green fluid, is excreted by the liver, stored in the gallbladder, and pumped into the small intestine as needed. Bile emulsifies or breaks down fat and prevents putrefaction of intestinal contents.

The overall goal of the liver's detoxification systems is to convert toxins into a water-soluble form for easy elimination from the body via the stool. The liver acts like a filter for the body. If the filter gets overloaded, it can no longer function effectively, and toxins will overflow into the body as a result. Alternative medicine offers several simple but effective techniques to remedy this situation by helping to cleanse, tone, and repair damaged liver cells, including a liver flush, coffee enemas, castor oil packs, and specific herbs, plants, and foods for liver support.

Liver Flush

A liver flush stimulates the elimination of wastes from the body, increases the flow of bile, and improves overall liver function, which is necessary if the body is to shed pounds. Here are some instructions for preparing and administering a liver flush:

1. Make 1 cup of freshly squeezed juice from organic lemons and/or limes. The number of lemons or limes needed will vary depending on the size of the fruit. Dilute with 1 cup of filtered water.
2. Add the juice of 1 clove of garlic and a small amount of ginger juice. Use a 1- to 2-inch piece of raw ginger root and either put it through a juicer or grate it, then press the shreds with a garlic press to get juice.
3. Add 1 tablespoon of high-quality, organic extra virgin olive oil and blend or shake thoroughly.
4. Drink this juice in the morning and don't eat any food for 1 hour afterward.
5. After an hour has elapsed, drink two cups of a detoxifying herbal tea. You can purchase detoxifying teas in health food stores or make your own by combining equal parts of dandelion, burdock root, fennel, and peppermint. Steep 1 teaspoon of this blend in 1 cup boiling water for 5 minutes, then drink.
6. Do the flush for 10 days, discontinue for 3 days, then resume for 10 days; this is one cycle. Repeat for another cycle.

Coffee Enema

Coffee contains specific chemicals that have been shown to protect the liver.[15] Research by Max Gerson, MD, of the Gerson Institute, who was inducted into the Orthomolecular Medicine Hall of Fame, led to the use of coffee enemas to stimulate liver detoxification. Easily done at home, a coffee enema can help purge the liver of accumulated toxins, dead cells, and waste products. The enema is prepared by brewing organic caffeinated coffee through an unbleached filter, letting it cool

How to Administer a Coffee Enema

It's best to do coffee enemas in the morning, since they can cause insomnia when used near bedtime, especially in individuals sensitive to caffeine. Eat a piece of fruit before the coffee enema to activate your upper digestive tract. Keep all equipment clean and sanitized. Coffee enemas can be useful in minimizing the headaches, fever, nausea, intestinal spasms, and drowsiness that often accompany detoxification programs.

1. Brew 4 cups of organic coffee and allow it to cool to body temperature.
2. Lubricate the rectal enema tube with K-Y Jelly, aloe vera gel, or another lubricant. Hang the enema bag above you, but no more than 2 feet from your body; the best level is approximately 6 inches above your intestines. Lying on your right side, draw both legs close to your abdomen.
3. Insert the tube several inches into your rectum. Open the stopcock and allow the coffee to run in very slowly to avoid cramping. Breathe deeply and try to relax.
4. Retain the solution for 12 to 15 minutes. If you have trouble retaining or taking the full amount, lower the bag; if you feel spasms, lower the bag to the floor to relieve the pressure. After about 20 seconds, slowly start raising the bag toward its original level. You can also pinch the tube to control the flow. Move to the toilet to release any excess liquid.

to body temperature, and delivering it via an enema bag (see "How to Administer a Coffee Enema," above).

Castor Oil Packs

Castor oil comes from the bean of the castor plant (*Oleum ricini*). The plant itself is quite poisonous, but the oil pressed out of the bean is safe to use, since the toxic constituents remain in the seeds. The Egyptians used castor oil as a laxative for cleansing the bowels and as a scalp rub to make hair grow and shine. Castor oil packs have been used traditionally for many conditions, including liver problems, constipation, and other ailments involving elimination, as well as nonmalignant ovarian fibroid cysts and headaches. The oil helps to draw out toxins, release tension, and improve blood circulation, especially in the lower abdomen. When used together with the healthy eating and exercise protocols discussed elsewhere in this book, castor oil packs can help break down stubborn fat deposits (see "Castor Oil Pack Instructions," page 40).

Dietary Recommendations to Support the Liver

Cruciferous vegetables (such as cabbage, brussels sprouts, cauliflower, and broccoli) are especially helpful for the liver. Brussels sprouts are

Lipotropic factors are substances that naturally prevent excess fat from accumulating in the liver. They help cleanse the liver by promoting the flow of fat and bile into the gallbladder. They also stimulate the growth of phagocytes (the bacteria-eating cells in the liver).

the best of the cruciferous vegetables for the liver, according to John Bastyr, ND, the founding father of Bastyr University of Naturopathic Medicine, in Seattle. Other helpful foods include onions, garlic, leeks, and chives. All of these foods for the liver contain sulfur.

Beets contain high levels of betaine, which a powerful lipotropic agent, meaning it increases the flow of bile, an emulsifier secreted by the gallbladder that helps to break down fat. Black radish and artichokes contain cynarin, which has liver-protective properties. Olive oil promotes the production of bile in the liver and also protects it from harmful microorganisms. Many aromatic cooking herbs and spices also aid the liver in its detoxification process. Outstanding among them is rosemary, which assists in the production and movement of bile through the liver and gallbladder. Dill, caraway, and fennel aid in phase II detoxification. All of these food choices are excellent as part of a weight-loss protocol.

Castor Oil Pack Instructions

1. Fold a flannel sheet to fit over your whole abdomen.

2. Cut a piece of plastic 1 to 2 inches larger than flannel sheet.

3. Soak the flannel sheet in gently heated castor oil. Fold it over and squeeze until some of the liquid oozes out, then unfold.

4. Prepare the surface where you will be lying, covering it with a large plastic sheet and an old towel to prevent staining.

5. Lie down on the towel and place the oil-soaked flannel sheet over your abdomen. Place the fitted plastic piece over the flannel sheet, then apply a hot water bottle over the area.

6. Wrap a towel under and around your torso.

7. Rest for 1 to 2 hours.

8. Rinse off the oil with a solution of 3 tablespoons baking soda to 1 quart water.

9. Repeat one to three times per week, or as instructed by your health-care practitioner.

Lipotropic Supplements to Support the Liver

Betaine, inositol, and choline are common lipotropic agents. Betaine is found primarily in beets, and beet root supplements (in capsule form) are used to ease bile congestion and improve bile flow to the small intestine; ox bile extracts are used for the same purpose. Inositol is found in fruits, meat, milk, and whole grains. Choline is present in high amounts in egg yolks, meat, milk, whole grains, and soybeans. Choline can chemically react with both water and fat, making it particularly suited for helping to transport fat-soluble toxins from the liver to the kidneys so that they may be excreted from the body.

Several amino acids are also helpful for supporting liver function. Methionine helps stimulate the flow of fats from the liver. Glutathione, a critical antioxidant (SEE QUICK DEFINITION), reduces free radical damage to cells, prevents depletion of other antioxidants, and activates immune cells. Glutathione is manufactured in the liver from glutamic acid and the amino acid N-acetylcysteine (NAC). Carnitine is manufactured in the liver from the amino acids methionine and lysine with the aid of vitamin C. The body uses carnitine to transport fats into the mitochondria (the energy centers of cells) for combustion and energy production. When liver function is impaired, both glutathione and carnitine levels may become low. Carnitine supplements help cleanse the liver of accumulated toxins. Taurine is needed by the liver to manufacture bile acids for the digestion of fats and is particularly useful in removing environmental chemicals (such as chlorine and petroleum solvents) from the body.

 An **antioxidant** is a natural biochemical substance that protects living cells against damage from harmful free radicals. Antioxidants work against the process of oxidation—the robbing of electrons from molecules. Oxidation can lead to cellular aging, degeneration, arthritis, heart disease, cancer, and other illnesses. Antioxidants react with free radicals and neutralize them before they can damage the body. Antioxidant nutrients include vitamins A, C, and E, beta-carotene, selenium, coenzyme Q10, pycnogenol (found in grape seed extract), L-glutathione, superoxide dismutase, and bioflavonoids. Plant antioxidants include ginkgo biloba and garlic.

Therapeutic Herbs for the Liver

Most herbs and plant foods contain important phytonutrients (phyto means "plant"), substances that have health-protecting qualities. Burdock, goldenseal, baptisia, smilax, Oregon grape root, globe artichoke (*Cynara scolymus*), and echinacea all contain phytonutrients that improve liver function. The herbs discussed below are especially notable for supporting liver function.

Milk thistle (Silybum marianum): For centuries, European herbalists have used the bioflavonoid silymarin, found in milk thistle, for restoring liver function. Bioflavonoids are plant pigments with beneficial properties; they protect against damage from destructive free radicals in the body and enhance the activity of vitamin C. Silymarin accelerates the process of regenerating damaged liver tissue, thereby freeing the organ to carry out its key functions. It has been proven effective against poisoning by acetaminophen and petrochemical solvents.[16] It's best to use milk thistle standardized to 70% to 80% silymarin content.

As with basal metabolism, the rate of **thermogenesis** will determine whether the body sheds or accumulates fat. *Thermogenesis* means, simply, to generate heat in the body during metabolism. The digestion of food, movement of the muscles, and other metabolic processes all produce heat as a by-product. In certain metabolic activities, however, heat is the primary product. This type of pure thermogenesis is one of the body's key weight-control mechanisms and serves as a kind of waste incinerator for excess calories. When this mechanism does not burn fat as it should, weight gain is sure to follow.

Katuka (Picrorrhiza kurroa): This tiny plant grows in the Himalayas at altitudes between 9,000 to 15,000 feet. Its active ingredient has been found comparable or superior to silymarin. It is very useful for rejuvenating the liver and also helps the immune system.[17]

Dandelion (Taraxacum officinale): As a liver and digestive tonic, as well as blood cleanser and diuretic, dandelion aids in detoxification of the body.[18] Given that chemical or heavy metal toxicity is frequently involved in obesity, dandelion can help cleanse the body and support the liver in its elimination functions. As a digestive tonic, dandelion also helps with the gastrointestinal complaints.

Green tea (Camellia sinensis): Green tea is rich in catechin, a bioflavonoid used by European naturopaths and medical doctors to treat chemical hepatitis, cirrhosis, and other environmental and viral forms of liver disease. Catechins can be taken as a nutritional supplement.[19] In addition, green tea specifically aids weight loss through thermogenesis (SEE QUICK DEFINITION).

The Stagnated Lymphatic System

Lymph is a clear to milky fluid that carries nutrients to cells. It also carries waste products and cellular debris that accumulate in the tissue spaces between cells to the bloodstream for elimination. Interspersed throughout the lymph channels are the lymph nodes, clusters of immune tissue that work as filters to remove foreign and potentially harmful substances from the lymph fluid. Each lymph node contains scavenger cells (macrophages and reticuloendothelial cells) that destroy toxins and microbes. Lymph nodes are clustered in strategic junctures of the body, such as the head and neck, the armpits, and the groin. The gastrointestinal tract, including the appendix, contains a tremendous quantity of lymph nodes known as gut-associated lymphoid tissue (GALT), which serves as a primary filter for the bloodstream.

Unlike the circulatory system, which uses the heart to pump the blood, the lymphatic system doesn't have its own pump. Instead, it

How Traditional Chinese Medicine Views the Liver

The idea of a congested or sluggish liver is an ancient concept in traditional Chinese medicine (TCM). The signs of a sluggish or congested liver can manifest as PMS, fatigue, lethargy, an inability to properly digest foods (particularly fats), multiple allergies, environmental and chemical sensitivities, constipation, arthritis, and obesity. TCM maintains that various emotions are connected to different organs. The liver is considered the reservoir of anger toward other people or toward the self. Anger affects the liver's ability to govern the flow of qi (SEE QUICK DEFINITION), blood, and vital nutrients to ligaments, tendons, sinews, joints, bones, and muscles. One of the main Chinese herbs used in liver ailments is gardenia, known as the "happiness herb" because it has an ability to loosen emotions that have been stuck due to chronic liver congestion. In TCM, the liver is associated with the wood element and is represented by the color greenish yellow. Leafy greens and other substances of that color are considered beneficial for toning and boosting liver function.

depends on movement of skeletal muscles during exercise, breathing, and normal day-to-day activities. As the muscles contract and relax, they push the lymph fluid along; backflow is prevented by valves throughout the system. Massage and other lymphatic drainage techniques can also enhance circulation of the lymph fluid. Because the lymph fluid is full of nutrients on their way to the cells and waste products that must be removed, any interference with this flow can create serious problems for the body.

Stagnant lymphatic fluid has a different consistency; instead of being clear and thin, it becomes thick and cloudy in the early stages of toxicity. If the lymph remains stationary, it will progress to a glutinous consistency similar to thick cream, and eventually cottage cheese. Viscous lymphatic fluid becomes an oxygen-deprived sludge that impedes the flow of nutrients to the cells and barricades toxic substances from exiting the extracellular spaces. Lack of nutrients to tissues combined with the stagnation of waste products leads to degenerative diseases, and it's also directly related to the development of cellulite and obesity. Stagnation of the lymph can be caused by allergenic and mucus-

 Qi or chi (pronounced CHEE) is a Chinese word variously translated to mean "vital energy," "essence of life," and "living force." In Chinese medicine, the proper flow of qi along energy channels (meridians) within the body is crucial to a person's health and vitality. There are many types of qi, classified according to source, location, and function (such as activation, warming, defense, transformation, and containment). Within the body, qi and blood are closely linked, as each is considered to flow along with the other. Qi may be stagnant (nonmoving), deficient (partially absent), or excessive (inappropriately abundant) from a given organ system. Qi has two essential qualities: yang (active, fiery, moving, bright, energizing) and yin (passive, watery, stationary, dark, calming).

What Clogs the Lymph?

A number of factors can contribute to a stagnant lymphatic system:

- Insufficient exercise: This is a major factor because exercise moves the muscles and creates pressure within the lymph vessels, forcing the fluid to flow.

- Overexposure to environmental chemicals or other toxins.

- Stress: Tension in the body can lead to structural misalignment in the neck, pinching the lymph vessels.

- Intestinal problems such as chronic constipation: If plugged up with mucus or fecal matter, the walls of the colon cannot serve as an outlet for the lymph. In order to effectively release lymphatic material, the inner lining of the colon needs to be healthy.

- Some dietary habits: Eating too many mucus-producing foods such as dairy, fatty foods (especially those containing hydrogenated oils), highly processed foods, and allergenic foods is particularly harmful.

- Structural misalignments, particularly in the neck and shoulder area.

- Medications.

- Impaired blood circulation due to chronic conditions such as diabetes or atherosclerosis.

- Surgical procedures (such as breast or abdominal surgery) that require the removal of adjacent lymph nodes. Radiation therapy can have the same effect.

- Hormonal imbalances.

- Infections or traumatic injuries.

- Antiperspirants: Since they are absorbed through the skin, antiperspirants can impair the functioning the lymph nodes located in the underarm area.

- Tight-fitting clothing, such as bras and exercise clothing.

forming foods, chronic constipation, musculoskeletal imbalances, lack of exercise, improper breathing, prescription drugs, and impairment of local or systemic circulation due to complications of diabetes or atherosclerosis.

A clogged lymphatic system is directly responsible for weight gain through several mechanisms:

- Cellulite formation: Fat can accumulate directly beneath the skin. In regions such as the upper hips, thighs, arms, and buttocks, pockets of fat can give the overlying skin a dimpled texture somewhat like an orange rind. This is commonly referred to as cellulite, and it's often due to a blockage in the body's lymph system. There is a direct correlation between decreased lymphatic flow and the development of cellulite.[20]

- Slowed metabolism: Clogged lymph slows the metabolism by decreasing the rate at which nutrients are delivered to the tissues and wastes are removed. This further increases the likelihood of weight gain.

- Fluid retention: Decreased lymph flow causes swelling and fluid retention, which leads to weight gain.

Therapies for Improving Lymphatic Drainage

It is of paramount importance to prevent stagnation of the lymphatic system. This ensures that the lymph fluid continues to circulate freely throughout the body and that the body is properly detoxified. Techniques that encourage lymphatic drainage include manual lymph massage, light beam therapy, dry skin brushing, exercise, and herbs.

Manual Lymph Drainage

Manual lymph drainage is a specially designed massage technique that uses gentle, stationary circular motions on the lymph nodes, palpating with the tips or the entire length of the fingers. These motions act like an external pump that pulls lymphatic fluid through the lymph channels and enhances the release of toxins. Lymph drain massage should not be confused with conventional massage techniques, as it relies on gentle and directed manipulations designed to induce lymph flow. The lymph should only be massaged lightly, as too much pressure can cause thickening. Lymph drain massage, commonly prescribed in Europe, is growing in popularity in the United States.

Your Lymph System at a Glance

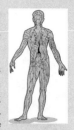

The lymphatic system is the body's master drain. It includes a vast network of capillaries that transport the lymph, a series of nodes throughout the body (primarily in the neck, groin, and armpits) that collect the lymph, and three organs (the tonsils, spleen, and thymus) that produce white blood cells (lymphocytes) to scavenge for toxins and microbes.

Lymph is the fluid that fills the spaces between cells in the body. This fluid contains nutrients to be delivered to cells and cellular debris (bacteria, dead cells, heavy metals, and waste products) to be removed. The purpose of the lymphatic system is to carry toxins away from the cells by collecting and filtering the lymph, neutralizing and disposing of bacteria or other invaders, and returning its contents to the bloodstream.

The lymph flows slowly through the body to the abdomen and chest (at the rate of 3 quarts per day), where it drains into the bloodstream through large ducts. Once in the blood, the toxins carried by the lymph are transported to the liver and kidneys, where they are broken down and excreted. Some of the lymph also empties directly into the colon, where it is eliminated with the feces. Unlike blood circulation, the lymphatic system does not have a pump (like the heart) to move it along. Rather, its movement depends on muscle contractions, general body activity, massage and other forms of compression, and gravity. The lymph system becomes most active during times of illness such as the flu, when the nodes (particularly at the throat) visibly swell with collected waste products.

Do-at-Home Lymph Massage

While not intended as a substitute for lymph drain massage, a self-massage technique may be helpful in stimulating the flow of lymph. Doing one leg at a time, elevate the leg and gently massage up from your ankle, around your knee, and up toward your hip, massaging the front and back of your leg. This technique moves lymph fluid in the direction it should naturally flow. The ideal time to perform this type of massage is at the end of the day's activities.

Light Beam Therapy

High-tech lymphatic drainage uses various types of light beam generators to break up lymph blockages. The light beam generator looks like a flashlight with a long, extendable hose. Practitioners use this handheld device to focus energy on areas of blocked lymph. The energy from the generator breaks the electrical bonds that hold clusters of lymph protein molecules together, thus unclogging stagnated lymph fluid. This therapy is often used to enhance the benefits of lymph massage. It is also very effective as a therapy for lymphedema, a condition where the overaccumulation of lymphatic fluid causes swelling.

Dry Skin Brushing

The skin is an organ of both absorption and elimination; oxygen, vitamins, and minerals, as well as toxic substances (through air and water contact), can find their way into internal organs through the skin, and more than a pound of waste products in the form of sweat are eliminated by the skin each day.

Dry skin brushing is based on acupuncture, which recognizes an estimated 3 million nerve points spread over the surface of the skin. By applying friction to acupuncture points, dry skin brushing stimulates these energy connections, invigorating the entire nervous system so that every organ, gland, muscle, and ligament benefits. Dry skin brushing (see "How to Perform a Dry Skin Brush," page 47) helps to physically move toxic lymph fluid through the lymph vessels. It also improves the skin's ability to eliminate toxins by exfoliating, or removing, dead skin cells and allowing the skin to breathe. This helps oxygenate the layer of tissue right beneath the skin and also reduces cellulite.

Herbal Wraps

Circulation of lymph can be stimulated by using body wraps or lotions containing essential oils made from herbs. Certain herbs, such as rosemary, eucalyptus, sage, and juniper, stimulate stagnant lymph and aid its circulation. Other herbs that as detoxifiers or as astringents, such as Irish moss, aloe powder, buckthorn, ginger, bayberry, seaweed, and

How to Perform a Dry Skin Brush

To perform a dry skin brush, you will need a moderately soft brush with natural vegetable bristles, preferably with a removable wooden handle. Nylon or synthetic bristles can be too sharp and possibly hurt the skin; they can also create a buildup of undesirable static electromagnetic energy. When starting, you will need to brush gently until your skin become conditioned; this usually takes just a few days.

Begin at your fingertips and work your way up the inner and outer surfaces of each arm. Work toward your heart, using short, brisk strokes. Then start at your feet and brush upward toward your groin, one leg at a time. Include the top and the sole of each foot and the front and back of each leg. Then brush your pelvis, belly, buttocks, and lower back; avoid your head and neck. The strokes should not irritate but be brisk enough to color the skin pink and cause a tingling sensation. Dry skin brushing is best done before a shower or bath. As you become accustomed to dry brushing, the entire process should take no more than ten minutes. It would be a good idea to brush your skin daily for three months, then twice weekly as a lifetime practice. Every two weeks or so, wash your brush with soap and water and dry it in the sun or in a warm place, as it will rapidly fill with dead skin cells and other impurities. For hygienic reasons, each person should have a separate brush.

white oak bark, can be added to enhance the wrap's healing potential. Prepare a body wrap by diluting the chosen essential oils with a vegetable oil, such as sunflower and almond, or gel, such as aloe vera or seaweed gel which can be purchased at health food stores or spas. Apply the mixture to your skin, then cover the area comfortably, not tightly, in plastic wrap. You should relax during the wrap, leaving it in place for about 45 minutes. Precautions: Never leave a wrap on overnight and do not use wraps if pregnant.

Exercise

The rate of lymph flow increases dramatically during physical activity because the contracting and relaxing motions of the muscles in any form of exercise helps to pump the lymph. Light bouncing on a mini trampoline is especially effective in helping to restore lymph flow.[21] (For more information on the mini trampoline, see chapter 2, page 62.)

Foods for a Healthy Lymph System

Ample quantities of fresh fruits and vegetables in ensure that the lymph fluid stays clear and moves easily through the body. Certain vegetables and fruits, such as cabbage, pineapple, grapes, papaya, and melons, have a particularly strong effect on the lymph, since they contain enzymes that break down excess or stagnant proteins in the lymphatic channels.

Herbs That Stimulate Lymphatic Drainage

Also known as goose grass or bedstraw, cleavers (*Galium aparine*) removes "damp congestion," the traditional Chinese medicine designation for pain and swelling often associated with excess weight. Cleaver extract (available at health food stores) can be added to vegetable juice or carrot-apple-ginger juice. If you can identify wild cleavers, make a spring tonic by combining cleavers with dandelion greens and chickweed. Other herbs helpful for the lymphatic system include prickly ash bark, burdock root, nettles, bayberry bark, acacia gum, aloe, bladderwrack, couchgrass, Irish moss, lemon balm, lobelia, oatstraw, and red clover. These herbs can help to thin the consistency of the lymph, allowing it to circulate more efficiently.

Success Story: Losing Weight through Lymphatic Cleansing

Linda, 54, was uncomfortable with her double chin. Her weight fluctuated between 180 pounds and 200 pounds on her 5 foot 6 frame. When her legs started to swell, she became concerned. She visited her family physician, who said all her blood values were in normal limits, but suggested that she lose weight. He recommended that she see a nutritionist to help design a healthy eating program. Linda decided to see a naturopathic physician in her area. (Licensed naturopathic physicians are highly trained medical doctors who are well schooled in nutrition and other natural therapies.) The naturopath quickly recognized the symptoms of stagnant and toxic lymph and immediately recommended a program for Linda to get her lymph fluid moving again.

"My legs seemed to be full of fluid, so I thought I had circulation problems," Linda remarked. "I'd never even heard of the lymphatic system. I just knew I was uncomfortable and needed help." Fluid retention is a common result when the body is overwhelmed with toxins. Linda's program was intended to restore the lymphatic system to normal functioning and move toxic wastes out of the body. The naturopath suggested that Linda commit to a diet of vegetable soup, salad, herbal tea, and one protein powder smoothie per day for two weeks. Meanwhile, Linda received lymph drain massage and light beam therapy.

After two weeks, Linda noticed that her appearance had already started to change. This acted as a wonderful motivation for her to continue on her protocol. The naturopath added a multivitamin-multimineral formula along with cleavers, barberry bark, and aloe vera juice. Linda also included 20 minutes of jumping on a mini trampoline as part of her daily routine. After six months, she felt like a new person. Her double chin was gone and her legs were no longer swollen. "Now I eat normally and my weight stays between 140 pounds and 145 pounds. Unclogging my lymph system turned my body around!"

Supporting the Portals: Kidneys, Skin, and Lungs

An effective detoxification protocol must include therapies that enhance the body's ability to expel waste products through all the detoxification pathways. The exit routes, or portals—the kidneys, skin, and lungs—must be supported to ensure that toxins are efficiently removed. If there is an imbalance in these organs, toxins can be reabsorbed, compromising detoxification and impeding the healing process.

Kidneys

The kidneys assist the body in removing xenobiotics (environmental estrogens), drug residues, nitrogenous wastes originating from protein metabolism, and a host of other water-soluble toxins. They also regulate sodium and potassium levels, as well as blood pressure. During detoxification, it's important to keep your urine diluted by drinking at least 2 quarts of filtered water per day. Concentrated urine contains high levels of toxins, especially during detoxification, and these can cause kidney damage. Periodic laboratory measurements of kidney and liver function during a detoxification program are a necessity.

Botanical diuretics can assist the kidneys in excreting waste. Some increase blood flow to the kidneys, while others work by inhibiting the reabsorption of water, which increases urinary output.

- Dandelion *(Taraxacum officinale):* Dandelion leaves are an excellent diuretic and also support the liver.
- Parsley *(Petroselinum sativum):* Much more than just a plate garnish, parsley is used to support kidney function because of its diuretic action. Include fresh parsley juice in vegetable juices and eat it regularly as a vegetable.
- Horsetail *(Equisetum arvense):* Also called scouring rush because it was used by native peoples to scour dishes, horsetail is an excellent diuretic and also contains the mineral silica, a critical nutrient for bone, muscles, and healthy hair, skin, and nails.

Skin

The skin is the largest organ of the body. Often referred to as the "third kidney," it's the first line of defense against external pathogens. The pores and glands of the skin are important organs of elimination through which toxic chemicals, such as formaldehyde, phenol, various insecticides, chlorine, and petroleum products can be excreted via either sweat or sebum (oil secreted by the skin). Although these chemicals may enter the body through inhalation or ingestion (for example, in tap water), they're also often absorbed through the skin or during bathing.[22]

Sauna (heat stress detoxification): Using a sauna can effectively clear the body of fat-soluble toxins. Studies of fat biopsies before and after a heat stress detoxification protocol revealed an average of 21.3% reduction in body levels of 16 toxic chemicals, including PCBs and PBBs.[23] The study found that people's toxin levels continued to decrease for up to four months after discontinuing heat and detoxification therapy. Detoxification programs that included fasting, drinking fresh juices, sauna therapy, exercise, and lymphatic drainage reduced body levels of various pesticides by up to 66%.[24]

Sauna brew: This herb tea is recommended for people using sauna therapy. The tea expedites sweating, especially if consumed as a hot tea before and during the sauna treatment, thereby enhancing the removal of toxins from the body. People have commented that this blend also tastes exceptionally good. Combine equal parts of cinnamon, ginger, boneset, yarrow, peppermint, and elder and use 1 tablespoon of the herb mixture per cup of tea. Pour 1 cup of steaming hot water over the herbs, cover, and allow to steep for 20 minutes.

Lungs

During the energy crisis in the 1970s, U.S. building construction practices changed; homes, offices, schools, and most buildings were sealed tightly and better insulated. This saves a great deal of energy but tends to trap indoor air pollution, including pollens and other allergens, oils, and dry-cleaning fluid (a known liver toxin). Toxic chemicals such as benzene (a carcinogen) are released from paint, new carpets, drapes, and upholstery. Formaldehyde vapors rise up from plywood, new cabinets, furniture, carpets, drapes, wallpaper, and paneling. All enter the body through the lungs.

Herbs for lung detoxification: Herbs are frequently used to target specific aspects of lung contamination and detoxification:

- Fenugreek and horehound help decrease production and thickness of mucus secretions.
- Wild cherry bark is an expectorant that helps remove mucus and reduce congestion.
- Mullein, elecampane, and grindelia strengthen lung tissue.
- Eucalyptus and thyme oils are antiseptics that kill microbial organisms; a combination of these herbs can be taken as a tincture.

Inhalation therapy: Steam inhalation can be very helpful for detoxifying the lungs. Add two to three drops of eucalyptus and thyme oils to a pot of boiling water, remove the pot from the stove, and place your head above the steam. Create a tent by covering your head with a towel and inhale the steam vapors, but be sure to keep your head far enough above the steam so as not to get burned.

two

Start Exercising

Red Alert!! Exercising is an absolute necessity for any weight-loss program!

If you are reading this book, you have an interest in moving toward a healthier life, which includes weight management. One of the most important steps you can take is to start exercising. Studies continue to show that even moderate levels of exercise can have dramatic health benefits, including preventing heart disease, diabetes, osteoporosis, depression, and many other health problems. Unfortunately, many Americans spend their leisure time doing little or nothing in terms of physical activity. This is one of the main causes of the American obesity epidemic.

Change Sedentary Habits

Starting to exercise is an absolute necessity for any weight-loss program. Healthy food choices and getting enough physical activity to burn off excess calories are the key to good health and maintaining a healthy body weight. You don't have to be a marathon runner; even moderate exercise like walking the dog or gardening can produce health benefits. Exercise can help build muscle, boost your energy levels, improve your cardiovascular fitness, reduce stress, and promote weight loss.

Isaac Newton's first law of motion, the law of inertia, states that an object at rest tends to stay at rest and an object in motion tends to stay in motion. This seems to hold true for people as well. If someone is used to a sedentary lifestyle of driving to work, sitting all day, going out to lunch, sitting during lunch, driving home, and lounging all evening in front of the TV, there seems to be no time for exercise. But once you start to include exercise into your daily life, you'll often look for more and more opportunities to keep moving. Park farther away from work, take the stairs, stretch before taking a shower, do isometric exercises while sitting at your desk—the opportunities for movement are endless!

The amount of exercise recommended to treat or prevent obesity is 60 to 90 minutes, seven days per week.[1] However, even 30 minutes a day can do the body a world of good. In addition, if periods of exercise are sprinkled in throughout the day in 15- or 20-minute segments, it still can be useful. Not only is exercise essential to weight loss, it actually stimulates the generation of mitochondria, the energy centers within the cells.[2] This is one of the reasons why the more you exercise, the more energy you have—and the more you want to exercise!

Exercise to Maximize Thermogenesis

Proper exercise increases the body's thermogenic (fat-burning) response, not only during the activity, but for long afterward. It does this by increasing the basal metabolism (SEE QUICK DEFINITION, page 54), which is a bit like the rate at which a car consumes gasoline while idling. The body burns calories constantly. Even during sleep, your heart is beating, your lungs continue to breathe, and every cell in your body is participating in metabolism. All of these functions require calories. Even moderate exercise can raise your metabolism and so that you burn additional calories for approximately 12 hours afterward. This can amount to as much as 15% of the calories burned during a workout, a significant amount when you're trying to lose weight.

The Oxygen Priority

Oxygen is vital for the proper function of cellular metabolism. The body extracts most of the energy it needs from fat and glucose. The energy in these substances is stored in chemical bonds that hold the molecules together. Oxygen reacts with the molecules, splitting them open and liberating their energy for use by the body. (To illustrate this, think of the chemical bonds as stretched rubber bands. When a bond is broken it releases stored energy, similar to how a stretched rubber band snaps when you suddenly let go of one end.) When oxygen is deficient, metabolism slows and less fat is broken down. Oxygen enters the body through the lungs, where it is absorbed by the blood and then transported to every cell. Regular exercise helps to increase the body's oxygen supply by strengthening the heart and increasing the capacity of red blood cells to absorb oxygen, improving delivery of nutrients to all parts of the body.[3]

> **QUICK DEFINITION** **Basal metabolism** refers to the number of calories used by the body at complete rest to maintain basic life processes, such as breathing and circulation. Basal metabolism, which is controlled by the thyroid gland (the largest endocrine gland, located near the front of the throat where it wraps around the windpipe right behind the Adam's apple), keeps the body at a normal, healthy resting temperature of 98.6°F. Using hormones, the thyroid sends chemical messages to every cell in the body, controlling body temperature, heart rate, and muscle movements. When the thyroid is dysfunctional or underactive—a condition called hypothyroidism—it sends out fewer hormones, causing basal metabolism to slow down. This slowing causes a number of problems, including general feelings of sluggishness and increases in body weight.

Resting heart rate is a measure of the strength of the heart. A strong heart beats fewer times per minute than a weak heart because it has a larger capacity to move blood and delivers a higher volume of blood with every beat. If the heart is weak, it has a harder time delivering enough blood to meet the body's oxygen demands, even during sleep. Aerobic exercise not only increases the strength of the heart, it also increases red blood cell count, allows for faster transport of oxygen through the body, and helps lower elevated blood pressure. Additionally, exercise improves cholesterol by increasing the amount of high-density lipoproteins (HDL, or good cholesterol) in the blood.[4] Exercise increases the capacity of the lungs, which also makes oxygen more available to cells, body tissues, and organ systems. This enhances metabolism and allows nutrients to be absorbed more efficiently. The good news is that it doesn't take long to bring down your resting heart rate. A regular walking program can decrease the heart rates of previously sedentary individuals within 18 weeks.[5] A brisk walk outdoors can also expose you to much-needed fresh air and sunlight, which helps to increase the body's production of the neurotransmitter serotonin, a brain chemical that helps to control appetite.

Identifying Your Exertion Cues

When starting an exercise program, don't try to do too much too quickly. It is important to monitor your vital signs before, during, and throughout exercise sessions. Be aware of your body's exertion cues and learn how to accurately measure them so that you can exercise safely.

- Monitor your resting and target heart rates, which will enable you to adjust your level of activity. Resting heart rate can be measured by simply placing your fingers across your wrist and counting the number of beats for 15 seconds, then multiply by four; this is the number of beats per minute. To determine your target heart rate, use the following formula: Subtract your age from 220, then multiply the result by .7; for example, for a 50-year-old person, maximum heart rate is determined by subtracting 50 from 220, which equals 170. Then, 170 is multiplied by 0.7 (70%) to reach the target heart rate of 119. Always take your heart rate before you begin your exercise, during the session, and after you have cooled down.

- Alternately, you could use a heart rate monitor, a device that will monitor and display your heart rate as you exercise. Once primarily worn by people recovering from heart disease, heart monitors have become very popular among athletes and fitness enthusiasts in recent years. Inexpensive models are available to anyone wanting to know if they are exercising safely.

- Notice your breathing. If your breathing is fast and labored, slow down. Once

you have gained some stamina, your breathing during exertion should be steady and even.

- Take the talking test. If you are able to comfortably carry on a conversation during exercise, you probably aren't overdoing it.

- Watch for signs of physical pain. If you experience any sharp or sudden pain or can't breathe comfortably, slowly come to a stop.

- Notice changes in body temperature. Drink water before, during, and after exercise to keep your body temperature from rising too much and to prevent dehydration. If you find that you are overheating during exercise, slow your pace, drink water, or reduce the layers of clothing you are wearing.

- Observe your general energy level. Although starting an exercise program may not be comfortable if you have been inactive, you should be able to enjoy the activity. Begin with a modest level of movement and exertion and gradually increase the duration, frequency, and intensity of the activity. Don't throw yourself into a highly demanding physical conditioning program and risk the possibility of injury.

 If you are recovering from heart disease, respiratory illness, or any other serious illness, consult your physician for recommendations on a safe exercise program.

The Muscular Advantage

Dieters who exercise have a tremendous advantage. Not only does exercise boost metabolism, it also builds lean muscle, which in turn increases

How to Stick with Your Exercise Program

Here are some tips from the President's Council on Physical Fitness and Sports, to help you stay on track with your exercise program:[6]

- Adopt a specific plan and write it down.

- Keep setting realistic goals as you go along and remind yourself of them often.

- Keep a log to record your progress and make sure you keep it up-to-date.

- Include weight and/or percent body fat measures in your log. Extra pounds can easily creep back.

- Upgrade your fitness program as you progress.

- Enlist the support and company of your family and friends.

- Update others on your successes.

- Avoid injuries by pacing yourself and including a warm-up and cooldown period as part of every workout.

- Reward yourself periodically for a job well done!.

 For more on the link between **toxins and weight gain**, see chapter 1, Detoxification, page 3.

calories burned by the body. Dieting without exercise is generally counter-productive, because curbing calories signals the body to slow the metabolism, and if too few calories are consumed, the body begins to metabolize muscle tissue. Slowed metabolism and loss of muscle tissue can both keep you from achieving your weight-loss goals. This emphasizes the importance of maintaining an adequate, well-balanced diet and a sound exercise program to allow your body to drop weight safely and permanently.

How Your Body Burns Calories

Intense, prolonged exertion, such as weight lifting, is fueled primarily by glucose, a simple sugar that the body makes from dietary carbohydrates and sugars. Conversely, fats are the preferred fuel for fast movements, such as running and jumping. These different types of activities also involve different types of muscle fibers. Weight lifting, for example, relies on slow-twitch fibers, while running relies on fast-twitch fibers.

The fact that fat is the preferred fuel of fast-twitch muscle fibers does not necessarily mean that an ideal exercise program for weight loss should focus on quick-action exercises rather than those that build strength. Strength-building exercise increases lean muscle mass, which is one of the best ways to increase how many calories your body burns. Muscle cells have high energy demands even at rest. Consequently, the more muscle you have, the more calories you'll use throughout the day.

Designing an Exercise Program

What does it mean to be physically fit? The media bombards us with images of very slender models, superbly conditioned athletes, and other extreme examples, but try to ignore these. Instead, visualize realistic and attainable fitness goals appropriate for you

The key to starting and staying with an exercise program is finding activities that you enjoy and will continue to do. Don't choose an activity just because it burns more calories or promises quick results. It's best to choose the right types of exercise for your fitness level. Also make sure you have exercise options that aren't weather dependent. For instance, if you choose walking, (one of the best types of exercise to start off with and stay with), look into a mall walking club nearby so you can continue your exercise in inclement weather. If you have difficulty developing a program and are not sure where to begin, consult a personal trainer for further guidance.

Before beginning any exercise program, consult your physician and have a thorough exam to rule out any health conditions that may preclude certain types of exercise. If you've been physically inactive for several years, it is best to undergo a detoxification program before you begin strenuous exercise. Over time, the toxins you're exposed to in air, water, and food accumulate in your liver, lymphatic system, and colon. Holistic health-care professionals advise clients to avoid strenuous exercise until they have adequately cleansed the body of toxins, because vigorous exercise can release accumulated toxins, which may overload your system. However, low to moderate exercise does not cause this effect.

Calories Burned by Moderate Activities

In the table below, the calories burned are for a 150- to 160-pound person. A lighter person would burn fewer calories, and a heavier person more.

Calories Burned by Day-to-Day Activities	
Activity	**Calories Burned**
Raking leaves for 30 minutes	150
Washing and waxing the car for 45–60 minutes	150
Stair walking for 15 minutes	150
Walking for 15 minutes	75
Social dancing for 30 minutes	150
Shooting baskets for 30 minutes	150
Shoveling snow for 30 minutes	300

From the Department of Health and Human Services, Centers for Disease Control and Prevention, www.cdc.gov/nccdphp/dnpa/physical/recommendations/adults.htm.

Including more physical activity throughout your day is a simple way to add moderate levels of activity to your routine and help you maintain a basic level of fitness. Activities such as unloading groceries, walking a flight of stairs three times a day, and washing the car by hand can help a person who weights 150 to 160 pounds burn as much as 10,500 calories in a month.These sorts of activities can help you establish a basic level of fitness. A strenuous exercise program may be too daunting and ultimately self-defeating; for many people, moderate activity may be a more realistic and attainable goal.

You may also find it easier to get started if you don't push yourself to do all of your daily exercise in one fell swoop. In fact, the American College of Sports Medicine and the U.S. Centers for Disease Control and Prevention suggest that exercise sessions will yield similar benefits whether completed all at once or divided into 10-minute bouts. Both structured and nonstructured physical activity, such as an exercise class or household chores, can add to the overall beneficial effects.[7] This knowledge can really help with time management and motivation, two of the excuses people often use to explain why they don't exercise! Social support can also help you overcome obstacles to exercising and lead to a better long-term outcome in weight loss.[8] Because exercise burns calories, it can help you achieve weight loss with less reduction in the amount of calories consumed. In other words, exercise is a great strategy for counterbalancing the sense of deprivation so often associated with weight loss.

Success Story: Exercise for Weight Loss at Any Age

Bill, a 58-year-old male, shares his weight loss and fitness story: "When I turned 40 years of age, I began to rethink my life. My marriage was ending and I did not like my appearance when I viewed recent photos of myself. At first I felt discouraged because I thought I was too old to get into great shape, but it was time to reinvent myself. I joined a gym for the first time in my life and began regular workouts. I also reevaluated my diet. Although I was already eating "pretty healthy," I took a closer look at what I ingested on a daily basis. I decided to live without sugar and to consume less fats and carbs as well. I did not wish to "diet" as so many Americans do. I wanted to change to a lifestyle that worked for me. Over the course of a year, my weight slowly dropped 20 pounds. I looked and felt great. In fact, as the years passed, I felt more toned and actually younger! I also learned that you are what you think. Attitude, diet, and exercise became my mantra. I felt much lighter on my feet. I started jogging, got back to swimming and biking, and took up roller-blading. I made a great discovery too. I found that the more I did, the more I could do. Exercise is truly the key. People do not believe my age. As a single person (even in my late 50s), I have learned that people of all ages find me attractive. I never dreamed I'd be dating and enjoying such a wonderful healthy active life at age 58!"

Although exact recommendations change throughout the years, there's no doubt that daily exercise is vital for both health and weight loss. According to the President's Council on Physical Fitness and Sports, a balanced physical fitness program incorporates the following elements:[9]

A warm-up: Begin gradually. Start with 5 to 10 minutes of basic warm-up exercises, which can include gentle stretching or a short, slow walk.

Cardiorespiratory fitness: Endurance athletes, such as long-distance runners or swimmers, have the stamina for their physically demanding sports because they have good cardiorespiratory fitness. Their heart and lungs are able to deliver oxygen and nutrients to the tissues and remove wastes over sustained periods of activity. The main thing is to get moving, be it walking, running, cycling, or any other aerobic activity. After warming up and breathing more deeply, begin the activity and gradually pick up the pace. This may mean moving from a slow walk to a brisker pace or increasing the speed on a treadmill. If it has been a long time since you've exercised regularly, begin slowly. Your first session may consist of 5 minutes of warming up and another 5 to 10 minutes of walking.

Muscular strength: A muscle's capacity to exert force for a brief period of time can be developed by participating in sports or by specific weight-training exercises. By regularly working individual muscle groups, they increase in strength. Join your local gym and learn how to use the free weights, or do more day-to-day activities that require regular lifting, such as chopping wood and gardening. Be certain you use proper lifting stances to protect your back and joints from injury. For best results, consult with a certified personal trainer, who can guide you in proper technique and help you design an individualized workout strategy based on your unique needs. Strive for at least two 20-minute sessions of free weights per week. Weight training helps change your body composition, increasing your ratio of lean muscle mass to fat, thereby improving your metabolism.

Muscular endurance: This is the muscle's ability to undergo repeated contractions or to continue applying force against a fixed object over a sustained period of time. Every week, try to fit in at least three 30-minute sessions of exercises such as push-ups, sit-ups, and similar calisthenics to develop endurance in all of your major muscle groups. Public parks sometimes have par courses that include equipment and instructions for many of these exercises at designated stations. Again, other activities involving vigorous work around the house, such as washing the car, can provide similar benefits.

Flexibility: Flexibility is the ability to move muscles freely through a full range of motion. Dancers rely on flexibility to maximize their performance, but everyone can benefit from increased flexibility, and it can help prevent injury. Try to incorporate 10 to 15 minutes of gentle, nonbouncing stretching exercises into your workouts. This can be done before you set off on a walk or bike ride and also at the end of the session. Yoga and tai chi are excellent for increasing flexibility.

Cooldown: Always be sure to cool down afterward; don't stop exercising abruptly without giving your body a chance to slow down. If you've just walked a mile in 20 minutes, take another 5 minutes to slow down and allow your body to gradually shift into low gear.

Although you'd ideally incorporate all of the elements above into your exercise program, remember that the first priority is simply to *get moving!* And don't forget that the key is to establish a routine you'll be able to stick with, so choose activities that are fun, satisfying, and not too strenuous at the outset. Here are some activities you might choose from:

- Cycling
- Walking
- Swimming and aquatic exercise
- Jumping on a mini trampoline
- Aerobics
- Jogging

- Running
- Ballroom dancing
- Yoga
- Tai Chi
- Qigong
- The Super Seven Home Workout (see page 67)
- *Anything* that will get you moving

Let's take a closer look at some the specific benefits of some of these easy and practical forms of exercise.

Pedal Your Way to Health

A stationary bicycle is a great choice for a home exercise program. It is easy to use, can accommodate all fitness levels, takes up a small amount of space, and provides adequate exercise. Plus, stationary bikes are gentle on the back and joints; unlike running or walking, they provide a nonimpact workout that is nonetheless effective in strengthening the heart and lungs.

Using a stationary bike can assist weight loss by burning calories, and as with other forms of aerobic exercise, it will increase your basal metabolism rate. Even moderate use of a stationary bicycle—30 to 40 minutes three to four times per week—can raise your basal metabolism rate, which in turn increases the amount of calories your body burns for approximately 12 hours afterward.

Running in Place on a Treadmill

Whatever your initial fitness level, a treadmill can provide the appropriate workout, from gentle to strenuous. Even a moderate treadmill program can help control weight, guard against heart disease, and reduce cholesterol levels by providing a regular cardiovascular workout. It also improves muscle tone, reduces stress levels for greater emotional stability,

Calories Burned by Vigorous Exercise

You must burn 3,500 calories to lose 1 pound. Here are some examples of the number of calories that are burned during vigorous exercise (the number of calories burned will vary according the weight of the individual):

Calories Burned by Various Forms of Exercise	
Activity	**Calories Burned/Hour**
Running/jogging	590
Bicycling	590
Swimming	510
Aerobics	480
Walking	460
Heavy yard work (chopping wood)	440
Weight lifting (vigorous effort)	440
Basketball (vigorous)	440

From the Department of Health and Human Services, adapted from the 2005 DGAC Report, http://www.health.gov/DietaryGuidelines/dga2005/document/html/chapter3.htm.

and improves mood and self-esteem. Somewhat surprisingly, walking on a treadmill also burns more calories than an exercising with a stationary bike, rowing machine, cross-country skiing machine, stair stepper, or a combination cycling and upper body machine. Specifically, the treadmill produced the "greatest cardiorespiratory training stimulus during a given duration of exercise,"[10] burning 700 calories per hour compared to 625 calories per hour for the stair stepper and 500 calories per hour for the exercise bicycle. In addition, the rate of perceived exertion was higher on the treadmill compared to the other exercise machines. Rate of perceived exertion refers to how strenuous a person feels an exercise is, compared to how much energy is used in terms of calories burned. Treadmills came out on top, burning 40% more calories at all levels of perceived exertion than the other exercise equipment.

Even a moderate program on a treadmill can help you control your weight.

Swimming and Aquatic Exercise

Water exercises make the muscles work harder because of the water's increased resistance, but with the benefit that the buoyancy diminishes shock and trauma to bones and joints. Swimming is one of the best water exercises and can be used as an aerobic exercise if continued for 20 minutes or more. Try different strokes to exercise different muscles and joints. Using flotation devices like kickboards and water wings can give more support to the body than unassisted swimming. If the lower half of your body needs special attention, walking in water is also highly recommended; the faster you walk, the greater the resistance the muscles encounter and the better the workout. There are also water aerobics classes available at gyms and health clubs.

Jumping on a Mini Trampoline

The contracting and relaxing motions of the muscles during exercise helps to pump lymphatic fluid and results in a dramatic increase of lymph flow. Light bouncing on a mini trampoline is especially effective at increasing the flow of lymphatic fluid because the rapid changes in gravity act as a powerful lymphatic pump, causing expansion of lymph ducts and channels for increased circulation. As you land on the mini trampoline, your body experiences twice the force of gravity, making it more effective than running for stimulating the flow of lymph.[11]

The mini trampoline is also a perfect exercise for weight loss. You can use it no matter what your fitness level, and you'll see results even if you do only 10 to 15 minutes per day. Jumping on the mini trampoline also helps to break down cellulite and gives fast results in terms of spot toning during weight loss. Plus, it's inexpensive and can fit in a very small space. Most mini trampolines have a flexible jumping surface measuring 26 to 28 inches in diameter and set 6 to 9 inches off the ground. If you place it by your TV or radio, you'll find that it's very easy to fit into your daily routine. Just jump on it during all the commercials!

Exercises from the East

Moderate to strenuous exercise, such as running or tennis, isn't the only way to increase metabolism and boost your body's ability to burn off calories. Proper breathing is also important. The lungs are capable of holding as much as 2 gallons of air, but most people breathe only 2 to 3 pints per breath. Ordinarily, air is very poorly exchanged at the base of the lungs, far down in the chest cavity. This is particularly true when a person breathes by expanding the chest, rather than expanding the abdomen. Breathing with the abdomen, also called diaphragmatic breathing, involves first expanding the abdomen during inhalation, then expanding the chest. Exhalation is also initiated from the abdomen, not the chest. Using this technique empties the lower portions of the lungs.

Here's a simple breathing exercise to help you expand your lungs and lose weight. It can also help you release stress and strong emotions. Next time you're upset or uptight, try this exercise; you'll be amazed how much it helps.

1. Sit in a comfortable position.
2. Place the palm of your hand over your navel and inhale normally, allowing your chest and abdomen to expand.
3. As you slowly exhale, pull your navel in toward your spine as far as you can, completely expelling all the air as your abdomen and chest contract.
4. Inhale again, gently pushing your abdomen out and keeping your chest and shoulders relaxed.
5. Exhale as before.
6. Listen to the sound of your breath; closing your eyes will help you concentrate.
7. Repeat this procedure for 5 minutes.

Repeat three times per day. This is a great way to take a mini break at work. You can even do it in when you're driving (of course, don't close your eyes!).

Taking such deep, full breaths occasionally throughout the day is a good way to increase oxygen intake, raise energy levels, and burn fat. Beyond helping to burn calories, focused breathing and similar simple practices have a balancing and harmonizing influence on every body system. Slow stretching exercises that emphasize correct methods of deep breathing can help also build muscle and shed fat. Exercises used for centuries by Eastern cultures, such as yoga, qigong, and tai chi, increase metabolism while developing strength, flexibility, and balance.

The meditative quality of yoga, qigong, and tai chi distinguishes them from conventional Western exercise techniques. Designed to integrate the mind and body, these Eastern techniques allow individuals to become better attuned to the inner functioning of their bodies. By performing the exercises in silence, listening to the breath, feeling the pulse of the heart, and sensing the flow of inner energy, these healing arts help people to better handle stress and maintain overall health.

To the untrained Westerner, these exercise systems may appear too slow and easy to aid with weight loss. However, when compared with activities such as running or lifting weights, yoga, qigong, and tai chi actually deliver considerable physiological benefits. For example, these systems help to expand the lungs, stimulate metabolism, improve blood circulation, and increase muscle flexibility and relaxation. Their effect on blood circulation is somewhat different from that of more vigorous forms of exercise, as they do not send a torrent of blood to the muscles. Instead, by focusing on breathing with the lower abdomen, blood flow is directed toward the internal organs.

Central to all these practices is the belief that sustaining a steady breath not only increases oxygen intake, it also increases blood flow, which helps circulate vital energy, known as prana or qi. This can help to vitalize a body that's physically strong but energetically zapped. While Western standards for physical fitness tend to focus solely on body weight and development of muscles, Eastern healing arts provide the body with additional benefits.

Yoga

Yoga is one of the most ancient systems of self-healing practiced today. It teaches the basic principle of mind-body unity: If the mind is chronically restless and agitated, the health of the body will be compromised. Conversely, if the body is in poor health, mental clarity will be adversely affected. The practice of yoga can help integrate mind, body, and spirit.

Classical ashtanga yoga is divided into eight branches (ashtanga means "eight limbs") that give guidance as to the proper diet, hygiene, detoxification regimes, and physical practices to help the individual integrate their personal, psychological, and spiritual awareness. The most well-known type of yoga is hatha yoga, which teaches certain asanas (postures) and breathing techniques to create profound changes in the body and mind. A key objective of yoga is harnessing and increasing the flow of prana, or life energy. The blockage of prana, whether due to improper diet, lifestyle stressors, or imbalance in one's physical, emotional, or spiritual health, can lead to illness. Breathing techniques and the duration certain postures are held work to remove blockages in the flow of prana and can improve oxygen intake.

Yoga can also help with a sluggish lymphatic system. The lymphatic system depends on movement of the body to transport fluid in and out of tissues. When a person is inactive or when their patterns of motion are imbalanced, lymphatic fluid can become stagnant, leading to disease and weight gain. Through yoga's stretches and postures, lymphatic fluid is pumped throughout the body, removing toxins and waste products from cells and delivering fresh nutrients. This is especially important during weight loss, when the body releases toxins that have been stored in fat.

In addition to improving circulation of blood, lymph, and prana, yoga corrects imbalances of hormones by regulating the chakras. According to yoga philosophy, the seven chakras are centers of spiritual and physical energy within the body. Interestingly, these locations of the chakras roughly correspond to those of the hormone-producing glands.

The safest and most reliable way to use yoga therapeutically is to follow a balanced program of postures to achieve an overall normalizing and health-inducing effect. It is best for the beginner to start with a simple program of basic postures. A structured course can teach the fundamental breathing techniques and postures, which you can then practice on your own. Find a local teacher or use yoga tapes or books as guides.

Tai Chi

Tai chi is a unique Chinese system of slow, continuous, flowing movements that create a sense of tranquility and vitality. It is gentle yet effec-

The Swimming Dragon

In Chinese medicine, the swimming dragon qigong exercise is considered to be effective for weight loss. It helps burn fat by stimulating the physiological furnaces in the body known as the "three burners," the primary regulators of metabolism. One burner directs breathing; the second affects digestion, sending energy to the stomach, spleen, liver, and pancreas; and the third oversees elimination, managing the intestines, bladder, and kidneys. Although these burners are not part of physical anatomy, Chinese medicine recognizes them as invisible organizing principles that keep the machinery of the body running smoothly.

The swimming dragon involves tracing three circles in the air with your hands following a continuous serpentine pattern. Each of the circles is traced at a level that corresponds to the location of one burner's region of influence. The top burner is traced near the head and chest, the middle burner near the chest and waist, and the lower burner near the waist and knees. As you trace these circles, the motion of your hands should be smooth, moving from left to right, and tracing one-half of each circle as you descend from top to bottom. As you move your hands from left to right, your hips should move in the opposite direction. It is helpful to watch yourself in a mirror when you attempt this for the first time. If done correctly, your body should move just like a serpent in water. Here are the step-by-step instructions:

1. Stand erect but relaxed, with your hands at your sides.

2. Bring your hands in front of your face, holding your fingers and palms together and pointed away from you.

3. Tilt your head and hands to the left, and begin tracing the first half of the first circle. As you do this, begin moving your hips to the right, keeping your thighs together.

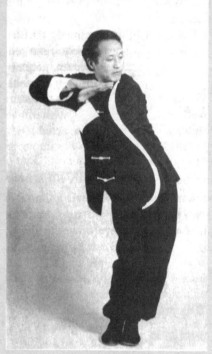

Photo by T.K. Shih

4. Trace three connected half-circles in a smooth serpentine motion, slowly bending your knees and lowering your body.

5. When you reach the bottom of the third half circle — near the height of your knees when standing — complete the circle and move upward, making another serpentine motion with your hands that is the mirror opposite of what you did on the way down. You have just traced the three circles.[14]

Each cycle of three circles should take 1 full minute. For beginners, one to three cycles is adequate. Eventually, you should work up to 20 cycles.

Instructional book, *The Swimming Dragon*, available from the Chinese Healing Arts Center (see Resources, page 275).

tive in stretching muscles and circulating the blood. Traditional Chinese medicine holds that tai chi stimulates and nourishes the body's internal organs by circulating qi, which also facilitates emotional and mental well-being. Tai chi has multiple benefits, strengthening cardiovascular fitness, building muscular strength, and improving posture.[12] In addition, tai chi improves the function of the immune system and enhances psychological motivation by helping to calm the mind and improve self image.[13]

Qigong

Qigong (also referred to as chi kung) is an ancient exercise that stimulates and balances the flow of qi along acupuncture meridians (energy pathways). Qigong cultivates inner strength, calms the mind, and restores the body to its natural state of health. Although less artistic and dynamic than tai chi, qigong is much easier to learn and can be done by the severely disabled as well as the healthy. Qigong practice can range from simple calisthenics-type movements with coordinated breathing to complex exercises that direct brain-wave frequencies, deep relaxation, and breathing to improve strength and flexibility and reverse damage caused by prior injuries and disease. The increased presence of mind developed through qigong practice can aid in the development of improved body image and the internal motivation needed to continue on a healthy lifestyle path that leads to weight loss.

The Super Seven Home Workout

The following exercise system is specially designed for weight-loss support by Titus Kahoutek and Jasson Zurilgen, Certified Personal Trainers/C.H.E.K. practitioners (see Resources for contact information).

This group of exercises will

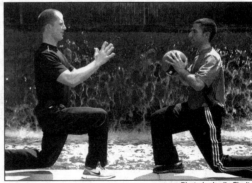
Photo by Joelle Fiorito

help you maintain tone and develop strength while on a weight-loss program. They'll also help you establish balance and core strength while increasing lean muscle mass, which in turn contributes to the overall fat burning efficiency of the body.

This set of exercise will help you burn calories in three ways: You can expect to burn 200 to 300 calories each time you do this workout. Then, after the workout you'll burn an additional 200 to 300 calories as your body goes through the recovery process. Finally, by building more muscle you raise your body's metabolism, which means you'll burn more calories even at rest.

Exercise 1: Dynamic Horse Stance

Benefits: This exercise truly benefits the whole body. It promotes strength and flexibility through the entire trunk and also improves coordination and control of your body. The primary areas affected are the glutes, abdominals, mid back (important in good posture), and shoulders.

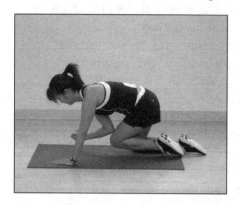 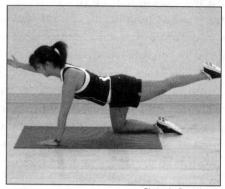

Photos by Brad Kevelin

Description: This exercise has a fairly loose form, which makes it an ideal warm-up for any exercise routine. Start on your hands and knees, placing your hands directly beneath your shoulders, and your knees directly under your hips. Bend your elbows about 20 degrees, or until your chest is parallel to the ground. Next, with your thumb pointed up, extend one arm out to a 45-degree angle while simultaneously extending the opposite leg out straight, inhaling as you do so. As you exhale, tuck your arm and leg back in until your elbow and knee meet.

Tips: Think of the hips as the foundation of this movement. Keep them parallel to the floor. The more stable the hips, the stronger foundation for the arm and leg to extend from.

Frequency: Two to three sets of 10 repetitions with a 10-second hold in the extended position.

Exercise 2: Lunges with Twist

Benefits: This is another highly effective exercise that incorporates multiple planes of movement as well as high cardiovascular demand. Doing this exercise will challenge your balance, coordination, and strength. It also helps burn fat. The muscle groups most affected are the thighs, hamstrings, glutes, and the muscles of the torso.

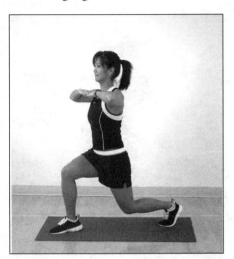 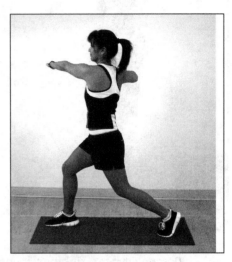

Description: Start in a lunge position. Position 1: Both knees should be bent about 90 degrees. If you have a limited range of motion in the knee joint, stay within a tolerable range of motion. Your front knee should be directly over the foot, and your hips should be centered so that your weight is evenly distributed between both legs. Once in this position, raise your elbows out to the sides up to shoulder height with your fingers pointed toward each other. Position 2: Stand up out of the lunge into a split stance. At the top of this motion, rotate your torso in the direction of the lead leg while keeping your head pointed straight ahead and your eyes level with the horizon. Going from position 1 to position 2 and back again is 1 repetition.

Tips: Vision is a major asset in stability and balance, so find a focal point at the far end of the room. Another thing that will help is to keep your belly button pulled in toward your spine. This activates the deep abdominal wall, which is a key component in protecting the spine.

Frequency: Two to three sets of 10 repetitions per side.

Exercise 3: Squats

Benefits: This exercise benefits the entire lower body.

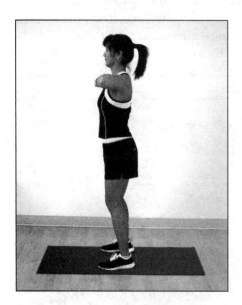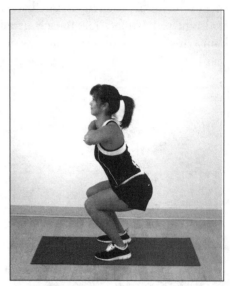

Description: Start this movement with your belly button pulled in toward your spine, feet square and a little more than shoulder-width apart. Sit back as if there were a chair under you until your thighs are parallel to the floor. (If you have any trouble with range of motion, stay in your pain-free zone but do use your maximum pain-free range). Your body weight should be evenly distributed between both legs. Once you reach your lowest position, press your legs into the ground and slowly rise back to a standing position.

Tips: There are many variations on this exercise, and it's easy to add extra load as needed. But be aware that increasing the load (by using weights, for example), increases the importance of engaging your deep abdominal muscles, which helps to burn belly fat.

Frequency: Two to three sets of 10 to 15 repetitions.

Exercise 4 : Wood Chops

Benefits: As with the previous exercises, this one really benefits the whole body in regards to strength, stamina, and coordination.

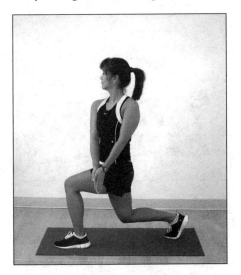 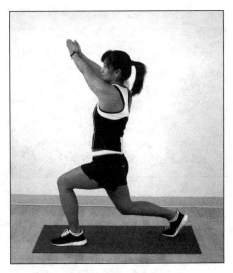

Description: Start in 90-90 lunge position (see exercise 2, page 69). (If you have any trouble with range of motion stay in your pain-free zone but do use your maximum pain-free range). About 60% of your weight should be placed on the back two-thirds of the front foot. With your arms straight, hold your hands together and point them down on the inside of the lead leg. Draw your belly button in toward your spine, pull your shoulders back, and look straight ahead. From this starting position, begin the movement by standing up in the lunge while simultaneously bringing your arms toward your outside shoulder. The end range of this movement is when you are in a standing lunge position with your arms extended over the opposite shoulder. One repetition of this exercise is when you have gone from the start position to the end range and back again.

Tips: This exercise is significantly more effective when the you perform the movement as precisely as possible. Measure your success by how well you perform the movement, not just by doing the reps. You can make this exercise more challenging by simply holding a weight in your hands.

Frequency: Two to three sets of 10 to 15 repetitions.

Exercise 5: Push-Ups

Benefits: The main muscle groups affected are the chest, triceps, and core.

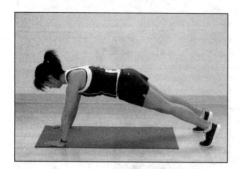 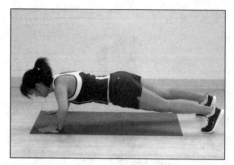

Description: Start in plank position with one arm extended (see exercise 7 for the plank position). Beginners start with your knees on the floor and progress to your toes as you get stronger. Make sure your deep abdominals are activated then begin to lower yourself toward the ground by opening your elbows away from each other. Most people let their chest collapse between their shoulder blades and their head fall forward. The true benefits of the exercise come when good posture is maintained throughout the movement. Go down until your elbows are at 90 degrees or until your form breaks down. At that point, press into the floor with a steady pressure until you're back at the starting position. Exhale as you press away from the floor. The round-trip back to the starting position counts as one rep.

Tips: Pay more attention to form than number of reps or the depth of movement.

Frequency: Three sets of 8 to 12 repetitions.

Exercise 6: Alternating Superman

Benefits: This is a great exercise that works the rear deltoids, mid and lower trapezius (essential for good posture), low back, glutes, and hamstrings.

Description: Start by lying facedown with your arms extended over your head and held about 45 degrees away from your body. With your hand extended and your thumb up, raise one arm and the opposite leg. Imagine a string attached to your thumb and heel that is lifting your arm and leg from the floor. Hold this pose for 8 to 10 seconds, then lower your arm and leg to the floor in a controlled motion. Repeat this movement with the other side to complete one set.

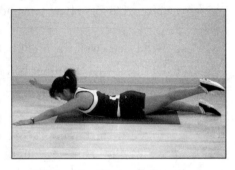

Tips: Imagine your trunk is a solid object that your limbs move from. By activating your deep abdominals prior to initiating the movement, you create a stable base of support for your arms and legs.

Frequency: Three to six sets.

Exercise 7: Plank

Benefits: Core strength

Description: This exercise is easy to do but hard to master. You simply activate your deep abdominals and hold your body off of the ground on your elbows and toes.

Tips: If you can't stabilize your low back or begin to feel pain or pressure in your low back, try tilting your pelvis in the direction of your belly button. If that doesn't work, drop your knees to the floor.

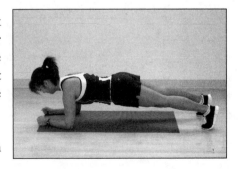

Frequency: Hold for as long as you can maintain form.

If I may leave you with one thing to think about as you incorporate fitness into your lifestyle, I would urge you to develop a positive relationship with exercise and physical activity. So many people just try to get through it, as if it were a chore. This attitude usually ends with poor results followed by frustration, until eventually exercise falls by the wayside. Instead consider your workout to be a time allotted for communicating with your own body. You'll soon start to notice how certain behaviors affect you and your performance:

- Did I sleep well the night before?
- Did I eat well the night before?
- Am I stressed or easily distracted?

These are just examples of the type of questions that you may come up with. With this newfound sensitivity to your body's signals, you will have more tools for making healthy decisions on a more consistent basis.

three

Healthy Eating

Low-calorie diets and exercise have been the typical solution to losing weight. With thousands of diets and a multimillion dollar industry dedicated to weight control, shedding a few pounds should be easy. Unfortunately, the weight lost by dieters is almost always regained. As a result, many dieters fall into the yo-yo trap, a repetitive cycle of weight loss and gain.

Whenever the body is deprived of food, whether from famine or dieting, it decreases its metabolic rate to compensate for fewer calories. Energy is stored so efficiently in fat tissues that someone of normal weight can survive for weeks without eating. The desire to binge after food restriction, although disheartening to dieters, is actually a built-in survival mechanism intended to click on in response to famine.

Rather than suffering through restrictive diets that seldom work anyway, learn how to eat in a healthy and balanced way; this can have a major and more lasting impact on your weight. Incorporating healthier eating habits

IN THIS CHAPTER

- The Healthy Eating Plan
- Benefits of a Whole Foods Diet
- Making the Transition to Whole Foods
- Dietary Fats — The Real Story
- Avoiding the Bad Fats
- Choosing the Right Fats

into your lifestyle will improve your overall health and help you achieve a healthy body weight for the rest of your life.

The Healthy Eating Plan

Both alternative and conventional medicine agree on many aspects of what constitutes an ideal diet for both weight loss and overall health:

- Reduced calorie intake
- Portion control
- Reduced total fat, saturated fat, trans fat, and cholesterol
- Increased monounsaturated, omega-3, and omega-6 fatty acids
- Increased dietary fiber, fruit, and vegetables
- Increased micronutrients (such as folate, B_6, and B_{12})
- Increased plant protein in lieu of animal protein
- Elimination of highly processed foods
- Adopting a more Mediterranean or prudent dietary pattern[1]

It's a simple approach: Consume less fat, animal protein, and processed foods, and eat more complex carbohydrates, especially whole grains rich in fiber, and at least five servings daily of fruits and vegetables. A whole foods diet is generously filled with a wide variety of different colored vegetables, fruits, and grains; raw seeds and nuts and their butters; beans; fermented milk products such as yogurt and kefir; and fish, poultry, and fermented soybean products, like miso and tempeh. It should also be lower in meats, animal fats, and cheeses. Eating well-balanced meals at regular times during the day (four to five hours apart) is also a good idea; this will stabilize your blood sugar and help you control your appetite. Avoid empty calories, which are foods that add almost no nutrition, but are extremely high in fat and calories, and lead to fast weight gain. These include soft drinks, candy, cakes and pastries, bagels, some salad dressings, mayonnaise and other condiments, and most processed and fast foods. In addition, empty calories actually do not satisfy hunger for an appreciable period of time, but often have the opposite effect and increase cravings which leads to more weight gain.

Before we get into the details of what constitutes a whole foods diet, let's take a look at the basic building blocks in all foods: carbohydrates, protein, and fats, also known as macronutrients.

Carbohydrates

Carbohydrates consist of simple sugars, complex carbohydrates, and fiber. They are the preferred source of energy for all bodily functions. The typical American diet includes more refined and processed foods than the diet of any other nation. It is estimated that refined sugars comprise one-fifth of all calories consumed daily by Americans.[2] When food is refined and processed, not only is fiber removed, simple sugars also often replace complex carbohydrates. A diet low in fiber and high in simple sugars is a major contributing factor to excess weight gain as well as diabetes, heart disease, and cancer. Foods rich in complex carbohydrates include vegetables, whole grains, brown rice, potatoes, legumes, milk, and dairy products. (Be sure to use foods raised or processed organically.)

Dietary fiber can have a major impact on weight gain as evidenced by the almost complete lack of obesity in cultures that consume a diet high in fiber.[3] Fiber has been shown not only to reduce serum cholesterol, but also to pull dietary fat from the body into the feces. Other benefits of fiber include increasing chewing time (which slows down the eating process, allowing you to feel full sooner), preventing constipation, and stabilizing blood glucose levels.[4] Whole grains (such as wheat, oats, rice, rye, barley, and millet) have the highest level of fiber, followed in turn by legumes, nuts and seeds, root vegetables (such as potatoes, turnips, beets, and carrots), fruits, and leafy, green vegetables.

Proteins

Protein is one of the most plentiful substances in the human body (second only to water). It is a major component in muscles, skin, hair and nails, the heart, the brain, and red blood cells. Specialized proteins such as enzymes, antibodies, and hormones play an extremely important role in the body, facilitating every aspect of metabolism and ensuring proper functioning of the immune system and other physiological systems. Proteins are necessary for growth and repair of body tissues and the regulation of bodily activities. Proteins are present in nearly every cell and fluid in

 QUICK DEFINITION

Amino acids are the building blocks of the 40,000 different proteins of the body, including enzymes, hormones, and the brain's chemical messengers, called neutrotransmitters. Eight amino acids cannot be made by the body and must be obtained through diet; others are produced in the body but not always in sufficient amounts. The amino acids that occur most commonly in the body are alanine, arginine, asparagine, aspartic acid, caritine, citrulline, cysteine, cystine, GABA, glutamic acid, glutamine, glycine, histidine, isoleucine, leucine, lysine, methionine, ornithine, phenylalanine, proline, serine, taurine, threonine, tryptophan, tyrosine, and valine.

the body. Structurally, protein is made up of linked amino acids (SEE QUICK DEFINITION, page 77).

Healthy sources of protein are foods that contain all the essential amino acids, the building blocks of proteins. These "complete" proteins are milk, eggs, cheese, meat, fish, poultry, and soybeans. Green leafy vegetables, grains, and beans (legumes) are a source of some essential amino acids, but not all, and are therefore referred to as incomplete proteins. However, when different incomplete proteins with varying amino acid profiles are consumed over the course of a day or two, the body can obtain all the needed amino acids. This doesn't require a great deal of attention to food combining, as was once thought to be the case. As long as you consume a wide variety of foods, protein probably isn't an issue. In fact, overconsumption of protein is a far bigger problem in the United States. Of the animal proteins, poultry and fish are healthier sources than red meat and dairy, which are higher in saturated fats and should be eaten less frequently and in small portions. The American Cancer Society suggests that a portion of meat should be no larger than 3 ounces per day, roughly the size of a deck of cards.[5] Controlling portion size of animal products protects against cancer and aids with weight loss. Again, be sure to choose organic sources for all dietary proteins.

Fats

Fat contains more than twice as many calories per gram as protein or carbohydrates. A Swiss study revealed that, unlike carbohydrates, approximately 90% of extra fat consumed during a meal is converted to body fat.[6] However, not all fats are created equal. Of the three kinds of fats—saturated, polyunsaturated, and monounsaturated—polyunsaturated are the healthiest because they are a dietary source of essential fatty acids, which are important nutrients for health and wellness. Additional information on incorporating healthy fats into your diet and avoiding the unhealthy ones is provided later in this chapter.

Alcohol and Cigarettes

These two nonfood items are so widely consumed that they warrant discussion here. Alcohol should be avoided or minimized, since it can promote weight gain; just 1 ounce of alcohol has as many calories as about ½ ounce of fat in the diet.[7] Cigarettes, which many people use to manage their weight, appear to steer extra fat to the abdomen. In addition, those who are prone to glucose intolerance should take special care to avoid both of these substances.

However, a sense of balance and moderation is important in approaching one's diet. If the majority of your meals are comprised of whole, fresh foods, then a little junk food or an occasional alcoholic drink or piece of candy won't hurt. But when too few whole foods are consumed compared with those lacking in nutritional value, the body's physiology is damaged.

Eating Lower on the Food Chain

While it is preferable that a whole foods diet be as plant-based as possible, it is not necessary to become a complete vegetarian, totally eliminating meats and other animal foods from the diet. There are many kinds of dairy products and animal foods with reasonable levels of fat. In addition, whole milk, eggs, and meats provide amino acids and other important nutrients necessary for health. Even so, eat meats and other animal products in moderation, and always choose the leanest meats possible, raised without the use of antibiotics and other drugs, as this will cut down effectively on calories, weight gain, and exposure to toxins.

There are many reasons to stick to a more plant-based diet. First, important antioxidant nutrients, including vitamin C, mixed carotenoids, vitamin E, and many cancer-fighting substances known as phytochemicals, are found in fruits, vegetables, and grains. These antioxidant nutrients are considered the best protection against diseases related to aging and environmental factors, from dandruff, bad breath, and wrinkling to cataracts, cancer, diabetes, and heart attacks. In many studies, antioxidants have been associated with increased immune response,[8] as well as a decrease in inflammation.[9] One study performed on over 19,000 people concluded that the concentration of the antioxidant vitamin C (ascorbic acid) was inversely proportional to their waist-to-hip ratio, meaning that lower vitamin C levels were associated with bigger bellies.[10] Antioxidants help to protect cell membranes from oxidative damage due to free radicals, while excess body fat increases free radical concentrations. So, as you increase consumption of fruits and vegetables, you are protecting your cell membranes while

Free radicals are a major molecular cause of damage to healthy cells. A free radical is an unstable molecule with an unpaired electron that steals electrons from other molecules, producing harmful effects, such as membrane destruction and changes in the cell nucleus that can lead to mutations. Free radicals form when molecules react with oxygen and are "oxidized." This occurs due to normal metabolic processes, as well as increased chemical, physical, or emotional stress. Environmental toxicity in food, air, water, and cigarette smoke increases the production of free radicals.

also facilitating weight loss. In addition, the high fiber content of plant foods helps keep the digestive tract clean by absorbing and eliminating many potentially dangerous toxins. Plant foods also tend to have a lower toxicity than animal foods to begin with, precisely because they are lower on the food chain.

Medical and scientific evidence points to the benefits of moving toward a plant-based diet. Dean Ornish, MD, of the University of California at San Francisco, demonstrated that a diet low in animal protein, along with exercise and stress reduction, can actually reverse heart disease.[11] The American Dietetic Association published research showing that a vegetarian lifestyle reduces the risk of heart disease, diabetes, colon cancer, hypertension, obesity, osteoporosis, and diverticular disease.[12] Although a strictly vegetarian diet that's not well-rounded may pose risks of insufficient consumption of some nutrients, overall the health benefits of a well-planned vegetarian diet far outweigh the potential risks.[13]

Repetition versus Variety in the Diet

The standard American diet, often called SAD with good reason, usually consists of a very limited number of foods: mostly wheat, beef, eggs, potatoes, and milk products. For example, a breakfast of eggs, sausage, white toast, and hash browns isn't really any different from a lunch of a hamburger on a white bun and fries, which is the same as a dinner of steak and potatoes or white pasta. All of these meals are high in fat and calories, low in fiber, filled with toxins, and very low in many essential nutrients—not surprising, as they're essentially devoid of whole foods, fruits, and vegetables.

Such repetition leads to nutrient deficiency, disease, and obesity. It also tends to produce allergies and hypersensitivities to those foods, which may be due to the interaction between the chemical makeup of a given food and the allergic response of a given individual.[14] Eating a varied diet minimizes these problems. The optimal diet should consist of more vegetables, fruits, and whole grains than any other foods.

Benefits of a Whole Foods Diet

A whole foods diet promotes health by decreasing fat and sugar intake and increasing fiber and nutrient intake. Generally, it leads to more satisfaction, less congestion and fatigue, and less overeating. Let's take a closer look at some of these benefits.

More fiber: Most animal products, like meat, cheese, milk, eggs, and butter, contain no fiber, whereas whole plant foods like brown rice, broccoli, oatmeal, and almonds have 6 to 15 grams per serving. Because sufficient dietary fiber can help balance insulin levels and create a feeling of satiety, consuming enough fiber can aid in weight loss. And as would be expected, studies have shown that low fiber intake is associated with weight gain.[15] Fiber is also an agent of transport in the digestive tract, moving food wastes out of the body before they have a chance to form potentially cancer-causing and mutagenic chemicals. These toxic chemicals can cause colon cancer or pass through the gastrointestinal membrane into the bloodstream and damage other cells.

Less fat: On a percentage-of-calories basis, most vegetables contain less than 10% fat, and most grains contain from 16% to 20% fat. By comparison, whole milk and cheese contain 74% fat. A rib roast is 75% fat, and eggs are 64% fat. Even low-fat milk and skinned, baked chicken breast still have 38% fat. Not only do animal foods have more fat, but most of these fats are saturated. In addition, a lower-fat, whole foods diet means fewer calories, since an ounce of fat contains twice as many calories as an ounce of complex carbohydrates. Studies have shown that a diet containing fewer calories can increase health and extend life.[16] A low-fat diet aids with initial weight loss and maintains a healthy weight over time, as evidenced by the Women's Health Initiative Dietary Modification Trial, which examined weight changes and dietary components in 48,835 postmenopausal women in the United States who were of diverse backgrounds and ethnicities. Approximately half of the participants ate a diet with decreased fat and increased amounts of vegetables, fruit, and grains. Weight loss was greatest among the women who decreased their fat consumption over the course of the seven and a half years of the study.[17]

Decreased sugar consumption: Eating a diet high in natural complex carbohydrates tends to be more filling and decreases the desire to consume processed sugars. As with fat, sugar is a hidden and unwelcome ingredient in many processed foods.

More nutrients: Plant foods are richer sources of micronutrients (vitamins and minerals) than animal foods. Compare wheat germ to round steak: ounce for ounce, wheat germ contains twice the vitamin B_2, vitamin K, potassium, iron, and copper; three times the vitamin B_6, molybdenum, and selenium; 15 times the magnesium; and over 20 times the vitamin B$_1$, folate, and inositol. The steak only has three nutrients in greater amounts — vitamin B$_{12}$, chromium, and zinc.

Increased variety: Eating a greater variety of plant foods introduces more colorful foods into the diet — red beets, orange citrus fruits, yellow squash, all manner of leafy green vegetables, blueberries, purple eggplant, and a rainbow of chard. Bright color variations are due to minerals, vitamins, and, most especially, phytonutrients, compounds that lend fruits and vegetables both color and important health-promoting functions in the human body. Some of the color variations in vegetables are due to carotenes, naturally occurring pigments that are converted into vitamin A in the body. Carotenes act as antioxidants and have been scientifically validated as a powerful tool in cancer prevention.[18]

More food satisfaction and less overeating: Foods that are dense in nutrients and fiber, such as vegetables, whole grains, and beans, require more chewing time. As a result, you'll eat more slowly and will have consumed less by the time the food reaches your stomach. If you feel satiated sooner, you'll eat fewer calories.

Making the Transition to Whole Foods

Eating better means living better. The dietary changes you make should not be threatening, limiting, or difficult to live with. Most Americans were raised eating meat, fried and processed foods, and refined carbohydrates like white bread, white rice, and sugary cereals. The transition to a more vegetable-oriented, whole foods diet may seem daunting. However, this change may be easier and more pleasurable than you imagine, and considering the enormous health benefits, it's certainly worth it. Consider it an adventure into exploring new foods rather than a restriction in dietary choices. Fill up on the good stuff and eat the bad stuff once a week—if you still want to! Here are some tips that will make the transition easier:

- Eat more high-fiber plant foods like grains, legumes, nuts, and seeds.
- When dining out, try more exotic vegetarian dishes. Most ethnic restaurants — Indian, Chinese, Thai, Japanese, Mexican, Latin

Low-Fat Fallacies

Low-fat and nonfat food products are marketed to individuals who are health and weight conscious. Ironically, manufacturers often add a variety of unhealthy and artificial ingredients to these foods. For example, various viscous substances are added to low-fat salad dressings to mimic the thickness and smooth texture of oil. "These fat-mimickers do not occur naturally and they cannot be metabolized by our bodies," explains Paul McTaggert, of Los Angeles, California, an expert in the biochemistry of food. "They stay in our systems, thick, gooey, and paste-like. [Salad dressing] is a good example of how a not-so-great product was made into a worse one, and marketed as a better choice for health and weight."

Low-fat foods often lack flavor. To make them more palatable, some manufacturers load them up with extra sugar, which boosts the product's calorie content while still maintaining a reduced fat content. Others use artificial sweeteners such as aspartame (NutraSweet) or saccharin. These sugar substitutes, while lower in calories, are no guarantee to weight loss and may actually cause weight gain. Researchers at Harvard's School of Public Health found that "sugar substitutes have not proved helpful in curbing weight." Studies have shown that saccharin use actually leads to weight gain rather than weight loss.[19]

American, African, Middle Eastern — offer wonderful dishes with vegetables and grains. You can also prepare many of these at home. Experiment with spices and seasonings and invest in vegetarian or ethnic cookbooks for the secrets to the exotic flavors possible in vegetarian cooking.

- If you eat meat, choose range-fed, hormone-free, additive-free meats.

- Cook protein foods by one of the following methods: bake, broil, poach, stir-fry, sauté, or steam. Avoid frying as much as possible, as it adds calories and may add to the toxic load in the body. Do not overcook meats, which diminishes their nutritional value.

- Don't be rigid about your diet. Move toward a whole foods diet gradually.

- Achieve rhythm in your diet. Eating regularly provides your body with a consistent intake of nutrients and avoids the stress associated with skipping meals and overeating.

- Fill your pantry and refrigerator with healthy food choices that are ready to eat. Put meals and salads in "grab and go" containers.

- Never leave the house without food. If you've been dieting off and on for years, this may seem wrong to you. But remember, eating healthy foods on a regular basis will help you avoid unhealthy eating patterns and poor food choices. Keep organic nuts in your glove compartment in the car in case you don't have time for a meal. If you live in a warm climate, keep a small cooler in your car and keep it stocked with healthy snacks, fruits, and salads anytime you're away from home.

At the Market

Choosing the ingredients for an ideal diet in today's marketplace requires diligence, a healthy dose of skepticism, and a certain amount of fortitude to resist slipping into old patterns of relying on convenience foods. In fact, the best strategy is to create new healthy lifestyle habits that are also convenient. The improvements you make in your food choices will pay off in better health. Here are some shopping guidelines to steer you down the aisles:

- Read labels: The label on the front of the package is the last place one is apt to find the truth about a product. Bold statements such as "100% Natural" or "98% Fat-Free" might be legal, but they could be deceiving. Go directly to the small print on the ingredient list and nutritional analysis. New labeling regulations now mean better and more accurate information for consumers.

- Think complex carbohydrates: The "main dish" approach centering on protein and a high-fat sauce is out. Replace those large portions of meat loaf and baby back pork ribs with whole grains, beans, and fresh vegetables, balanced with moderate amounts of lean animal proteins if you wish.

- Buy organic foods: Organic farming doesn't use synthetic fertilizers, pesticides, herbicides, growth regulators, and livestock-feed additives. Instead, organic farmers raise food naturally using crop rotations, animal manure and green compost crops, organic fertilizers, mineral-bearing rock, and biological pest controls.

- Buy foods that are in season: By definition, foods grown out of season must be treated or manipulated to grow using artificial means. Often nonseasonal foods are imported from countries where pesticides banned in the United States continue to be used. Seasonal foods are healthier, more abundant, and less expensive.

- Eat a rainbow of colors: Instead of being concerned with getting all the right vitamins and minerals in perfect ratios, focus on eating a colorful diet. By making an effort to eat at least three different colors of vegetables or fruits at both lunch and dinner, you will ensure the best exposure to appropriate nutrients.

Dietary Fats — The Real Story

Low-fat dieting is a national obsession and has given rise to whole new lines of low-fat or nonfat products. But sometimes adding fats to your diet will help you lose weight—if they're the right fats. Certain fats, particularly the essential fatty acids, are vital for the healthy functioning of our bodies (including the maintenance of proper body weight), while hydrogenated fats like margarine may contribute not just to weight gain, but to a host of serious medical conditions. The relationship of dietary fat to body fat is grossly misunderstood. Although eliminating unhealthy fats from the diet is important, eating the right kinds can actually help with weight management.

Why We Need Fats

Fats are needed to support the functioning of the brain, nervous system, and immune system. They comprise the building blocks of hormones, assist in the absorption and transport of certain vitamins in the body, and are vital to maintaining a healthy metabolism, which controls how quickly the body burns calories. As you learned in chapter 2, metabolism is an important determinant of body weight. In order to avoid accumulating pounds, the amount of calories we eat must be balanced by the amount we burn via metabolism. When we burn fewer calories than we eat, the excess calories get stored as body fat; conversely, if we burn more calories than we eat, we lose weight. Low-fat diets attempt to tip the body's calorie balance in favor of weight loss by cutting out calorie-rich fats. However, because metabolism slows when fat intake is reduced, dieters can still end up burning fewer calories than they ingest, particularly since many low-fat foods are notoriously high in calories from added sugars (see "Low-Fat Fallacies," page 83) and this can affect insulin levels.

Fat-free and very low-fat diet programs tend to be high in carbohydrates (starches and sugars), which often serve as the primary energy source in such diets. However, too many carbohydrates will actually cause you to accumulate fat rather than lose it, since carbohydrates are converted to sugar in the body. If there is more sugar in the blood than the body can use, the excess gets stored as body fat. Dietary fats,

A Quick Guide to Fats

Fat or oil (lipid is the biochemical term) is one of the six basic food groups. Fats and oils are made of building blocks called fatty acids. Structurally, a fatty acid is a chain of carbon atoms with a certain quantity of hydrogen atoms attached; the more hydrogen atoms attached, the more "saturated" the fat. Fats come in three natural forms (saturated, monounsaturated, and polyunsaturated) and one synthetic form (called hydrogenated or trans fats).

Saturated Fats — Saturated fats are solid at room temperature and are primarily found in animal foods and tropical oils, such as coconut and palm oils. A fatty acid that has its full quota of hydrogen atoms is a saturated fatty acid. The body produces saturated fats from sugar, which is one reason why low-fat foods do not decrease body fat—their high sugar content is converted into stored fat in the body. Although high fat intake from animal sources has been associated with heart disease, some amount of saturated fat in the diet is necessary to help the body's cells remain healthy and resistant to disease.

Unsaturated Fats — Unsaturated fatty acids (both monounsaturated and polyunsaturated) are liquid at room temperature. Most vegetable oils are unsaturated. Unsaturated means some of the carbon molecules are not filled with hydrogen.

- Monounsaturated Fats: When a fatty acid lacks only two hydrogen atoms, it is a monounsaturated fatty acid. Monounsaturated fats are considered healthier than polyunsaturated fats because of their ability to lower blood levels of "bad" cholesterol and maintain or raise levels of "good" cholesterol. Canola oil and olive oil are naturally high in monounsaturated fats. Olive oil is the best oil for cooking, because it does not break down easily into singlet oxygen molecules (free radicals) like most oils do when they are heated. Olive oil is probably the most widely used oil, both for

on the other hand, tend to moderate blood sugar levels, which helps to control weight gain.

Fats also help manage weight by controlling appetite. Since fat takes longer to digest, it slows the emptying time for the stomach, which makes you feel satisfied for a longer period of time. For example, one study compared a bagel breakfast to an egg breakfast. The egg breakfast resulted in a greater feeling of satiety and significantly reduced additional food intake for the entire day. The study concluded

 For more on **carbohydrates and weight gain,** see chapter 5, Strengthen Your Sugar Controls, page 124.

that the egg breakfast could sustain greater weight loss than a bagel breakfast.[20] A great tip is to eat two organic soft- or hard-boiled eggs for breakfast, with romaine lettuce leaves or fresh pineapple chunks instead of bread.

cooking and raw on salads, on a worldwide basis.

- Polyunsaturated Fats: Oils high in polyunsaturated fats include flaxseed and canola oils, as well as pumpkin seeds, purslane, hemp oil, walnuts, and soybeans, which contain omega-3 and omega-6 essential fatty acids. A fatty acid lacking four or more hydrogen atoms is a polyunsaturated fatty acid. They can be found in both healthy and unhealthy fats and oils.

Hydrogenated and Trans Fats — These terms refer to a synthetic process in which natural oils are broken down into a semi-solid fat by adding a hydrogen atom to an unsaturated fat molecule. This process is widely used to prolong the shelf life of commercial baked goods, packaged foods, most salad oils and dressings, margarine, and cooking oils. The molecules that make up these fats, called trans-fatty acids, are known to interfere with the healthy functioning of our bodies due to their unusual molecular shape.

Essential Fatty Acids (EFAs) — Unsaturated fats required in the diet are called essential fatty acids. Omega-3 and omega-6 oils are the two principle types of EFAs and a balance of these oils in the diet is necessary for good health. The primary omega-3 oil is alpha-linolenic acid (ALA), found in flaxseed and canola oils, as well as pumpkin seeds, walnuts, and soybeans. Fish oils, such as salmon, cod, and mackerel, contain the other important omega-3 oils, DHA (docosahexaenoic acid) and EPA (eicosapentaenoic acid). Linoleic acid is the main omega-6 oil and is found in most vegetable oils, including safflower, corn, peanut, and sesame. The most therapeutic form of omega-6 oil is gamma-linolenic acid (GLA), found in evening primrose, black currant, and borage oils. Once in the body, omega-3 and omega-6 are converted to prostaglandins, hormonelike complex fatty acids that affect smooth muscle function, inflammatory processes, and constriction and dilation of blood vessels.

Essential Fatty Acids: The Good Fats

Fatty acids are the chemical molecules that make up all fats. The body needs a regular supply of certain fatty acids, appropriately called essential fatty acids (EFAs—see "A Quick Guide to Fats," above), in order to stay healthy. The body cannot synthesize these from other nutrients, but must obtain them directly from food. Individuals who are deficient in essential fatty acids may experience a number of health problems, including weight gain. Unfortunately, many people don't get the EFAs that they need. This can be due to a low-fat diet, or to a diet high in the wrong fats.[21] Essential fatty acid deficiencies contribute to weight gain by increasing appetite and reducing energy levels, which tends to support a more sedentary lifestyle, which in turn leads to more weight gain. On the other side of the equation, sufficient EFAs will boost the metabolic rate, increase energy production, and help move cholesterol out of arteries and tissues.

Diagnosing an Essential Fatty Acid Deficiency

The first step in seeing if your weight problem is linked to your intake of fats is to identify any essential fatty acid deficiencies. Then proper dietary changes and nutritional supplementation can be recommended. In addition to taking a patient's symptom history and assessing their dietary habits, alternative medicine practitioners use a number of laboratory tests that can provide detailed and practical information on EFA status.

Pantox Profile: This test includes a comprehensive lipid panel as well as an analysis of serum levels of antioxidant micronutrients. Using a small blood sample, the test measures the status of more than 20 nutritional factors, specifically lipoproteins (cholesterol and triglycerides), antioxidants, and iron balance. The test must be ordered by a health-care professional.

BodyBio Blood Chemistry Report and Fatty Acid Analysis: The BodyBio Blood Chemistry Report provides information on levels of 44 different biochemicals in the blood. The BodyBio Fatty Acid Analysis reveals the status of 67 fatty acids in the blood by studying the membranes of the patient's red blood cells to determine which fatty acids are present and in what quantities. Together, these tests provide a picture of the whole biochemistry specific to the patient. The fatty acid analysis charts 12 to 16 weeks of an individual's lipid metabolism, useful for accurately determining the fats, vitamins, and minerals the patient requires.

Individualized Optimal Nutrition (ION) Profile: Using blood and urine samples, the ION Panel measures 150 biochemical components. It is useful for physicians needing detailed biochemical assessments of patients with immune disorders, heart disease, multiple chemical sensitivities, or obesity. The ION test checks for nutritional status of fatty acids, vitamins, minerals, amino acids, cholesterol, thyroid hormones, glucose, and antioxidants.

Functional Intracellular Analysis (FIA): This is a group of tests that measure the function of key vitamins, minerals, fatty acids, antioxidants, amino acids, and metabolites at the cellular level. They also assess carbohydrate metabolism in terms of insulin function and fructose intolerance.

Avoiding the Bad Fats

Most of the negative reports about fat have to do with saturated fat and cholesterol. Diets high in these two substances are considered to be a leading cause of obesity and heart disease. However, the medical establishment's focus on saturated fats and cholesterol is not altogether warranted; these represent only a portion of the larger causal mechanism pushing up the rates of obesity and heart disease. For example, consider that traditional cultures who follow diets very high in saturated fats and cholesterol, such as the Atiu-Mitiaro peoples of Polynesia and the Eskimos of Greenland, are virtually free of heart disease.

Certainly, there are a multitude of factors responsible for obesity and heart disease, and insufficiency of EFAs may be a big part of the problem. Despite having an overabundance of body fat, overweight people often have low levels of EFAs. In addition, the quality of dietary fats varies greatly. The oils most commonly consumed are denatured hydrogenated oils, produced through chemical refinement of fats and oil products. This overprocessing, heating, and chemical extraction increase shelf life, but it also effectively eliminates healthy EFAs.

Hydrogenated Fat

The process for hydrogenating oils was invented in Europe in the late 1800s, and in 1909 Proctor and Gamble acquired the U.S. rights to this process for transforming liquid vegetable oils so that they would be semisolid at room temperature. This technique led to the development of margarine, shortening, and other trans fats (SEE QUICK DEFINITION, page 90). In a naturally occurring fat, most double bonds between molecules are in a "cis" configuration, which means that both hydrogen atoms are on the same side of the carbon chain. The process of hydrogenation rearranges the hydrogen atoms, moving one of them to the other side of the carbon chain. This straightens out the molecule, creating the "trans" configuration, which makes it more like plastic, with a higher melting point. That's why these fats stay solid at room temperature. The advantage of hydrogenated fats is that they're more stable, not going rancid as easily. Commercially, this is a great boon, giving products made with these fats a longer shelf life. However, the costs in terms of human health are devastating.

Trans fats are taken up by the body in the same way as cis fats. However, once they are incorporated into the cell membrane, the difference in the structure of their chemical bonds interferes with a host of metabolic processes, including the production of cellular energy and important anti-inflammatory substances. Foods high in trans fats include French fries, microwave popcorn, chocolate bars, commercial peanut butter (but not the organic kind), most fast foods, and many commercial baked goods—the same foods that lead to obesity. Trans fats are associated with a host of other negative health effects, including heart disease,[22] colon cancer,[23] allergies,[24] and type 2 diabetes.[25]

Due to the ever-increasing scientific evidence on the detrimental health effects of consuming trans fats, the Danish government banned oils and fats that contain more than 2% industrially produced trans fats.[26] In the United States, the FDA implemented a labeling law on January 1, 2006, whereby all packaged foods must list trans fat content on their Nutrition Facts panels. However, if a food contains less than 0.5 gram per serving, it may say that the product contains zero trans fats. This loophole can fool consumers into believing that products don't contain trans fats when they actually do. Read labels carefully. If the words *partially hydrogenated* or *shortening* appear in the ingredients, the product contains trans fats! If you follow the "no paragraphs" approach to eating approach discussed in chapter 10, page 243, you will truly be consuming zero trans fats, which is the best goal to go for! The substitution of trans fats for good, healthy omega-3 and omega-6 fats in the American diet is a harmful mistake that values shelf life above health. Make every effort to avoid all trans fats and partially hydrogenated oils! (For more information, visit www.bantransfats.com.)

Olestra and other Fake Fats

Olestra, often marketed under the name, Olean, is a fake fat developed by food conglomerate Procter and Gamble. It is a sucrose polyester, a molecule of sugar to which many fatty substances are added. The resulting molecule is so large that it cannot be efficiently broken down

 QUICK DEFINITION Although some **trans fats** occur naturally in minute quantities in certain foods, most of them are man-made, created by a process wherein vegetable oil is chemically and structurally altered by being combined with hydrogen to lengthen shelf life. This process transforms some of the fatty acids in the oil into trans-fatty acids (TFAs). Trans-fatty acid composition of commercially prepared hydrogenated fats varies from 8% to 70%, and until very recently, trans fats comprised about 60% of the fat found in processed foods. It is estimated that Americans consume over 600 million pounds of TFAs annually in the form of frying fats. TFAs can increase the risk of heart disease when consumed as at least 12% of the total fat intake. TFAs also reduce production of prostaglandins (hormones that act locally to control all cell-to-cell interactions) and interfere with fatty acid metabolism.

by the body. It passes through without being absorbed, but since it is a fatty substance, it carries a lot of important fat soluble nutrients out of the body along with it. Olestra can also cause diarrhea, loose stools, and other gastrointestinal problems. Since it is calorie free, it is widely used in chips and other snack foods that are labled as low fat or lite. Food products that contain olestra used to have to be labeled with the following warning: "Olestra may cause abdominal cramping and loose stools. Olestra inhibits the absorption of some vitamins and other nutrients. Vitamins A, D, E, and K have been added." The United States is the only country that allows the use of olestra. In 2003, the FDA allowed the label warning to be dropped. Olestra has been banned in the UK and Canada, due to the wide range of side effects that it can cause.[27]

Homogenization

Another process that damages fat is homogenization, a technique used to make milk uniform in texture. Homogenization breaks up fat globules found in the cream fraction of milk into very small particles, which remain suspended in the milk rather than floating on top of it. Due to homogenization, natural whole milk, which will have a layer of cream on top, is virtually unknown and unobtainable in the United States today.

While we have become accustomed to drinking milk without a cream layer, what we don't know is that we increase our fat buildup and risk of heart disease with each glass. The problem is that the tiny globules of fat that result from homogenization allow the deadly enzyme xanthine oxidase to get into the body. In the bloodstream, xanthine oxidase damages artery walls, causing lesions to occur on the lining.[28] These lesions attract cholesterol deposits, which eventually clog the artery.

All milk fat, excluding that from humans, contains xanthine oxidase. However, in milk's natural state, the normal-sized fat globules from cream are too big to easily pass through the lining of the intestines and enter the bloodstream. Since xanthine oxidase is chemically bound to these fat molecules, the enzymes go wherever the fat globules go. When the fat is a normal size, xanthine oxidase is expelled out of the body, along with the fat.[29] Homogenization, however, makes the globules small enough to squeeze through the intestinal lining and into the blood.

Oxidation

In addition to hydrogenation and homogenization, fats can also be damaged by oxygen in a process called oxidation. During oxidation, fats become rancid and form new substances—oxysterols and peroxides—

which are free radicals (unstable, toxic molecules that cause considerable damage to the body's cells). Oxidized oils are loaded with free radicals, which may cause a variety of chronic, degenerative diseases.[30]

Oxidation occurs very rapidly when oil is heated during cooking. The most common source of oxidized fats is food cooked in deep-fat fryers, a mainstay of fast-food restaurants. The oils used in these fryers are subjected to very high heat for prolonged periods; consequently, they are almost always rancid and contaminate the foods cooked in them with free radicals. Oils and fats also oxidize simply by being exposed to air. This means that as soon as oil is pressed from nuts or seeds it becomes vulnerable to oxidation. In their natural state, many unsaturated fats contain antioxidants that protect them from oxidation, but these are often removed or destroyed when oils are refined. They then become more vulnerable to oxidation from prolonged exposure to air. For these reasons, it's best to purchase the freshest oils possible, and to store them in a cool dark place. Light can also contribute to oxidative damage, so oils packaged in dark or opaque containers are safer. And bear in mind that the higher the cooking heat, the greater the oxidation.

Choosing the Right Fats

The average American gets approximately 40% of their calories from fat. A major source of this is animal fat, specifically beef, dairy products, fish, and chicken. The current recommendation from groups such as the American Heart Association and the American Cancer Society is to reduce daily fat consumption to 30% of total caloric intake. While this is a step in the right direction, many health-care experts believe that for long-term health and weight control, fats should constitute only 15% to 20% of your daily calories. They should also be selected carefully, making sure to exclude all harmful fats.

In general, choose vegetable and seed oils that are cold-pressed. This means that the oils were extracted from their sources with a minimum of heat, a process that protects the oils from damage. You should always check the expiration date of any oil you buy; many high-quality oils have a short shelf life (three to four months). In addition, look for dairy products that have not been homogenized. Most of the butter available is made from homogenized milk, but in response to increased consumer demand, many stores are also beginning to carry raw butter, made from unhomogenized milk.

Many people are surprised to find that they experience an immediate drop in weight as soon as they begin to replace the unhealthy fats with healthy ones. Here are some general dietary recommendations for supplying your body with nourishing, healthy fats:

- Use liberal amounts of unprocessed sesame oil blended with coconut oil; other good choices are cold-pressed avocado, almond, and grapeseed oils.

- Avoid margarine and hydrogenated oils.

- Increase your consumption of ground raw nuts and seeds (especially sesame seeds), sea vegetables, fish, tempeh, poultry, avocados, and legumes.

- Incorporate more freshly ground black pepper, cayenne, thyme, turmeric, and ginger into your diet; these foods contain substances that will help stabilize fats in the cell membranes.

Adding Essential Fatty Acids to Your Diet

Essential fatty acids can be obtained from foods and edible oils, as well as from supplements. Because of their delicate chemical structure, EFAs are particularly prone to oxidation, so they should not be used for cooking or subjected to heat. It's best to use an alternate cooking method, such as steaming, and then toss or drizzle the food with a healthy oil, such as flaxseed or extra virgin olive oil. Here is a guide to the two major groups:

Omega-3 Fatty Acids

The primary omega-3 fatty acid is alpha-linolenic acid, found in plant oils such as flaxseed, safflower, peanut, sunflower seed, walnut, sesame, and olive. Docosahexaenoic acid (DHA) and eicosapentaenoic acid (EPA) are also omega-3 fatty acids; they come from fish oils, such as salmon, cod, and mackerel. Beans, especially great northern, kidney, navy, and soy, also supply omega-3 fatty acids.

At 58% alpha-linolenic acid, flaxseed oil is a particularly good source of omega-3 fatty acids. It is also a flavorful oil and can be used with lemon juice on salads or drizzled on vegetables and grains after cooking. The recommended dosage of flaxseed oil is 1 to 2 tablespoons daily (capsules are also available). Absorption of the oil is enhanced if it's taken with a spoonful of cottage cheese. In addition to the oil, the flaxseeds themselves can also be sprinkled on foods, from oatmeal to casseroles (the seeds should be freshly ground to help release the oil).

Flaxseed oil is especially prone to oxidation and can easily turn rancid in the presence of light or air, even in its capsule form. Refrigerate it in tightly sealed, dark glass bottles.

Olive oil is another good source of omega-3 fatty acids and also contains high quantities of monounsaturated fats. Studies have demonstrated that monounsaturated fats are excellent for lowering blood cholesterol levels. Olive oil consumption has been shown to help cells resist aging and stay healthy by increasing the antioxidant capacity of cell membranes, and decreasing the breaking apart of strands of DNA. This is exciting research that may help to explain the many benefits of a diet high in olive oil.[31] You can use olive oil liberally on salads. As with flaxseed oil, olive oil should always be kept in a tightly sealed container.

Omega-6 Fatty Acids

There are two forms of omega-6 fatty acids: linoleic acid and gamma-linolenic acid (GLA). Linoleic acid is found in flaxseeds, pumpkin seeds, walnuts, and wheat germ. GLA is difficult to obtain from food sources and is best taken as a supplement. GLA is useful for increasing the body's resting metabolism; that is, the rate at which it burns calories while not exercising. Resting metabolism is what maintains the body's internal temperature, with heat generated primarily in areas of dense brown fat. Brown fat is one of the types of stored body fat and is different from common body fat (known as yellow or white fat). We do not gain brown fat in the same way as yellow fat; rather, we are born with a given amount of brown fat and slowly lose it as we age. GLA raises the rate of heat-generating activity within brown fat, a process known as thermogenesis. A rise in the body's thermogenesis level causes more calories to be burned off as heat energy and fewer of them to be stored as fat.

Normally, the body can convert linoleic acid into GLA. However, stress, alcohol, aging, hypothyroidism, illness, and a diet high in saturated fats or damaged oils can block this conversion, resulting in a GLA deficiency. Evening primrose, which contains both omega-3 and omega-6 fatty acids, is a good source of GLA (suggested dosage is 500 mg daily).

Medium-Chain Triglycerides (MCTs)

MCTs are a form of natural fat found in certain seeds. Like GLA, medium-chain triglycerides, or MCTs, have been shown to promote weight loss, and they also tend to accelerate metabolism while lowering blood levels of cholesterol. Additionally, they improve absorption of vitamin E, calcium, and magnesium, protect against hypoglycemia (low blood sugar), and benefit those with digestive disorders. A good source of MCTs is grapeseed oil, available at most health food stores; use it uncooked on salads. Because MCT oils don't spoil easily and have a high burn-point, they are also good for cooking.

Another extremely healthy source of MCTs is coconut oil (65% MCT), which has a long shelf life and a high melting point of 76 degrees. It was popular as a cooking and baking oil in the United States until tropical oils, and saturated fats in general, fell out of favor due to a belief that saturated fats increase heart disease. However, the fact is that people who consume large amounts of coconut oil as part of their normal diet have not shown increases in health problems. For example, the Polynesian population of Tokelau eats a diet of steamed vegetables, fresh fish, and yams, and their primary source of fat is coconuts. Yet, in addition to being relatively free of heart disease, these islanders have an extremely low incidence of obesity.[32] That is because there is a big difference between commercial refined coconut oil and the all-natural, unprocessed coconut oil consumed by these people.

Refined commercial coconut oil is made from copra (the dried meat of the coconut), which is refined, bleached, and deodorized. Chemical solvents are used to get a higher yield of oil from the copra, which is then deodorized using high heat, and bleached with sodium hydroxide to remove free fatty acids and prolong shelf life. Additionally, refined coconut oil is often hydrogenated or partially hydrogenated, making it high in unhealthy trans-fatty acids. Virgin coconut oil is produced in a very different manner. Only fresh coconut meat, not copra, is used. It is either dried at minimal heat or processed while fresh, without the use of any chemical extracting agents. This maintains all the essential fatty acids, as well as a substance called lauric acid, which is highly anti-viral. The fresh oil that is extracted is very stable on its own and has a shelf life of several years.

Virgin coconut oil has been a staple cooking oil for thousands of years in tropical climates. When used as a cooking oil, it remains stable at high temperatures and does not form free radicals like most vegetable oils. One of the most exciting aspects of virgin coconut oil is that research shows its MCTs can actually aid weight loss. Virgin coconut oil lowers levels of lipids (fats) in the body,[33] and leads to a leaner body mass.[34] Diets high in coconut oil decrease the body's storage of yellow fat,[35] and may act by directly inhibiting genetic messages that instruct the body to store fat.[36] Medium-chain triglycerides help with weight control in several ways. They have been shown to increase thermogenic (fat-burning) activity in the body,[37] increase the amount of calories that the body burns, and support a feeling of satiety.[38] As an added benefit, virgin coconut oil is rich in lauric acid (a nutrient also found in mother's milk), which supports the body's immune system through its antimicrobial and antiviral properties.[39]

When choosing coconut oil, be aware that quality can vary greatly. One of the main differences between virgin coconut oil and refined coconut oils is the scent and taste. The best coconut oil will be labeled "organic virgin coconut oil" and will be in a glass jar. As soon as you open the top, you will be greeted by a delicious coconut aroma. That will assure you that you have found the "good stuff." You can eat it on a spoon (1 tablespoon per day) or use it as a cooking oil.

four

Heal Your Emotional Appetite

Although weight gain is often the outcome of underlying physiological problems, such as a toxic liver, a blood sugar imbalance, or food allergies, each of these physical causes also has a distinct emotional dimension. For example, anger tends to occur with a toxic liver, moodiness with a blood sugar imbalance, and anxiety with a food allergy. However, these emotions are not simply the effects of the physical illness, they can also be the cause: anger can make the liver become toxic, and a toxic liver may induce anger. Mainstream medical science has largely failed to appreciate the relationship of the emotions and health.

In contrast, ancient traditional medical systems, such as traditional Chinese medicine and Ayurvedic medicine, have long recognized that emotional well-being is inextricably linked with physical health. Consequently, disease cannot be reduced to either a psychological or physiological problem; both of these influences are always involved. Combining the physical and emotional in a comprehensive approach to health is considered by alternative medicine practitioners to come under the broad category of mind-body medicine.

Mind-body treatments enable you to examine what may be unconsciously driving you to gain weight and help raise your consciousness regarding what you choose to eat and why. Relieving stress and alleviating depression can help achieve permanent weight loss. In this chapter, we'll look at ways that you can heal your body with your mind by examining the emotional components of your weight problem and exploring ways to alleviate stress. Weight loss involves both physical and emotional transformation, a process that must take place in every dimension of life.

Success Story: Emotional Balance Leads to Weight Loss

Ilene tried every diet plan on the market, but with no success. She suffered from high blood pressure and had been on medication for 25 years, but with no improvement in her condition. When her weight reached 250 pounds (she was 5 foot 6), her doctor told her she was beginning to develop diabetes. He wanted to prescribe additional medications to help control the diabetes, but Ilene was reluctant to become dependent on yet another drug. Consequently, she decided to seek out a second opinion from a nutritionally oriented physician.

When she met with the doctor, he determined that Ilene's condition stemmed from a nutritional deficiency and an addiction to sugary, greasy junk foods. He immediately started her on a recovery program that included nutritional supplements and mild exercise. While these remedies were important to help Ilene break her sugar addiction, a key aspect of her treatment program involved exploring emotional issues. The new doctor helped Ilene understand that there was a genuine and concrete link between her health and some very painful emotional issues in her life. She discovered that she had been eating to comfort herself and that fat literally and figuratively covered up her uncomfortable feelings.

To help with her psychological issues, Ilene learned guided imagery techniques. In guided imagery, a therapist suggests images to the person and instructs them to visualize the image in their mind. The person is then asked to discuss what thoughts and feelings arise in response to the image, which helps to draw out buried emotional conflicts. Ilene found out that she needed to make changes in the choices she made, both through improvements in diet and lifestyle and by becoming more sensitive about what was going on with her emotionally. Once she had that realization, it became much easier to give up certain foods and adopt new habits. The treatments helped Ilene develop a new attitude toward food and a new outlook on life, which enabled her to control her food cravings and eat a healthier diet. Consequently, after three months of treatment, Ilene's high blood pressure began to subside and her blood sugar problem disappeared. After nine months, she had lost 70 pounds. She had also come to understand that weight management is an ongoing process of uncovering deeply buried feelings, allowing her to get in touch with what her body really wants and needs.

Feeding the Emotional Appetite

Getting at the real sources that are driving you to gain weight may be one of the greatest challenges of achieving a healthy body weight. Like Ilene, many individuals who look inside themselves for the answers discover that they have been struggling against a buried emotional conflict. Unresolved or unexpressed emotional issues may drive people to food cravings and bingeing. Any attempts at weight loss will prove unsuccessful until these issues are resolved. Food may act as a tranquilizer, a reward, or a substitute for affection. Most people eat for reasons other than hunger from time to time. Occasional "emotional eating" during times of anxiety or celebrations is perfectly normal. But when it becomes a habit of overeating, significant weight gain, and poor dietary choices, emotional eating can seriously affect health. Food can become an escape mechanism to avoid addressing underlying psychological problems.

Research clearly links eating disorders to emotional and psychological disturbances. For example, binge eaters suffer higher levels of depression and anxiety and lower self-esteem than those who don't binge.[1] Obese patients often report having a history of psychiatric complications, alcoholism, marital problems, physical and sexual abuse, or stress related to their physical health and financial and legal matters.[2] Many use overeating as a way to cope with emotional distress. Other studies have found a clear correlation between emotions such as boredom, anxiety, hostility, and anger (particularly unexpressed anger) and the development of weight problems.[3]

Six Myths about Stress

Six myths surround stress. Dispelling them enables us to better understand our problems and then take action against them. Let's look at these myths.

Myth 1: Stress is the same for everybody. Completely wrong. Stress is different for each of us. What is stressful for one person may or may not be stressful for another; each of us responds to stress in an entirely different way.

Myth 2: Stress is always bad for you. According to this view, zero stress makes us happy and healthy. Wrong. Stress is to the human condition what tension is to the violin string: too little and the music is dull and raspy; too much and the music is shrill or the string snaps. Stress can be the kiss of death or the spice of life. The issue, really, is how to manage it. Managed stress makes us productive and happy; mismanaged stress hurts and even kills us.

Myth 3: Stress is everywhere, so you can't do anything about it. Not so. You can plan your life so that stress does not overwhelm you. Effective planning involves setting priorities and working on simple problems first, solving them, and then going on to more complex difficulties. When stress is mismanaged, it's difficult to prioritize. All your problems seem to be equal and stress seems to be everywhere.

Myth 4: The most popular techniques for reducing stress are the best ones. Again, not so. No universally effective stress reduction techniques exist. We are all different, our lives are different, our situations are different, and our reactions are different. Only a comprehensive program tailored to the individual works.

Myth 5: No symptoms, no stress. Absence of symptoms does not mean the absence of stress. In fact, camouflaging symptoms with medication may deprive you of the signals you need for reducing the strain on your physiological and psychological systems.

Myth 6: Only major symptoms of stress require attention. This myth assumes that the "minor" symptoms, such as headaches or stomach acid, may be safely ignored. Minor symptoms of stress are the early warnings that your life is getting out of hand and that you need to do a better job of managing stress.

Adapted from *The Stress Solution* by Lyle H. Miller, Ph.D., and Alma Dell Smith, Ph.D., available at www.apahelp center.org, thanks to the American Psychological Association.

Food Cravings and Stress

Stress is widely recognized as a contributing factor in many diseases. In fact, two-thirds of all office visits to family physicians are due to stress-related symptoms.[4] Chronic stress directly affects the immune system, and if not effectively dealt with, it can seriously compromise health.[5]

Stress can be defined as a reaction to any stimulus or interference that upsets normal functioning and disturbs mental or physical health.

It can be brought on by internal conditions, such as illness, pain, emotional conflict, food allergies, or psychological problems, or by external circumstances, such as bereavement, financial problems, job loss, relocation, and electromagnetic fields. When it becomes chronic, stress is often unrecognized, since the person begins to accept it as a fact of life without being aware of how it is actually compromising all bodily functions and preparing the foundation for illness.

Stress often elicits a feeling of anxiety or fear. On a physiological level, the adrenal glands begin releasing the hormones cortisol, adrenaline, and noradrenaline into the bloodstream. This normal flight-or-fight response rouses the body into action, causing an immediate increase in heart rate and breathing and a rise in blood pressure. Under severe stress, such as a life-threatening situation, the rush of adrenal hormones raises energy levels so that we can respond to the emergency. It supports a spurt of strength to allow the person to flee from or survive dangerous situations.

During a fight-or-flight response, the body channels all of its resources to the muscles. Under prolonged or chronic situations, the body begins to extract energy from protein cannibalized from the kidneys, liver, stomach, and bones. It also conserves energy by shutting down "non-emergency" functions, such as the digestion and absorption of nutrients.

Among the more serious impacts of chronic stress is impaired digestion, which causes nutritional deficiencies. Over time, the body will

Stress and the Adrenal Glands

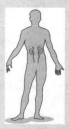

The adrenal glands, part of the body's endocrine system, are located atop the kidneys. The glands are composed of two types of tissue: the adrenal medulla and the adrenal cortex. The adrenal medulla, comprising 10% to 20% of the gland, is located in the interior portion and is responsible for the production of the hormones epinephrine (adrenaline) and norepinephrine (noradrenaline). These hormones are released in direct response to the sympathetic nervous system, which is responsible for the fight-or-flight response to stress or physical threats. The adrenal cortex, the outer layer, surrounds the medulla and accounts for 80% to 90% of the gland. It is responsible for the production of corticosteroids (also called adrenal steroids). Over 30 different steroids have been isolated from the adrenal cortex, including cortisol and cortisone.

Secretion of cortisol (as well as other adrenal steroids such as DHEA, adrenaline, and aldosterone) occurs in daily cycles, peaking in the morning and having the lowest values at night. Cortisol promotes protein building, regulates insulin and glycogen synthesis, and helps produce prostaglandins (hormonelike fatty acids involved in inflammatory processes). Under conditions of stress, high amounts of cortisol are released. Imbalances in cortisol secretion are also linked with low energy, inflammation, muscle dysfunction, impaired bone repair, thyroid dysfunction, immune system depression, sleep disorders, and poor skin regeneration.

QUICK DEFINITION
A **neurotransmitter** is a brain chemical with the specific function of enabling communications to happen between brain cells. Chief among the 100 identified to date are acetylcholine, gamma-aminobutyric acid (GABA), serotonin, dopamine, and norepinephrine.

attempt to compensate for these deficiencies by demanding more food. This can cause insatiable hunger and relentless food cravings and lead to excessive overeating. The net effect is that much of the food eaten in response to stress is converted into body fat. And although some people eat less during periods of stress, others overeat, especially comfort foods—the very foods that tend to add fat to the body.

Stress also causes biochemical changes in the brain that induce cravings for sweets. The production of cortisol, one of the hormones secreted by the adrenals during stress, can cause an imbalance in a brain chemical called neuropeptide Y. Flucuations in neuropeptide Y levels can predispose people to become obese, particularly when combined with the consumption of high fat foods.[6] Other brain chemicals (neurotransmitters—SEE QUICK DEFINITION) are also affected by stress:

- Serotonin helps produce sleep, regulate pain, and influence mood. It's called the "feel good" neurotransmitter. Low levels of serotonin may cause carbohydrate cravings.[7]

- Dopamine regulates physical movements and muscular control and influences mood, sex drive, and memory retrieval. Low levels are linked to depression and increased appetite.[8]

- Norepinephrine causes the brain to be more alert. It helps carry memories from short-term to long-term storage and enables a person to maintain a positive mood. Low levels are linked to mood disorders and increases in appetite; high levels induced by stress are linked to rebound weight gain after dieting.[9]

- GABA works to stop excess nerve signals

- Acetylcholine is required for short-term memory and muscle contractions.

Success Story: Balancing Brain Neurotransmitters to Support Weight Loss

Susan Groh, MD, addresses weight loss through an alternative medicine perspective. (See Resources for Dr. Groh's contact information.)

Rather than just prescribing weight loss "drugs," she performs a unique individualized evaluation of each patient. The diagnostic tests are more in-depth than those used in conventional medicine, and they assess the underlying cause of the patient's weight-loss resistance. Then, she designs a holistic program to balance brain neurotransmitters linked to both mood and weight gain, with a focus on reducing abdominal fat. This helps to reverse generalized inflammation, high cholesterol, glucose intolerance, insulin resistance, and cardiovascular risk factors. Her protocol includes regular physical activity, a healthy diet plan, and appetite suppression, which is achieved by using amino acids, vitamins and minerals that increase the individual's production of neurotransmitters. A weekly support group and/or individual spiritually oriented sessions help reinforce adherence and improve outcomes.

The following case represents a typical patient profile:

Mary, a 54-year-old woman, was fifty pounds overweight. She visited Dr. Groh specifically for guidance with weight loss. During the intake visit, Dr. Groh spent time with Mary, focusing on "being present" to her life at that moment. Mary had chronic low-grade depression, didn't smoke, found it difficult to exercise due to low motivation, had a glass of wine with dinner, liked to eat sweets, and regularly ingested a lot of simple carbohydrates at night. Mary reported that she actually felt increased fatigue after eating, instead of getting the energy boost she would like to experience. She found that hot flashes, loss of ambition, difficulty with memory and weight-gain issues had worsened along with menopause. Her family history included obesity and type 2 diabetes, although her initial medical exam did not reveal any irregularities in blood pressure or heart/lung functions. Standard blood tests were also all within normal range.

Dr. Groh proceeded to order additional tests that would take a more in-depth look at Mary's physiological activities:

- Free T 3, Free T 4, TSH: Levels of Free T 3 T4 low end of normal range; TSH suboptimal at high end of normal. Indicates suboptimal thyroid function, especially with low energy levels, mild depression, and difficulty with weight loss.

- 7- Hydroxy Pregnenelone: Levels too low to yield any reading. Indicates hormone imbalance, which can cause memory problems, low-grade depression, and weight gain.

- DHEA Sulfate: Low end of normal range, suboptimal. Indicates adrenal insufficiency, which is supported by symptoms of fatigue, weight gain, and poor memory.
- Hemoglobin A 1 C: Levels slightly elevated. Indicates that patient may be pre-diabetic; supported by family history.
- Glucose Tolerance Test: Fasting blood sugar normal when test started, but rose after glucose challenges; insulin level: high. Indicates insulin resistance and glucose intolerance.
- Triglycerides and VLDL (very low density lipoprotein): Elevated levels. Indicates a high level of fat that is carried in the blood, which can be due to high carbohydrate consumption and indicates a pre-diabetic condition.
- Vitamin D: Low levels. Indicates a need to increase vitamin D through supplementation with a goal of achieving a level of 80 or above. Low vitamin D is linked to increased risks of breast and colon cancer, depressed mood and other affective disorders, as well as low bone density and osteoporosis.

After reviewing both the clinical symptoms and blood work, Dr. Groh noted that Mary was glucose intolerant, insulin resistant, and prediabetic. Her eating habits and sedentary lifestyle were supporting the development of these syndromes. Mary's suboptimal hormone levels were also indicative of poor memory and mild depression, as well as difficulty in maintaining a healthy weight level.

Dr. Groh met with Mary to outline a therapeutic protocol. She suggested that Mary start taking Armour Thyroid, which is a prescription natural thyroid medication. She discussed the risks and benefits of this intervention, and suggested that calcium, vitamin D levels, and bone density should be monitored at the start of this therapy and periodically thereafter. Armour Thyroid helps to improve mood and supports weight loss. Dr. Groh then focused on enhancing Mary's natural production of neurotransmitters, including serotonin, dopamine, epinephrine, and norepinephrine. Among other functions, these neurotransmitters control mood and appetite regulation. Toward this end, Mary's supplement program included:

- Multivitamin-multimineral with sufficient quantities of vitamin D, vitamin C, calcium, vitamin B_6, folate, and selenium.

- Amino acids: L-lysine, 5-hydroxytrptophan, tyrosine, L-cysteine and *Mucuna pruriens* (a natural source of dopamine).
- Herbs/nutraceuticals for blood sugar balance: chromium, vanadium, arginine, carnitine, CLA, *Gymnema sylvestre*, bitter melon, and cinnamon.

The dosages of these supplements vary according to individual patient needs.

Mary was instructed to return in one week for monitoring and to begin the support group workshop. The counselor suggested that Mary work on psychological issues about using weight as "armor" in dealing with emotional challenges, which can increase resistance to weight loss. Mary reported that after one week on the supplement program she already had more energy and was feeling a lot more positive and less depressed and fatigued. After 1 month, Mary lost 5 pounds; at 2 months, 3 more pounds; and after 3 months, 3 additional pounds. She was down one dress size. Mary felt that she was much better at avoiding nighttime carbohydrate cravings, had a lot more motivation, and realized that she was not "on a diet," but had entered a whole new life stage of healthy living.

Are You Stressed-Out?

So how can you be sure whether you're stressed-out? If you answer yes to more than five of the questions below, it indicates that you may have too much stress in your life. In parentheses after each question are some potential underlying causes for the problem.

- Do you often grind your teeth? (digestive dysfunction, parasites)
- Is your breath shallow and irregular? (low metabolic energy, food allergies)
- Are your hands and feet cold? (hormonal imbalance, adrenal or thyroid weakness)
- Do you have trouble sleeping or tend to wake up tired? (liver dysfunction, food allergies)
- Do you often have an upset stomach? (food allergies)
- Do you get mad or irritated easily? (liver dysfunction)
- Do you feel worthless? (low metabolic energy, chronic fatigue)

The Personal Is the Political

As you explore your emotional issues, it is important to keep in mind that your inner desires and feelings regarding body weight are shaped by what you see and hear every day. Consequently, to really get at the source of what's driving you, you must be able to recognize how your inner desires are influenced by social factors. You need to distinguish between your own feelings and those that come from the outside in the form of social pressure, whether overt or more subtle.

Many people try to lose weight in pursuit of a sexier, slimmer image. While we are all entitled to pursue such an end, often the yearning to "look good" is motivated by a need to conform with someone else's ideal. Ask yourself why you feel the need to slim down. It is important not to confuse a yearning to satisfy someone else's demands or cultural stereotypes with your own desire to be healthy and live at your peak physical level.

Remember that the image of the perfect female body is a cultural construct and has changed many times throughout history. In Baroque paintings, beautiful women were portrayed as quite round and "Rubenesque." In modern society, however, the concept of "thin is in" has been the recent vogue, with images of supermodels such as Twiggy abounding in the 1970s. Yet this idealized image of the superthin model is not about anything real or beautiful. Because of the diet culture and the commercial interests that bombard us with images of ultrathin models, we learn to hate our own bodies and, in turn, are led to destructive and self-defeating eating behaviors. The reality is that most of us can never attain the cultural ideal, no matter how hard we try. This same artificial perfect physique image also applies to men. Freeing yourself from such ideals may be the best thing you can do to restore your health.

- Do you constantly worry? (hormonal imbalance)
- Do you have problems concentrating and articulating your thoughts? (low metabolic energy, digestive or hormonal imbalance)
- Do you frequently fidget, chew your fingers, or bite your nails? (food allergies, digestive disturbances)
- Do you have high blood pressure? (food allergies, digestive disturbances)
- Do you eat, drink, or smoke excessively? (low metabolic energy, poor diet)
- Do you sometimes turn to recreational drugs just to get away? (low metabolic energy, poor diet)

Are Your Adrenal Glands Stressed?

Because your adrenal glands are called on to respond to stress, repeated or chronic and prolonged stress overtaxes them and interferes with their normal function. This leads to fatigue, sleep disturbances, and other health problems, including weight gain. If stress is a problem for you, consider having an Adrenal Stress Index (ASI) test. This is a laboratory test that used by holistic health-care practitioners to pinpoint whether an imbalance in the adrenal glands might be contributing to hormonal imbalance and weight gain. It evaluates how well the adrenal glands are functioning by tracking hormone levels over a 24-hour cycle, which reflects the body's internal clock, or circadian rhythm. Four saliva samples taken at intervals throughout the day are used to monitor the adrenal rhythm. Saliva levels of hormones have been shown to closely mirror blood levels, and a saliva test is also less invasive. These samples are used to determine whether two main stress hormones (cortisol and DHEA) are being secreted in proper proportion to each other and at the right times. Based on the results, a physician can prescribe the appropriate treatment to restore the balance of hormones and correct their circadian rhythm. For information on where to get the Adrenal Stress Index test, see Resources, page 272.

Mind-Body Therapies for Stress Control

The best way to avoid weight gain in response to stress is to avoid stressful situations. However, since almost everyone faces stress, it is important to learn techniques that can offset its negative effects. Damage results from a negative emotional response to stress, rather that from stress itself. There are many natural techniques that reduce the stress response, including meditation, acupuncture, flower essences, and aromatherapy.

Develop Deliberate Eating Habits

A good way to control weight gain, and not just in response to stress, is to develop more deliberate eating habits. This requires focusing on the reasons why you are reaching for a snack or other food. It involves consciously exploring the many nuances of the feelings associated with the desire to eat and distinguishing actual physical hunger from a desire to gratify an emotional need. Pause before you reach for any food and ask yourself this series of questions:

- Am I really hungry?
- Do I feel upset?
- Is the food I want nutritious, or merely flavorful?

Mind-Body Therapies for Stress Control

- Develop deliberate eating habits
- Cognitive therapy and social support
- Guided imagery
- Neuro-linguistic programming
- Hypnotherapy
- Meditation
- Acupuncture and therapeutic touch
- Breathing exercises
- Yoga and qigong
- Flower essence therapy
- Aromatherapy

If you catch yourself about to eat in response to stress, or in response to boredom or anything other than actual physical hunger, drink 8 ounces of water instead. The moment of reflection, along with the water, will help stop the overeating behavior.

To further enhance your awareness of your eating habits, keep a daily food diary that includes notes about what you ate; how you felt before, during, and after eating; how many times you ate; any cravings you may have experienced; and whether you succumbed to them or not. Writing down this information will make you a more sensitive observer of your food choices and habits and allow you to assess long-term patterns in your behavior.

Cognitive Therapy and Social Support

It has been estimated that the average human being has approximately 50,000 thoughts per day. Unfortunately, up to 85% of this internal dialogue tends to be negative—angry, fearful, pessimistic, or anxious.[10] There are effective ways to reprogram your thinking for successful weight loss. The basis of cognitive therapy is to identify—through maintaining a journal and by introspection—this negative, self-defeating inner dialogue of thoughts (what cognitive therapists refer to as "automatic thoughts"). Positive, coping thoughts can then be used to counter the negative thoughts. The goal is to pull yourself out of reflexive self-destructive mental behavior that may be exacerbating your problem and to bolster the positive, self-reliant aspects of your personality. Cognitive therapy does not focus on the root causes of psychological problems; rather, it seeks to support health by interrupting the flow of negative thoughts. Countering each negative thought with a list of positive responses to the same situation enables the mind to reframe the situation.

It is easy to feel overwhelmed during times of transition as you struggle to incorporate changes, such as new ways of eating, into your life. Resist the temptation to isolate yourself, and remember why you are undergoing this process. As you continue to make choices for a healthier life, realize that any periods of discomfort are temporary. If you do not already have one, establish a support network of friends and family to help you get through the rough spots. You might also consider recruiting a dieting buddy or a workout partner to help you stay the course when your motivation begins to flag. Investigate joining a support group; you may find that being in the company of like-minded people experiencing similar changes and difficulties may bolster your own progress and help keep things in perspective. And, because cognitive therapy has been shown to be useful to support weight loss,[11] if you find you're having difficulty achieving reasonable results, consider working with a cognitive therapist.

Guided Imagery

Many alternative health-care practitioners use guided imagery as a tool for healing. Mental images affect important body processes, such as immune function, blood flow, and heart rate.[12] Using the power of the mind and the imagination, guided imagery and visualization can elicit positive physiological responses. By directly accessing emotions, imagery can help an individual understand the needs that may be represented by a health issue and can help develop ways to meet those needs. Imagery is also one of the quickest and most direct ways to become aware of emotions and their effects on health, both positive and negative. Imagery is simply a flow of thoughts that one can see, hear, feel, smell, taste, or experience internally.

Neuro-Linguistic Programming

Neuro-linguistic programming (NLP) helps people detect unconscious patterns of thought, behavior, and attitudes that contribute to their health problems. These unconscious patterns are then reprogrammed in order to alter psychological responses and facilitate the healing process. "Neuro" refers to the way the brain works and how thinking demonstrates consistent and detectable patterns; "linguistic" refers to the verbal and nonverbal expressions of thinking patterns; and "programming" denotes how these patterns are recognized and understood by the mind and how they can be altered.

NLP was developed by studying the thinking processes, language patterns, and behavioral patterns of accomplished individuals. Body cues —eye movement, posture, voice tone, and breathing patterns—coincided with certain unconscious patterns of a person's emotional state.

Guided Imagery for Weight Loss

Here's a short exercise in guided imagery. Wholeheartedly participating in this exercise can stimulate hormonal regulators that can help you control your appetite and make better food choices. The best time to use guided imagery techniques is just before sleep or immediately upon awakening.

Simply sit comfortably in a quiet location where you will not be disturbed. Breath deeply for a few minutes, paying attention to your breath. Imagine yourself looking at your clothes. In your imagination, you can visualize them in your closet or in a store. See yourself choosing a piece of clothing. Instead of the size you are now wearing, imagine that it is the size you would be at your goal weight. (Be realistic; don't imagine a size 4 if you are now a 3X; start with a size 16.) See yourself putting on the clothes and looking at yourself in the mirror. See the clothes fitting perfectly. Allow yourself to experience the emotion of pleasure at looking so good in the clothes. Hold onto that pleasurable emotional state as you gently open your eyes.

NLP practitioners ask questions to discover how a person relates to issues of identity, personal beliefs, life goals, and their health. They then observe the person's language patterns, eye movements, postures, muscle tension, and gestures. These relay information about how the person relates to their condition in both conscious and unconscious ways, revealing what limiting beliefs may exist. These belief structures can then be altered using NLP. The practitioner will ask the person to see herself in a positive state. The brain's natural response is to duplicate the positive images or beliefs by triggering the necessary immunological responses to guide the body toward the desired goal.

People who have difficulty losing weight have often adopted negative beliefs. They perceive themselves as helpless, hopeless, or worthless, expressed in statements like "I can't get healthy" or "I'll never lose weight." NLP helps to move the person from their state of discomfort to a desired state of health by facilitating reprogramming of these beliefs.

Hypnotherapy

Hypnosis can help change emotional attachments to eating the wrong kinds of food. Hypnosis works by helping to attain a state of consciousness where a person is open to suggestion. It can aid in adjusting emotional programming and can replace one set of associations with another. The hypnotherapist acts as a facilitator, helping the client form new belief patterns. Three conditions are essential to successful hypnotherapy:

1. Good rapport between hypnotist and subject.
2. A comfortable environment, free of distraction.

3. A willingness and desire by the subject to be hypnotized.

People who benefit most from hypnotherapy are those who understand that hypnosis is not a surrender of control; it is only an advanced form of relaxation. Many people have used hypnosis to successfully lose weight,[13] but it isn't a magic bullet. An effective hypnotherapy program must also include healthy food choices and exercise. That said, hypnosis can be a key tool in developing the motivation needed to stay on track.

Meditation

Meditation is a safe and simple way to balance your physical, emotional, and mental states. In the broadest sense, meditation is any activity that keeps the attention focused in the present. When the mind is calm and focused in the present, it is neither reacting to past events nor preoccupied with future plans, two major sources of chronic stress. There are many forms of meditation, but they can be categorized into two main approaches, concentration meditation and mindfulness meditation.

To still the mind and allow greater awareness or clarity to emerge, concentration meditation focuses the "lens of the mind" on one object, a sound or mantra, the breath, an image, or a specific thought. The breath is one of the most popular objects of focus in this type of meditation. As the person focuses on the ebb and flow of their breath, the mind is absorbed in the rhythm and becomes more tranquil. Mindfulness-based meditation entails turning off the mind's internal dialogue and simply receiving whatever exists in the environment without judgment. The meditator attempts to experience each unfolding moment fully, whether this involves visual observation, sounds, taste, aromas, or sensations. When

Five Healing Steps You Can Take Now

Christiane Northrup, MD, of Yarmouth, Maine, honors the dictum "do unto yourself as you (usually) do unto others" in offering these five easy steps as a way to prevent emotional turmoil:

- Say no: Draw boundaries and get rid of the "shoulds," guilt trips, and people-pleasing habits.

- Listen to your body: Rest when you are tired, eat when you are hungry, and realize that your body has an innate, internal wisdom and always knows exactly what you need.

- Let go of whatever is not working: To heal, you must be willing to let go of things that no longer serve you (bad relationships, old ideas and beliefs, a stressful job) and make room for healthy things (physical well-being, positive people, new opportunities).

- Accept yourself "as is": Pat yourself on the back for coming as far as you have, and realize that healing only begins when you love yourself for who you are today, right this moment.

- Say yes to feeling good: Believe you can feel better and take steps to make it so.[14]

SAD No More

People who receive little natural light during the day often experience an imbalance in their serotonin and melatonin levels — specifically, a rise in melatonin and a corresponding decline in serotonin. When low light exposure is chronic, it can lead to a specific type of depression called seasonal affective disorder (SAD). Often called "winter depression," SAD frequently occurs during the fall and winter months, when days grow shorter and natural light is limited.

The symptoms of SAD's winter doldrums are no doubt familiar to many. In fact, the National Institute of Mental Health estimates that over 10 million Americans experience SAD every year and another 25 million have milder depressive symptoms on a seasonal basis. What does SAD feel like? Typically, there is chronic depression and fatigue, which may leave you bedridden; hypersomnia (substantially increased sleep duration) and reduced quality of the sleep, leaving you feeling less refreshed; and cravings for carbohydrates and candy and other sweets, which can lead to significant weight gain. Individuals with SAD may experience elevated metabolism, which helps them burn more calories, but this is offset by increased appetite, especially for starchy and sweet foods. Over the span of several months, this often leads to weight gain of 5 to 10 pounds.

One way to restore serotonin levels is by stimulating the pineal gland, which produces serotonin and melatonin, through light therapy. When light enters the eye, electrical impulses travel along the optic nerve to the brain, where they trigger the pineal gland to secrete hormones. Light stimulates the pineal to produce serotonin, while darkness causes it to produce more melatonin. Light therapy counteracts the effects of winter depression and assists in weight loss by helping to maintain healthy levels of serotonin and melatonin. The oldest form of light therapy is natural sunlight: the sun is the ultimate source of full-spectrum light, which means it contains all possible wavelengths of light, from infrared to ultraviolet. Obviously, one solution is to spend the winter in the tropics and leave your SADness in New York or Ottawa. But if that isn't an option, full-spectrum lightbulbs, which provide a warmer, more natural light that closely resembles sunlight, can be particularly effective in overcoming symptoms of SAD and controlling appetite.[15]

distracting thoughts and judgments arise, the person simply witnesses whatever goes through the mind, not reacting or becoming involved with thoughts, memories, worries, or images. This helps the meditator gain a more calm, clear, and nonreactive state of mind.

Transcendental Meditation, a popular form of concentration meditation, is the most well-documented regarding the physiological effects of meditation, with over 500 clinical studies conducted to date.[16] Research shows that during TM practice, the body gains a deeper state of relaxation than during ordinary rest or sleep.[17] Brain-wave changes during TM indicate a state of enhanced awareness and coherence, and TM has actually been found to increase intelligence, creativity, and perceptual ability and reduce blood pressure and rates of illness by 50%.[18] TM also lowers blood levels of cortisol, which, as you read above, is responsible for many of the deleterious physiological changes seen with stress.[19]

Acupuncture and Therapeutic Touch

To help patients cope with stress, as well as correct other imbalances that may be contributing to weight gain, practitioners of mind-body medicine often adjust a patient's energy fields. These fields, generally ignored by mainstream practitioners, link the emotions, consciousness, and physical body. The energy field that emanates from the body is widely recognized in most ancient healing cultures. It is called qi or chi in China and prana in India.

In the Chinese model, qi is considered to be the life force that flows along specific pathways, called meridians, throughout the body (see "A Glossary of Traditional Chinese Medicine Terms," page 114). Points of heightened energy along the meridians are called acupoints. Sometimes the flow of qi in the body can become blocked, causing illnesses to develop. An acupuncturist uses the acupoints to stimulate the flow of qi and thus restore health to the body. In addition to its physical effects, acupuncture has a positive psychological effect as well. Acupuncture's effects are equivalent to those of drug-based therapies in cases of depression, insomnia, and other nervous disorders, and its action is swift and lasting without the side effects of drugs. Acupuncture is also a proven means of combating food cravings and controlling weight.[20] Acupuncture points, especially on the ear, have been used to help control carbohydrate cravings and regulate appetite.

Therapeutic touch is another method used in manipulating the body's energy fields to promote relaxation and, in turn, induce weight loss. The technique was first developed in 1972 by Dolores Krieger, Ph.D., RN, a professor of nursing at New York University. It is based on the idea that the therapist exudes a healing force that can affect the patient's recovery and cure.

Despite the name, therapeutic touch generally involves no physical contact between patient and practitioner. Instead, the practitioner places their hands two to six inches away from the patient and, with slow and rhythmic hand motions, determines where the blockages in the patient's energy field lie. The practitioner then works to replenish the energy flow where necessary, release any congestion, and remove obstructions. Therapeutic touch has been shown to alter enzyme activity, increase the healing of surgical wounds, and increase the manufacture of red blood cells.[21]

A Glossary of Traditional Chinese Medicine Terms

Traditional Chinese medicine (TCM), which originated over 5,000 years ago, is a comprehensive system of medical practice that heals the body according to the principles of nature and balance. A Chinese medicine physician considers the flow of vital energy (qi) in a patient through close examination of the patient's pulse, tongue, body odor, voice tone and strength, and general demeanor, among other elements. Underlying imbalances and disharmony in the body are described in terminology analogous to the natural world (heat, cold, dryness, dampness, or wind). The concept of balance, or the interrelationship of organs, is central to TCM. In TCM, imbalances are corrected through the use of acupuncture, moxibustion, herbal medicine, dietary therapy, massage, and therapeutic exercise.

Acupuncture is an integrated healing system developed by the Chinese and introduced in the United States in the mid-1800s. The treatment is administered by an acupuncturist using hair-thin, stainless steel needles, generally presterilized and disposable; these are lightly inserted into the skin at any of over 1,000 locations on the body's surface, known as acupoints.

Acupoints are places where qi can be accessed by acupuncturists to reduce, enhance, or redirect its flow.

Meridians are specific pathways in the human body for the flow of qi. In most cases, these energy pathways run up and down both sides of the body and correspond to individual organs or organ systems, designated as Lung, Small Intestine, Heart, and so on. There are 12 principal meridians and 8 secondary channels. Numerous points of heightened energy, or qi, exist on the body's surface along the meridians; these are the acupoints.

Moxibustion involves burning a dried herb called moxa (usually mugwort) over the skin at a specific acupuncture point. The moxa may be attached to a special acupuncture needle or stand in a free-standing cone set on a slice of ginger. The slow burning provides a penetrating heat. The purpose is to warm the blood and qi, particularly when a patient's energy picture is cold or damp.

Breathing Exercises

Breathing patterns often reflect the body's emotional state. For example, shallow chest breathing and hyperventilation are part of the body's natural response to stress. People who suppress unpleasant feelings and thoughts may also unknowingly restrict their breathing. Proper breathing can help facilitate an emotional release. Breathing techniques are utilized in most forms of meditation, as well as in yoga and qigong.

Yoga and Qigong

Yoga is a form of stretching and movement that combines breathing techniques with a series of postures (called asanas). Yoga relaxes the mind and body and stimulates the body's endocrine glands. It is an ideal exercise to use during a weight-loss program, especially if exercising is a new habit. Gentle beginner yoga moves help to increase circulation while they relax the body and mind, and they improve fat burning as well!

Qigong, which literally means "breath mastery exercise," is an ancient Chinese exercise technique that integrates breathing exercise with movement and meditation. Similar to yoga, qigong helps to calm the mind and maintain the optimum functioning of the body's self-regulating systems. Qigong exercise can range from simple calisthenic-type movements with breath coordination to complex exercises where brain-wave frequency, heart rate, and other organ functions are altered intentionally by the practitioner. It also stimulates and balances the flow of qi, the vital life energy that courses through the body.

 For more on **diaphragmatic breathing, yoga**, and **qigong**, see chapter 2, Start Exercising, pages 63–67.

Flower Essence Therapy

Flower essence therapy is used to treat a variety of illnesses, including weight gain, by calming the emotions. The treatments consist of subtle liquid preparations made from the fresh blossoms of flowers, shrubs, and trees. The approach was pioneered by British physician Edward Bach in the 1930s, when he introduced the 38 Bach flower remedies, all based on English plants. Flower essences are made by floating fresh blossoms in springwater and letting them sit in the morning sun for a few hours. The blossoms are removed, leaving the mother essence of the flower, which is then diluted to a dosage level. Drops of the essences can be placed under the tongue, ingested in a tonic, or diluted in a bath. Though their impact is subtle, they often prompt a shift in view from within, engendering recognition of feelings that exist below the level of ordinary awareness. Flower essences can help alleviate emotions such as apprehension, worry, loneliness, depression, and fear. They can also act as a catalyst for calmness and mental clarity; this is how they enhance our ability to recognize and understand what's driving our behaviors.

Flower essences are especially effective in treating addictive behaviors and can help people gain greater control over their unconscious food habits. A variety of flower preparations are used to treat addictions. (See "Flower Essences for Weight Loss," page 117.) Although you can use flower essences on your own, a trained flower essence practitioner can help tailor a treatment program specific to your needs and offer counseling as you work through emotional issues.

Success Story: The Power of Flower Essences

Patricia, 39, was 5 foot 4 and weighed 156 pounds. She suffered from allergies, fatigue, constipation, and feelings of low self-esteem. To cope with her tiredness and constipation, she drank 8 to 10 cups of strong coffee every day. She'd been on many diets and her weight had fluctuated between 110 and 160 pounds since high school.

Patricia decided to visit a nutritionist to help her with her health issues. The nutritional evaluation revealed that her adrenal glands were completely exhausted, due to chronic stress and overuse of coffee. The nutritionist suggested a comprehensive program of moderate exercise, healthy eating, and nutritional supplementation. She also introduced Patricia to a unique therapy she had never tried before, flower essence therapy. The nutritionist put together a group of remedies that would be useful for Patricia specifically. These included Morning Glory, Agrimony, Chestnut Bud, and Walnut to help wean her from coffee. She also suggested that Patricia add lavender and chamomile oils to baths.

Patricia was happy to find that the flower essence therapy helped her discover a different source of energy—one that made her more sensitive to the nuances in her body. As Patricia began to address painful emotional issues, the therapist suggested Tansy, Impatiens, and Pink Yarrow, which helped offset fatigue and offset mild depression. After about a year of nutritional supplements and flower essence therapy, Patricia lost 25 pounds. Ultimately she reached her ideal weight of 120 pounds and stayed within a few pounds of this weight for the next five years. Patricia found that the flower essences gave her more energy, a new outlook, and an increased sensitivity to her own body and its signals. In her words, "It was a slow, gradual change from the inside out."

Aromatherapy

Aromatherapy can be an effective technique to calm the emotions, achieve mental clarity, and control appetite. Like flower essence therapy, aromatherapy involves inhaling fragrances; however, instead of water-based essences, aromatherapy relies on oils extracted from the leaves, flowers, branches, or roots of plants. Due to the tiny size of their constituent molecules, essential oils can easily penetrate bodily tissues (either through the surface of the skin or by inhalation); this particularly effective absorption of the oils is the reason why aromatherapy can influence central nervous system activity.[22]

Essential oils that can support weight loss include birch bark, fennel, juniper berry, myrrh, oregano, and tangerine. Here are some others you may find useful, depending on your situation:

- Bergamot quells the urge for sweets or caffeine.
- Cajeput gets rid of intestinal parasites.
- Chamomile stimulates the immune system and calms jangled nerves.
- Juniper promotes lymph drainage.
- Lime aids digestive and liver problems.

There are several different methods for administering aromatherapy treatments:

- Diffusion: Diffusers disperse microparticles of essential oils into the air. They can be used to help respiratory conditions or to simply change the air with the mood-lifting or calming qualities of the fragrance.
- External application: Oils applied externally are absorbed through the skin. Convenient methods of external application include baths, massages, hot and cold compresses, and topical application of diluted oils.

Essential oils in a hot bath can stimulate the skin, induce relaxation, or energize the body. In massage, the oils are worked into the skin and, depending on the oil and the massage technique, can be used either to calm or to stimulate an individual.

Flower Essences for Weight Loss

Here are a few suggestions for how to therapeutically match flower essences with conditions that impact weight:[23]

Flower Essence	Effective For
Agrimony	Eating habits that stem from frustration
Black-Eyed Susan	Denial of gluttonous behaviors
Chestnut Bud	Breaking unhealthy and repetitive eating patterns
Impatiens	Tendency to gulp and swallow food
Iris	Cravings for sweets
Milkweed	Bingeing
Morning Glory	Addiction to junk food, bingeing, and desire for stimulants, such as caffeine
Pink Monkey Flower	Eating habits motivated by low self-esteem and shame
Pink Yarrow	Overeating to dull painful emotions
Rosemary	Stagnant digestion
Snapdragon	Oral fixations, such as continuous biting, crunching, and chewing as a sublimation for feelings of misplaced libido or unexpressed anger
Tansy	Sluggishness and lethargy

■ Floral waters: Weaker than essential oils, these can be sprayed into the air or sprayed on skin that is sensitive to the touch.

■ Internal application: Ingestion of essential oils is advantageous for certain organ disorders. It is essential, however, to receive proper medical guidance for internal use of oils.

Part II
Correct Imbalances

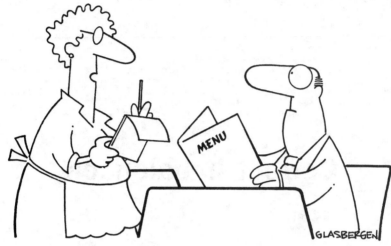

"Our diet spaghetti is exactly the same as
our regular spaghetti, except you plant,
cultivate, harvest and grind your own wheat."

five

Strengthen Your Sugar Controls

Action Alert! This is one of the most important steps toward attaining and maintaining a healthy weight: *Stop* eating sugary foods! If you would like to understand the whys and wherefores about this important dietary "must-do," read on.

Insulin is a hormone that manages the body's use of sugar. When insulin balance is disrupted, starches and sugars are turned into fat rather than being burned as fuel. If left unchecked, the condition can result in serious conditions, including obesity, diabetes, and heart disease. Proper diet, nutritional supplements, and other alternative therapies can help to restore insulin balance. That, in turn, keeps blood sugar levels in check, controls appetite, and helps to maintain a healthy weight.

In this chapter, we'll take a look at the role of insulin and other hormones involved in sugar imbalance and weight gain. I'll explain the concepts of hypoglycemia, insulin resistance, and metabolic syndrome, and outline the tests available for assessing sugar controls.

> **IN THIS CHAPTER**
>
> - Success Story: Balancing Insulin Reverses Weight Gain
> - Insulin, Appetite, and Your Weight
> - Insulin Resistance and Metabolic Syndrome
> - Glycemic Index and Glycemic Load
> - Success Story: Correcting Sugar Imbalance Leads to Weight Loss
> - Alternative Medicine Therapies for Sugar Control

In addition, I'll outline alternative medicine therapies to help you regain your sugar and insulin balance and control your weight.

Success Story: Balancing Insulin Reverses Weight Gain

Lucy, 42, was tired, lethargic, and about 40 pounds overweight. Even though she exercised regularly and thought she was eating a healthy diet, Lucy couldn't seem to lose her extra pounds. Upon questioning, we found that she had greatly reduced her dietary intake of meat and protein, believing that they were unhealthy for her (particularly the fat content in meat) and was eating a high-carbohydrate diet. The first step in determining Lucy's problem was to do a fasting blood glucose level. This is a simple blood test, performed after the person has fasted for 12 to 18 hours, to determine the amount of insulin circulating in the bloodstream.

The normal range for a fasting blood glucose test is from 70 to 110 mg/dl (milligrams per deciliter). Many natural health-care practitioners believe that an ideal number to strive for is 100 mg/dl. Lucy's level was 160 mg/dl, which indicates insulin resistance, or a prediabetic condition. Because of this insulin imbalance, Lucy had low blood sugar (hypoglycemia) and felt compelled to eat carbohydrates every two to three hours because of fatigue.

It was also important to evaluate Lucy's thyroid function. An underactive thyroid (hypothyroidism) can be a factor in weight gain by slowing down the body's metabolism, the rate that the body converts food into energy. We performed a blood test and also used her basal body temperature to assess thyroid function. Lucy's basal body temperatures were low at 96.1°F, 96.5°F, and 96.1°F (normal body temperature is 98.6°F), which may indicate an underactive thyroid. Basal body temperature may be low, even if thyroid blood tests are normal, a situation that warrants further examination, as blood tests aren't always accurate in diagnosing hypothyroidism.

The first step in treating Lucy's insulin imbalance was to change her diet. Due to her overindulgence in carbohydrates, she was instructed to eliminate simple carbohydrates completely for six weeks. We explained that this would be difficult initially because her body would still be producing high amounts of insulin, which would make her crave carbohydrates and sugary foods. She was limited to less than 40 grams of carbohydrates a day (as a comparison, ½ cup of rice is about 22 grams).

Lucy was encouraged to eat animal proteins (beef, chicken, and sea-food), tofu, leafy vegetables, cucumbers, onions, and celery.

Understandably, Lucy had difficulty sticking with this restricted diet the first month, but she did somewhat better the second month. When her fasting blood glucose level was rechecked, it had dropped to 145mg/dl—better but still too high. Because Lucy's compliance with the diet was inconsistent, it took about nine months to get her insulin level down to a relatively normal reading of 128 mg/dl.

We then designed a protocol to help normalize Lucy's thyroid function. This included a natural thyroid supplement (made from desiccated animal glands), and iodine-containing products such as kelp and bladderwrack. (Iodine is a component of thyroid hormones and also plays an important role in the body's use of these hormones.) Eating more protein also supports the thyroid, since it assures adequate levels of the amino acid tyrosine, an essential nutrient for the production of thyroid hormones. With these therapies in place, Lucy's basal body temperature slowly increased to 97.1°F. We also instructed Lucy to begin an exercise program that included yoga, especially the shoulder stand and the fish, asanas that specifically help the thyroid gland.

Lucy now feels much more energetic, and she's complying with her diet. She's really excited about the 30 pounds of weight that she lost during the first year!

Insulin, Appetite, and Your Weight

You probably know that sugar is high in calories and contributes to weight gain. For example, scientific studies have implicated sugary soft drinks as one of the causes of the rising epidemic of obesity in children.[1] Excessive consumption of foods high in sugar or starch can permanently damage your ability to utilize these substances as energy sources. As the body loses its capacity to process sugar or starch, it resorts to converting and storing these substances as body fat. The net result is that whenever you eat sugar, you gain weight, even if you cut down on overall calories.

At the core of your body's ability to use sugar is the hormone insulin. Insulin is the body's chief sugar regulator and a key appetite hormone, affecting your choice of what, when, and how much you eat. In healthy people, insulin controls appetite by keeping sugar (glucose) levels in the blood fairly constant within a narrow range.[2] However, the physiological mechanism that regulates insulin can be thrown off balance when it is forced to work overtime on processing excess sugars and starches, causing too much insulin to enter the blood, which leads to high insulin levels, obesity, and increased risk for diabetes.

How Sugar Becomes Fat

All carbohydrates (meaning both sugars and starches) and some of the proteins we eat are transformed into glucose, which is one of the body's key energy sources. Immediately after a meal, glucose levels rise in the bloodstream and the pancreas (the gland where insulin is manufactured) releases insulin to match the rise in glucose. The insulin reduces the levels of sugar circulating in the bloodstream by helping transfer it into the body's cells, where it is broken down and used as a fuel. Insulin acts like a chemical key that opens up the cell membranes, allowing glucose to enter. As glucose is absorbed by the cells, blood sugar levels decline, and when they become low, we feel hungry and eat, thus beginning the cycle all over again. In a healthy person, levels of glucose and insulin in the blood rise and fall gradually.

Glucose that is not burned as a fuel is converted into glycogen, a type of starch that is stored in the liver and muscles. Some of the excess glucose is also converted into fat (specifically triglycerides). Under normal circumstances, most glucose is burned as fuel and only minimal quantities are converted into body fat. However, this mechanism is thrown out of balance by the consumption of too much sugar.

A rapid rise in insulin not only brings about a glucose "crash," it also keeps blood sugar at a low level by preventing glycogen from being converted back into glucose. At the same time, the triglycerides manufactured from excess glucose can't be reconverted into glucose. This results in a low blood sugar level (hypoglycemia), which causes you to feel fatigued, light-headed, irritable, nervous, and depressed. This causes a sugar craving that must be satisfied in order to feel good again, fueling an addictive cycle.

With time, high blood levels of insulin triggered by the consumption of sugar and refined carbohydrates (white flour, white rice, and other processed grains) leads to a downward spiral of metabolic changes that adversely affect health. These include hypoglycemia, insulin resistance, metabolic syndrome, diabetes, and, of course, obesity.

Hypoglycemia

Most metabolic processes are complex feedback loop mechanisms, and this is true for the balance of blood sugar, which is regulated by insulin

and glucagons (SEE QUICK DEFINITION). Both of these hormones are produced in the islets of Langerhans in the pancreas, and they operate in a
give-and-take manner to maintain blood sugar at a normal level. If there
is a high level of glucose in the blood, insulin is secreted, which alerts
cells to take up the glucose so that the amount in the blood is lowered.
If there is a low level of glucose in the blood, glucagon is secreted, which
signals the liver to turn its stores of gly-
cogen back into glucose. Hypoglycemia
can be caused by a number of factors
that may interfere with either of these
processes. These include genetic factors
(but this is rare), alcohol consumption
(especially on an empty stomach), glucose-lowering drugs used for diabetes,
and chronic consumption of high-sugar
meals, which causes an oversecretion of
insulin, stimulating cells to quickly take
up glucose, leading in turn to a sudden
lowering of blood sugar level.[3]

 Glucagon is secreted by the
pancreas and helps to unlock
the body's fat stores to be
burned as fuel. If too much insulin is
present in the bloodstream, due to a
steady diet of carbohydrates for example, glucagon is blocked and the body's
fat stores aren't available as an energy
source. As a result, the person may feel
lethargic, and may crave carbohydrates
as a result.

Symptoms associated with hypoglycemia include weakness, sudden
fatigue, rapid heartbeat, anxiety, dizziness, confusion, and inability to
concentrate. In the extreme, hypoglycemia may lead to seizure, coma,
and even death.[4] Eating will often alleviate symptoms. Many people frequently experience the early stages of hypoglycemia, one of the driving
forces causing a craving for sweet snacks. However, this just fuels the
downward spiral toward blood sugar dysregulation, more weight gain,
and other illnesses. Next time you crave something sweet or starchy in
response to fatigue, choose 10 almonds instead. Chew them slowly and
follow with a cup of water. The protein, healthy fat, and minerals in the
almonds turn off the craving.

Insulin Resistance and Metabolic Syndrome

Insulin resistance is a condition that occurs when the cells no longer
react to insulin, making it difficult for them to absorb glucose. The
pancreas responds by releasing even more insulin into the blood, which
only worsens the problem, as the rising insulin simply further increases
the cells' resistance. Over time, the body loses its ability to burn glucose, causing energy levels to spiral downward. Controlling weight
then becomes increasingly difficult, as insulin, unable to get glucose

into the cells, converts more and more sugar into fat. In addition, the body losses it ability to burn fat; in fact, this is one of the main clinical markers for insulin resistance.[5] As the cells become increasingly starved of glucose, a cycle of carbohydrate cravings ensues. Once set in motion, the seesawing of glucose and insulin in the blood can cause periodic overwhelming temptations to gorge on starchy, sugary foods. Under these conditions, typical efforts at weight loss may prove useless. If left untreated, the swing of glucose and insulin becomes progressively worse, leading to dangerous and debilitating ailments, including heart disease and diabetes.

Obesity as determined by waist circumference has a very high correlation to insulin resistance.[6] High insulin levels lead not only to fat accumulation but also to salt and water retention, making you feel bloated and adding pounds. This condition also increases the appetite.

Metabolic syndrome, also referred to as syndrome X or insulin resistance syndrome, is defined as a grouping of symptoms that individually and collectively increase risk for a number of illnesses. The symptoms include insulin resistance, obesity, high triglycerides, low HDL (good cholesterol), high blood pressure, high blood glucose, and a tendency to form blood clots.[7] as well as low testosterone (in men) and elevated uric acid (gout). Astounding as it sounds, one-fourth of adults in the United States have metabolic syndrome, which is made worse by being overweight and by a sedentary lifestyle. Having even just a few of these symptoms can classify a person as having metabolic syndrome, which increases risk of heart disease,[8] diabetes,[9] and cancer,[10] as well as inflammatory markers linked to these and other disorders.[11]

The U.S. National Cholesterol Education Panel has established guidelines indicating that anyone who has any three of the following conditions has metabolic syndrome:[12]

- Abdominal obesity: waist circumference greater than 35 inches in women and 40 inches in men
- Elevated fasting blood sugar level: between 110 and 126
- High triglyceride levels: over 150
- Low levels of HDL ("good") cholesterol: less than 50 in women and 40 in men
- High blood pressure: 130/80 or higher

Assessing Your Risk of Metabolic Syndrome

To determine whether you're at risk for metabolic syndrome, take the following test.

Do you have a family history of any of the following: diabetes, obesity, high blood pressure?
Yes ❑ or No ❑

Is your blood pressure higher than 135/85?
Yes ❑ or No ❑

Are your triglycerides greater than 150?
Yes ❑ or No ❑

Is your fasting glucose outside the range 115 to 125?
Yes ❑ or No ❑

Is your waist measure greater than 40 inches (men) or 35 inches (women)?
Yes ❑ or No ❑

Do you have low testosterone or any sexual dysfunction?
Yes ❑ or No ❑

Is your HDL 40 or below?
Yes ❑ or No ❑

Do you have elevated uric acid (gout)?
Yes ❑ or No ❑

Are you overweight (BMI 25 or more)?
Yes ❑ or No ❑

Are you inactive, seldom exercising?
Yes ❑ or No ❑

For women:

Do you have a history of gestational diabetes (diabetes with pregnancy)?
Yes ❑ or No ❑

Have you delivered a baby of 9 pounds or more?
Yes ❑ or No ❑

Do you have a history of polycystic ovarian syndrome (PCOS)?
Yes ❑ or No ❑

If you answered yes to three or more questions on the test, you are at risk for metabolic syndrome.

If these guidelines indicate you have metabolic syndrome, or even if you're just overweight, you should have your levels of C-reactive protein measured; this substance is a marker for inflammatory response, and heart disease risk. Abdominal fat contributes to a high level of C-reactive protein, which in turn contributes to increased abdominal obesity, as well as the development of type 2 diabetes.[13]

Causes of Insulin Resistance

Although genetics may predispose some people to sugar imbalances and insulin resistance, other factors that contribute to this condition play a far greater role. These include poor dietary choices (too many simple and refined carbohydrates), food allergies, an underactive thyroid (discussed in chapter 6, Overcome a Sluggish Thyroid), stress, emotional influences (discussed in chapter 4, Heal Your Emotional Appetite), and a sedentary lifestyle (discussed in chapter 2, Start Exercising).

Too Many Simple and Refined Carbohydrates

A diet high in certain types of carbohydrates is one of the principal causes of both insulin resistance and metabolic syndrome. Carbohydrates, which consist of both sugars and starches, are an excellent energy source for the body because they can be completely converted into glucose. In contrast, only 10% of dietary fats and 50% of proteins get converted into glucose. Carbohydrates come in two forms: simple and complex. Simple carbohydrates (such as table sugar, honey, fructose, and corn syrup) are just what their name implies, simple, small molecules. They're made up of single sugar molecules or two sugar molecules joined together. When you eat them, they break down immediately and are quickly absorbed by the blood. Complex carbohydrates, found in vegetables, beans, and whole grains, are long chains of sugar molecules, often attached to protein, fats, vitamins, or minerals. These molecules break down slowly in the digestive tract and are gradually absorbed into the bloodstream. The result is a prolonged feeling of fullness and a sustained energy level.

Physicians and nutritionists are particularly concerned about refined carbohydrates (white flour, white rice, and so on), complex carbohydrates that have been stripped of their fiber-rich outer covering and nutrient-dense germ during processing. Refined carbohydrates are the main ingredient in most junk foods and sweets, such as pizza, cookies, pastries, doughnuts, soda, ice cream, and candy bars. Once in the body, the refined carbohydrates in these foods quickly convert into glucose and go almost directly into the bloodstream, requiring very little digestive activity.

When you eat simple carbohydrates, your pancreas is faced with a sudden flood of glucose and often cannot gauge how much insulin is needed. It goes into high gear and overresponds in order to cope with what it interprets as a sugar emergency. Sugary foods provoke a strong insulin response, so eating a lot of them eventually causes the pancreas to chronically overreact to the amount of glucose in the blood. This is very destructive to health and definitely affects weight. When sugary foods are eaten alone rather than in combination with other nutrients, such as protein, the situation is worse. This is a good example of why the type of food eaten is more important to weight maintenance than the calories eaten. Complex carbohydrates, abundant in grains, vegetables, and most fruits, are broken down slowly and do not cause the same kind of alarm reaction that simple and refined carbohydrates do.[14]

Food Allergies

Food allergies can also disrupt blood sugar balance. The body's first reaction to an allergenic food is often hypoglycemia or some other manifestation of insulin imbalance. Epidemiologic studies have discovered that there is a correlation between obesity (measured by body mass index) and allergic reactions.[15] In addition, overweight people who suffer from indigestion and other gastrointestinal complaints are more likely to report food allergies.[16]

The connection between sugar disorders and food allergies is often ignored in conventional medicine. However, performing a challenge test will often reveal the connection. A challenge test involves eliminating common foods for one week, and then reintroducing them into the diet, ideally one food at a time. When people reintroduce problematic foods, they often experience allergic reactions that have symptoms much the same as those of hypoglycemia. Common foods that can cause this reaction include wheat, milk, eggs, corn, beef, peanuts, and orange juice.

Watch Out for Hidden Sugars

Finding out whether a food product contains sugar requires more sleuthing today than it once did. Only a few manufacturers currently include the word *sugar* in the ingredients lists of their sugar-containing products. Instead, in an attempt to avoid this stigma, which could negatively impact sales, many food producers hide the sugars in their products behind a host of chemical synonyms. Take note that any product listing any of the following ingredients really does contain sugar:

- Dextrose
- Sucrose
- Glucose
- Fructose
- Dextrin
- Corn sweetener
- Lactose
- Maltodextrin
- Maltose
- Malt
- Sorghum
- Modified cornstarch
- High-fructose corn syrup
- Fruit juice concentrates

Hormones and the Thyroid

Hormone imbalances, particularly in women during perimenopause and menopause, affect insulin levels and the function of the thyroid, potentially leading to weight gain. In this menopausal period, bursts of the female hormone estrogen are released, leading to a condition called estrogen dominance. These bursts of excess estrogen cause insulin to be released, and sugar is converted into fat as a result. Estrogen dominance also depresses the function of the thyroid, which slows the rate of fat metabolism, leading to additional weight gain.

Stress

Stress and sugar imbalances are closely interrelated. Normally, a stressful situation triggers the fight-or-flight response in our bodies, which helps increase our energy level to handle the emergency. The response begins with the adrenals releasing the hormones cortisol, adrenaline, and noradrenaline into the bloodstream. This adrenaline rush rouses the body into action, causing an immediate increase in heart rate, respiration, and blood pressure. The liver reacts by releasing stored sugars (glycogen) to provide the needed energy.

This is all well and good for an emergency situation. But when your blood sugar levels are moving violently up and down several times every day because of chronic stress, your adrenals can become exhausted. Blood sugar levels become erratic, leading to sugar cravings. Also, many people crave comfort foods, typically sweet or starchy foods, when under stress.

Analyze Your Insulin Function

There are a couple of approaches to diagnosing problems with insulin function and sugar imbalances—evaluating your eating patterns and undergoing testing—and ideally you'd do both. It's important to evaluate what you eat, how various foods make you feel, and what these eating patterns may reveal about your insulin function. Diagnostic tests are also available to measure blood glucose levels and to evaluate insulin response.

Do You Have a Problem with Sugar?

If you are unable to manage your weight, there's a very good chance that this is related to an insulin or sugar imbalance. To get a better idea of whether this is the case, ask yourself these questions:

- Do I eat when nervous?
- Am I intensely hungry between meals?
- Am I irritable before meals?
- Do I feel a little shaky when hungry?
- Does my fatigue disappear after eating?

- Do I faint or have heart palpitations if meals are delayed?
- Do I get afternoon headaches?
- Do I crave coffee or candy in the afternoon?
- Do I regularly have intense cravings for sweets or snack foods?

If you answer yes to three or more of these questions, a sugar imbalance is probably a factor in your weight-control issues.

Examining Eating Patterns

The first step many holistic practitioners take when attempting to understand and address problems with obesity is to request that patients write down everything they eat for a week. It's important to note both physical and emotional feelings before and after eating, and to attempt to distinguish between appetite, which has to do with a particular food's appeal, and hunger, which is a more acute need felt within the body.

After a week of keeping your food journal, examine it with the following questions in mind:

- Do you eat at regular mealtimes or at different times each day?
- Do you eat set meals, or do you graze throughout the day?
- Do you snack between meals?
- What kinds of foods do you eat at meals or as snacks? Do you consume lots of carbohydrates (breads and pasta)? Fruits? Are you getting adequate protein (meat, chicken, fish, beans, eggs, dairy, or soy products)? Do you consume fatty foods at every meal? Do you drink caffeinated beverages (coffee, tea, or sodas) every day?

- Do you eat sweets every day?
- Do you regularly binge on sweets?

Looking carefully at your eating patterns in this way should give you an idea of your relationship to sugar and whether or not it is a factor in your weight problems. You can gather more information with a simple experiment: Consciously avoid eating any sugar at all for 24 hours. Note how you respond, physically, mentally, and emotionally. Were you more irritable or anxious than usual? Did you feel fatigued? Did you feel more or less alert?

Measure Your Blood Glucose

There are several diagnostic tests available that measure blood sugar level. Normal glucose metabolism should reflect a gradual increase and an equally gradual decline in both glucose and insulin over time. Two tests are commonly used. The first is a fasting blood glucose level, taken after fasting overnight, and the second measures how the body handles excess sugar after consuming a high-glucose drink.

Fasting plasma glucose (FPG) test: In this test the patient fasts overnight, then has blood drawn in the morning before eating anything. A normal level ranges between 70 to 110 mg/dl. If the initial value taken after fasting overnight is greater than 110 mg/dl and less than 126 mg/dl, this indicates a sugar regulation imbalance that may develop into full diabetes if left unchecked.

Oral glucose tolerance test (OGTT): This test is done in a laboratory or physician's office. First the patient fasts overnight. A blood sample is drawn to determine blood sugar level before the test begins. Then the patient drinks a high-glucose liquid (usually with 75 grams of sugar). Blood is drawn again at various time intervals: 30 minutes, 1 hour, 2 hours, 3 hours, and so on. A normal result would show an immediate rise in blood glucose following the high-glucose drink, followed by a fairly rapid decrease to a normal level. If there is dysregulated blood sugar control, blood glucose levels do not return to normal quickly, but take a much longer time. This can be due to either a lack of insulin or insulin resistance. More specifically, if the glucose level 2 hours after drinking the high-sugar solution is 110 mg/dl or less, glucose tolerance is normal. Above that, glucose tolerance is impaired: 110 mg/dl to 126 mg/dl indicates somewhat impaired glucose tolerance; 126 mg/dl to 140 mg/dl requires intervention; and greater than 140 mg/dl indicates insulin resistance or prediabetes. A level over 180 mg/dl may indicate diabetes, and over 200 mg/dl indicates full diabetes.

Although the above guidelines are commonly used, the American Diabetes Association has suggested that the cutoff for impaired glucose tolerance should be reduced from 110 to 100 mg/dl, which would classify a larger number of people as having impaired glucose tolerance. Lowering the cutoff level would be beneficial, alerting more people that they may have a problem and allowing them to take corrective measures to reverse the glucose imbalance before their condition becomes

Sugar on the Brain

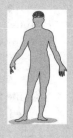

Although we generally feel satisfaction or relief after eating a sugary snack, the sensation does not come directly from the glucose that enters the bloodstream, but rather from the corresponding surge in insulin. This is because, in addition to managing glucose, insulin is used by the body to transport the amino acid tryptophan, a building block of the neurotransmitter serotonin, to the brain. Serotonin is sometimes referred to as the "happiness chemical" due to its influence on mood. High levels of serotonin in the brain produce feelings of self-confidence, calm, satisfaction, and composure. However, when levels start to decline, we feel anxious, cannot concentrate, and become depressed.

When tryptophan is scarce, serotonin is also in short supply. This creates an intolerable condition for the brain, which demands immediate action, hence our cravings for sugar. Sugar causes quick satisfaction by initiating the release of insulin, which delivers tryptophan to the brain and restores serotonin levels. In effect, sugar works like an antidepressant. (Prozac, or fluoxetine, so commonly prescribed for depression, also works by elevating levels of serotonin.)

Because of this, you can get addicted to sugar as if it were a drug, becoming dependent on it to elevate your mood. Unfortunately, individuals who experience violent swings in their glucose levels frequently experience sudden and extreme changes in temperament. After giving in to a food craving, they feel a fleeting sensation of bliss, but it's all too often followed by a black mood. They become angry at others or themselves for no apparent reason and often punish themselves for failing to stick to their diet. Although such emotional responses may often be perceived as psychological in origin, for those suffering from a blood sugar imbalance the problem has a distinct biochemical basis.

more serious.[17] The therapies that must be initiated to reduce diabetes risk include eating a healthy diet and exercising — also two of the most important recommendations for weight loss.

Glycemic Index and Glycemic Load

"Glycemic index" and "glycemic load" have become buzzwords in the weight-loss industry, but there is a lot of confusion about what they actually mean. In addition, as with most systems and rules about weight loss, it still boils down to the same basic message: eat a lot of whole, natural foods and stay away from processed and junk foods! Glycemic index offers a comparison of the insulin effect of different foods using values determined by the amount of insulin released in response to consuming 100 grams of a specific food. Glycemic load takes water and fiber content into account. This is usually a more realistic number in terms of how the body actually uses food that is consumed. For example, watermelon has a high glycemic index but a low glycemic load because it contains so much water and fiber; you'd have to eat a lot of watermelon to get 100 grams exclusive of its water and fiber content.

The effect of a given food will vary depending on factors other than its glycemic index. These include what other foods were eaten at the same time, how the food is prepared, and how an individual metabolizes the food. Scientific research is divided in terms of the usefulness of the glycemic index as a parameter for choosing foods that lead to weight loss. Paying attention to the glycemic index can be helpful in reducing consumption of processed and junk food. However, some studies have surmised that focusing on glycemic load does not provide any added benefit over other healthy eating plans in promoting weight loss.[18]

If you decide to use the glycemic index as a guide to choosing foods, you can use the following chart for guidance. Charts that include more foods are available on the Internet, such as the International Table of Glycemic Index and Glycemic Load Values, available from *The American Journal of Clinical Nutrition* at www.ajcn.org/cgi/reprint/76/1/5.pdf. Keep the following points in mind when assessing glycemic index values:

- Low glycemic index = 55 or less; medium = 56 to 69; high = 70 and above.
- Foods with a high rating (70 and above) cause a greater insulin response. These include white bread in all its forms (including bagels and English muffins), processed flaked cereals, instant hot cereals, low-fat frozen desserts, raisins and other dried fruits, whole milk and whole-milk cheeses, peanuts and peanut butter, hot dogs, and luncheon meats.
- Foods with a low rating (55 or less) do not cause a high insulin spike. These include most fresh vegetables, leafy greens, pitted fruits and melons, 100% whole-grain breads, minimally processed whole-grain cereals, sweet potatoes and yams, skim milk, buttermilk, most legumes, most nuts, poultry, shellfish, whitefish, and lean cuts of beef, pork, and veal.
- Cooked foods rank higher on the index than raw foods. Similarly, fruits and vegetables that have been juiced or pureed are higher on the index than whole fruits and vegetables.
- The glycemic index does not necessarily reflect the nutritional value of a food. Some foods that have a low glycemic index, are high in empty calories (indicated by * in the chart). Some foods that have a high glycemic index are nonetheless very nutritious and low in calories (indicated by ++ in the chart).

Glycemic Index

Food	Glycemic Rating	Glycemic Index
Bakery products		
Pound cake*	Low	54
Danish pastry	Medium	59
Muffin (unsweetened)	Medium	62
Cake	Medium	65
Cake, angel food	Medium	67
Croissant	Medium	67
Waffles	High	76
Doughnut	High	76
Beverages		
Soy milk	Low	30
Apple juice	Low	41
Carrot juice	Low	45
Pineapple juice	Low	46
Grapefruit juice	Low	48
Orange juice	Low	52
Crackers		
Shortbread	Medium	64
Water biscuits	Medium	65
Ryvita	Medium	67
Wafers	High	77
Rice cakes++	High	77
Breads		
Multigrain bread	Low	48
Whole-grain bread	Low	50
Pita bread, white	Medium	57
Pizza, cheese	Medium	60
Hamburger bun, white	Medium	61
Rye bread	Medium	64
Whole wheat bread	Medium	69
White bread	High	71
White rolls	High	73
Baguette	High	95

Glycemic Index

Food	Glycemic Rating	Glycemic Index
Breakfast cereals		
All-Bran	Low	42
Oat meal	Low	49
Oat bran	Medium	55
Muesli	Medium	56
Whole wheat flakes	Medium	57
Shredded Wheat	Medium	69
Golden Grahams	High	71
Puffed wheat	High	74
Puffed rice	High	82
Corn flakes	High	83
Cereal grains		
Pearl barley	Low	25
Rye	Low	34
Wheat kernels	Low	41
Rice, instant	Low	46
Rice, parboiled	Low	48
Barley, cracked	Low	50
Rice, brown	Medium	55
Rice, wild	Medium	57
Rice, white	Medium	58
Barley, flakes	Medium	66
Millet++	High	71
Dairy foods		
Yogurt, low-fat (sweetened)	Low	14
Yogurt, low-fat (artificially sweetened)	Low	13
Milk, chocolate	Low	24
Milk, whole	Low	27
Milk, fat-free	Low	32
Milk, skimmed	Low	32
Milk, semiskimmed	Low	34
Ice-cream, low-fat*	Low	50
Ice-cream, full-fat*	Medium	61

Glycemic Index

Food	Glycemic Rating	Glycemic Index
Fruits		
Cherries	Low	22
Grapefruit	Low	25
Apricots (dried)	Low	31
Apples	Low	38
Pears	Low	38
Plums	Low	39
Peaches	Low	42
Oranges	Low	44
Grapes	Low	46
Kiwifruit	Low	53
Bananas	Low	54
Fruit cocktail	Medium	55
Mangoes	Medium	56
Apricots	Medium	57
Apricots (canned in syrup)	Medium	64
Raisins	Medium	64
Pineapple	Medium	66
Watermelon	High	72
Pastas		
Spaghetti, protein-enriched	Low	27
Fettuccine	Low	32
Vermicelli	Low	35
Spaghetti, whole wheat	Low	37
Ravioli, meat-filled	Low	39
Spaghetti, white	Low	41
Macaroni	Low	45
Spaghetti, durum wheat	Medium	55
Macaroni and cheese	Medium	64
Brown rice pasta	High	92
Root vegetables		
Carrots, cooked	Low	39
Yam	Low	51
Sweet potato	Low	54

Glycemic Index		
Food	**Glycemic Rating**	**Glycemic Index**
Root vegetables (continued)		
Potato, boiled	Medium	56
Potato, new	Medium	57
Potato, canned	Medium	61
Beet root	Medium	64
Potato, steamed	Medium	65
Potato, mashed	High	70
Chips	High	75
Potato, microwaved	High	82
Potato, instant	High	83
++Potato, baked	High	85
Parsnips	High	97
Snack foods and sweets		
Peanuts	Low	15
*Chocolate bar, 1 ounce	Low	49
Jams and marmalades	Low	49
Popcorn	Low	55
Mars bar	Medium	64
*Table sugar (sucrose)	Medium	65
Corn chips	High	74
Jelly beans	High	80
Pretzels	High	81
Dates	High	103
Soups		
Tomato soup, canned	Low	38
Lentil soup, canned	Low	44
Black bean soup, canned	Medium	64
Split pea soup, canned	Medium	66
Vegetables and beans		
Artichoke	Low	15
Asparagus	Low	15
Broccoli	Low	15
Cauliflower	Low	15

Glycemic Index		
Food	Glycemic Rating	Glycemic Index
Celery	Low	15
Cucumber	Low	15
Eggplant	Low	15
Green beans	Low	15
Lettuce, all varieties	Low	15
Peppers, all varieties	Low	15
Snow peas	Low	15
Spinach	Low	15
Young summer squash	Low	15
Tomatoes	Low	15
Zucchini	Low	15
Soybeans, boiled	Low	16
Peas, dried	Low	22
Kidney beans, boiled	Low	29
Lentils, green, boiled	Low	29
Chickpeas	Low	33
Green beans, boiled	Low	38
Black-eyed peas	Low	41
Chickpeas, canned	Low	42
Baked beans, canned	Low	48
Kidney beans, canned	Low	52
Lentils, green, canned	Low	52
Broad beans	High	79

Success Story: Correcting Sugar Imbalance Leads to Weight Loss

Marjorie, 32, had a group of symptoms that included chronic fatigue, emotional stress and depression, PMS (premenstrual syndrome) symptoms, and obesity. Although only 5 feet tall, she weighed 180 pounds. Marjorie's nutritionist suggested that she take a glucose tolerance test to determine if she had sugar imbalances. It was not a surprise to find that she had insulin resistance, which was compounding her health issues and causing her body to store extra fat. It is typical for people with insulin resistance to store fat around their midsection, which was true in Marjorie's case. She also had high cholesterol and triglycerides, which are markers for metabolic syndrome, along with high blood sugar.

Marjorie craved sugar, was addicted to carbohydrates, always felt hungry, and had a ravenous appetite. Her nutritionist discussed the importance of making changes in her diet, and because Marjorie was motivated to make a change, she was willing to give it a try. She started on a high-protein, low-carbohydrate diet. By limiting her intake of carbohydrates, this dietary plan helped stabilize levels of both glucose and insulin. Majorie ate three meals a day consisting of proteins and vegetables, with limits on the high-glycemic vegetables like peas, carrots, turnip, and squash. She totally eliminated sugar, grains, dairy products, beans, and potatoes. Because she was prediabetic, Majorie was instructed to have between-meal snacks of moderate amounts of nuts and fruit to keep her blood sugar levels stable. Majorie was also given a supplement program that included vanadyl sulfate, a dietary form of vanadium and chromium picolinate (both minerals that regulate glucose); essential fatty acids and the amino acid carnitine (which both help burn fat); and the herbs bilberry and *Gymnema sylvestre* (to reduce blood sugar).

After six months on this program, Majorie lost 30 pounds and her cholesterol and triglyceride levels both dropped to normal readings. She was extremely happy about the way she felt, especially since both her energy level and emotional state improved tremendously.

Alternative Medicine Therapies for Sugar Control

A number of natural therapies can help stabilize blood sugar levels and normalize insulin function. Diet is the primary way to control blood sugar fluctuations, but additional therapies may also be helpful, including supplements, herbs, and exercise. Lifestyle changes have been scientifically proven to be the best treatment for insulin resistance and prediabetic conditions. The Diabetes Prevention Program, a well-known multicenter trial, studied over 3,200 people with impaired glucose tolerance. Patients who followed the prescribed protocol of a healthy diet and 30 minutes per day of mild exercise reduced their risk of developing full-blown type 2 diabetes by 58%, which is two times better than

Alternative Medicine Therapies for Sugar Control

- Dietary Recommendations
- Nutritional Supplements
- Herbal Remedies
- Exercise

risk reduction accomplished by taking the oral diabetes drug Glucophage (metformin).[19] In addition, lifestyle changes lead to weight loss, increased energy, and an overall better quality of life.

Dietary Recommendations

Maintaining a healthy, sensible diet is crucial for restoring blood sugar balance, as well as for losing weight. Many diet programs suggest ways you can cut calories; however, simply reducing caloric intake can be self-defeating and cause greater harm to sugar-regulating mechanisms. If you have been dieting and suddenly give in to the temptation of a slice of chocolate cake, your system will overreact, releasing double and triple doses of insulin and quickly converting the additional calories into fat. The rebound weight gain that follows this response is sometimes called the yo-yo effect.

Advanced Glycation End Products (AGE)

Diet can also help avoid buildup of advanced glycation end products. These are protein complexes that bind with glucose in the blood and accumulate in the body by cross-linking to one another. As they build up, they cause damage to cell membranes, especially in the blood vessels that supply nutrients to the eyes, nerves, and kidneys. Research is discovering that these complexes cause many of the known complications of diabetes, including neuropathies and cardiovascular disease, and are also involved in Alzheimer's and other diseases of aging. The best way to avoid the buildup of advanced glycation end products is to follow all the recommendations for balancing blood sugar, including eating a diet high in organic vegetables and fruits and doing moderate exercise daily.

Increasing your vegetable consumption has measurable positive effects and is a much better approach. Eating raw vegetables has been shown to improve body weight control and insulin resistance by increasing the amount of glucose that cell membranes are able to absorb.[20] Anthocyanins, a group of colorful pigments widespread in the plant kingdom, have powerful antiobesity effects that actually regulate the expression of genes controlling insulin resistance and the development and function of fat cells (adipocytes). The chemicals found in a healthy diet filled with colorful vegetables change the messages sent to fat cells so that they store less fat and more readily break down fat.[21]

Here are some basic dietary rules to restore blood sugar health. Even if your glucose tolerance isn't impaired, following these guidelines is a good idea, as this will help you avoid problems with sugar metabolism in the future:

- Eat whole, fresh, and unprocessed foods as much as possible.
- Avoid simple or refined carbohydrates and sugar products

Artificial Sweeteners: Beware of Sugar-Free Products

Almost any item that is touted as "sugar-free" is sweetened with some kind of artificial sweetener. These include saccharin (Sweet'N Low), aspartame (NutraSweet and Equal), sucralose (Splenda), and a host of other potentially toxic chemicals. Madison Avenue advertisements entice people to use various artificial sweeteners as a means to lose weight. However, this is not an effective approach. Studies show that the use of artificial sweeteners has several adverse consequences, including tricking the body into desiring more calories rather than less.[22] In addition, a long list of negative effects have been linked to the use of artificial sweeteners. Here are just a few:

■ Saccharin: possible link to cancer.[23]

■ Aspartame: headaches or migraines, dizziness, seizures, nausea, numb-ness, muscle spasms, weight gain, rashes, depression, fatigue, irritability, tachycardia, insomnia, vision problems, hearing loss, heart palpitations, breathing difficulties, anxiety attacks, slurred speech, loss of taste, tinnitus, vertigo, memory loss, and joint pain.[24]

■ Sucralose: bloating, nausea, diarrhea, headache, anxiety, hives, skin rash.

■ Tagalose (Naturlose): flatulence, bloating, nausea, and diarrhea.

■ Acesulfame-K (Sweet One, Sunett): not adequately tested.

■ Sugar alcohols (sorbitol, xylitol, mannitol, maltitol): appear to have less negative effects than the others, although bloating, gas, and diarrhea have been reported. Xylitol even seems to demonstrate some positive effects.

(see "Watch Out for Hidden Sugars," sidebar page 129) and replace them with complex carbohydrates, such as whole grains, beans, and vegetables; complex carbohydrates are easier on the pancreas and promote insulin balance.

■ Eat five or six smaller meals throughout the day; this helps stabilize the release of blood sugar.

■ Eat adequate amounts of protein (meat, chicken, fish, eggs, dairy, beans, soy products, and nuts) at each meal; proteins take longer to break down in the body, thus stabilizing blood sugar levels.

■ Avoid foods made with hydrogenated oils (trans fats) and be sure to incorporate adequate amounts of healthy fats, such as olive, sesame, coconut, and flaxseed oils; healthy fats help slow the release of sugar into the bloodstream.

■ Reduce your intake of fruit juices and dried fruits, and drink vegetable juices (except carrot) and herbal teas instead; fruit sugars can cause a rapid rise in blood sugar levels.

Stevia and Xylitol

Stevia

Stevia (*Stevia rebaudiana*) is a plant native to Paraguay and Brazil, although it grows easily in many areas of the world. It has been used for its sweet taste for centuries and is a traditional medicinal herb for obesity and blood sugar disorders. Stevia is extremely sweet — 200 to 300 times sweeter than table sugar. It does not affect blood glucose levels and is considered safe for diabetics. In Japan, stevia has been the sugar-free sweetener of choice, over saccharin, aspartame, and other artificial sweeteners, in soft drinks and foods since 1977. It has been enjoyed by millions of people worldwide with no reports of toxic effects in adults or children.

Stevia has an interesting political history in the United States. In 1996, right around the same time that the artificial sweetener aspartame was proposed for FDA approval, the FDA indicated that stevia could not be used as a sweetener, calling it an "unsafe food additive."[25] This was an unusual move by the FDA, because under FDA guidelines natural substances used before 1958 with no reports of adverse effects are considered to be generally recognized as safe (GRAS). There were also dramatic reports of FDA personnel raiding warehouses that were storing stevia, confiscating the stevia, and even threatening to burn books that were about how to use it as a sweetener![26] Shortly after stevia was banned as a sweetener, several FDA board members left for higher-paying positions with Monsanto, the company that promoted Nutrasweet (aspartame) as the sugar-free sweetener of choice in the U.S. market.

Studies have uncovered additional attributes of stevia, beyond imparting a sweet flavor, including decreasing blood sugar in patients with type 2 diabetes,[27] probably by enhancing both insulin secretion and insulin utilization.[28] It has been shown to improve insulin resistance[29] and also has anti-inflammatory and immune supportive actions.[30] Stevia is available in the United States as a dietary supplement but cannot be listed as a sweetener. It is available in many forms, including the whole leaf (green), a liquid extract (brown), and a powder (white). The white powder is also sold in convenient little packets that make it very user-friendly, since it is used the same way as artificial sweeteners such as saccharin and aspartame. Be aware that the green and brown preparations use the whole leaf, while the white powder may contain isolated compounds such as stevioside.

 There are some reports that the isolated component, stevioside, can adversely affect fertility in rats.

Xylitol

Xylitol occurs naturally in some vegetables, fruits, mushrooms, and cereal grains and in corncobs. For commercial purposes, it's usually extracted from birch tree wood chips or corn to produce a white powder used as a sweetener. Although xylitol has a very sweet taste, it does not raise blood sugar or insulin levels.[31] Research has shown that xylitol also has antimicrobial actions that decrease bacteria associated with tooth decay[32] and ear infections.[33] Cautions: Although xylitol is recognized by the FDA as a safe food additive,[34] ingesting large amounts (over 30 grams per day) can cause gastrointestinal symptoms. There is one report of severe hypoglycemia in a dog that ate a large quantity of xylitol chewing gum.[35]

Sucralose

Sucralose, also known as SPLENDA, is a totally artificial substance that is not found in nature. Other non-nutritive sweeteners include saccharin, aspartame, and ace-sulfame-k. SPLENDA is manufactured by pharmaceutical giant Johnson & Johnson by adding three atoms of chlorine to each molecule of a starting substance, which may be extracted from various compounds, including sucrose(sugar) or raffinose (a substance found in beans and onions). The process of manufacturing sucralose involves the use of many chemicals, including trityl chloride, acetic anhydride, thionyl chloride in the presence of dimethylformamide, 4-methylmorpholine, and methyl isobutyl ketone. The end product, sucralose, is a man-made chlorocarbon chemical that has a sweet taste. This is a far cry from the manufacturer's premise that sucralose is really a "no-calorie sugar." The fact is, the chemical composition of sucarlose more closely resembles pesticides than natural sugar. Although the FDA claims that sucralose is safe at normally consumed dose levels, there are many concerns and unanswered questions about the safety of sucralose, especially for long-term use. Very few human trials have been done to examine the effects of sucralose; the longest trial lasted only three months. In addition, most of the research was done by the manufacturer. Individuals have reported symptoms after ingesting sucralose that include:

- Skin — Redness, itching, swelling, blisters, rash
- Lungs — shortness of breath
- Head — Swelling, eyelids, lips, tongue, throat; headaches
- Nose — Stuffy, runny, sneezing
- Eyes — Red, itchy, swollen, watery
- Stomach — Bloating, gas, pain, nausea, vomiting, diarrhea, or bloody diarrhea
- Heart — Palpitations or fluttering
- Joints — Joint pains or aches
- Neurological — Anxiety, dizziness, spaced-out sensation, depression

(For more information, visit http://www.truthaboutsplenda.com.)

It is prudent to avoid using sucralose until studies are done on the potential for adverse effects after long term use.

- Reduce your intake of caffeinated beverages, which elevate blood levels of sugar and insulin.
- Avoid artificial sweeteners and products containing them. Xylitol and stevia (see page 143) are probably the best sweeteners for those with sugar imbalances.

Nutritional Supplements

The following nutritional supplements can help control your appetite and strengthen your body's natural glucose-regulating mechanisms.

Chromium is a trace mineral that helps to regulate insulin production and stabilize blood sugar. Many Americans may not be getting enough chromium in their diet due to depletion of soil chromium levels, eating high levels of sugar, and increased urinary excretion of chromium when under stress. People with sugar dysregulation disorders such as type 2 diabetes have low levels of chromium.[36] Chromium has been recognized for decades as a nutritional factor that improves glucose tolerance.[37] Chromium helps insulin bind to the receptor sites on cell membrane, which decreases insulin resistance.[38] This action may be due to chromium's ability to increase the activity of kinase, an enzyme that is important for signaling the cell to react to insulin.[39]

Studies have repeatedly demonstrated the essential role of chromium in balancing blood sugar, improving insulin metabolism, protecting cell membranes,[40] and losing weight. There are several forms of chromium supplements, including chromium picolinate and chromium polynicotinate (chemically bound to niacin). The recommended dosage is 200 mcg per day, although health-care practitioners may recommend higher doses. In addition to supplements, an excellent source of chromium is brewer's yeast, available in powder form at most health food stores.

Vanadium is a trace mineral that research has shown to be involved in the regulation of insulin levels. Several glucose- and insulin-related imbalances are helped by supplementing with vanadium, which enhances glucose transport across cell membranes.[41] The insulin-like effects of vanadium are believed to be due to the activation of several key components found in insulin-signaling pathways.[42] Vanadium also helps the body to break down fat cells, and it may significantly decrease elevated plasma glucose levels.[43] A trace amount of vanadium is found in a wide variety of foods, including gelatin, cereals, parsley, corn, soy, mushrooms, and seafood. Supplements are usually offered in the form of vanadyl sulfate. Since vanadium is a trace mineral, very small amounts are required; usually between 10 to 50 mcg per day. One small study found a positive effect on weight loss after the subjects took 100 mg of the mineral daily for four weeks.[44] However, until more safety data is available, it is not advisable to take high amounts of this trace mineral.

Alpha-lipoic acid (ALA) has been prescribed by German physicians for over 30 years to help patients with type 2 diabetes. It is called the "universal antioxidant" because it is soluble in both water and fat.[45]

Food Sources of Nutrients for Controlling Blood Sugar

Certain nutrients are required by the body for glucose metabolism, specifically chromium, manganese, zinc, B complex vitamins (particularly pantothenic acid or B_5), inositol, and vitamin C. The following are dietary sources of these nutrients (foods are listed in descending order of importance):

- Chromium: brewer's yeast, whole wheat and rye breads, beef liver, potatoes, green peppers, eggs, chicken, apples, butter, parsnips, and cornmeal

- Manganese: pecans, Brazil nuts, almonds, barley, rye, buckwheat, split peas, whole wheat, walnuts, spinach, oats, raisins, beet greens, brussels sprouts, cheese, carrots, broccoli, brown rice, corn, cabbage, peaches, and butter

- Zinc: fresh oysters, ginger root, lamb chops, pecans, split peas, beef liver, egg yolk, whole wheat, rye, oats, lima beans, almonds, walnuts, sardines, chicken, and buckwheat

- B complex vitamins: brewer's yeast, beef and chicken liver, mushrooms, split peas, blue cheese, pecans, eggs, lobster, oats, buckwheat, rye, broccoli, turkey and chicken (dark meat), brown rice, whole wheat, red chile peppers, sardines, avocado, and kale

- Inositol: navy beans, barley, wheat germ, brewer's yeast, oats, black-eyed peas, oranges, lima beans, green peas, molasses, split peas, grapefruit, raisins, cantaloupe, brown rice, peaches, cabbage, cauliflower, onions, sweet potatoes, watermelon, strawberries, lettuce, tomatoes, and eggs

- Vitamin C: acerola cherries, red chile peppers, guava, red sweet peppers, kale, parsley, collard and turnip greens, green peppers, broccoli, brussels sprouts, mustard greens, cauliflower, red cabbage, strawberries, papayas, spinach, oranges, lemons, grapefruit, turnips, mangoes, asparagus, cantaloupe, Swiss chard, green onions, and tangerines

ALA decreases insulin resistance[46] as well as enhancing the recycling of other antioxidants such as vitamin E, vitamin C, coenzyme Q10, and glutathione. Supplementing with ALA provides a significant boost in the body's ability to break down glucose,[47] which leads to weight loss. ALA helps reduce insulin resistance through several mechanisms, including decreasing the accumulation of triglycerides in muscle tissues and activating enzymes that regulate cell metabolism.[48]

Alpha-lipoic acid has been found to be as effective as irbesartan (Avapro) at reducing inflammation in patients diagnosed with metabolic syndrome.[49] In addition, ALA is much safer than the prescription drug and yields many additional benefits. Alpha-lipoic acid is naturally produced by the body and is found in red meat. As a supplement, the dosage of ALA varies widely. Many research studies have used ALA intravenously in high doses of up to 1,000 mg per day. Oral supplements may range from 300 mg to 800 mg per day, although 20 to 50 mg per day is recommended for overall antioxidant protection.

CAUTION Most people do not experience adverse effects due to ALA, but skin rashes and symptoms of low blood sugar are possible. If a person is deficient in vitamin B$_1$ or biotin, these vitamins should be taken along with ALA.[50]

Fiber, often found in high quantities in foods that contain complex carbohydrates, acts to lower blood glucose levels and diminish hunger. In addition, a high-fiber diet increases the number of insulin receptor sites on the cells, making them more sensitive to insulin. This allows the pancreas to produce less insulin to achieve the same glucose-lowering effect.

Pectin and guar gum are two forms of fiber that are especially effective in controlling blood sugar levels because they reduce the biochemical demand on the pancreas. Dietary fiber slows the rate of food passage through the intestines (called transit time), creating a more gradual rise in blood sugar levels after a meal. A good source of pectin is fresh fruits, especially apples. Guar gum is a component in many of the fiber blends available at health food stores.

Herbal Remedies

Gymnema sylvestre has been traditionally used in the ancient Indian healing system called Ayurveda to treat sugar control problems, including diabetes. The Hindi name for gymnema, *gurmar* translates to "sugar destroyer," which describes the herb's ability to block and decrease the desire for sweet taste. Gymnema and components extracted from the herb, such as gymnemic acid, have been studied for a variety of sugar-balancing effects. This herb's ability to lower blood sugar was published in medical journals as early as 1930.[51] It may accomplish this through several mechanisms,[52] including raising insulin levels by helping to regenerate pancreas cells.[53]

In addition, gymnema helps cells absorb glucose and slows the liver's glucose production.[54] Studies have shown gymnema's effectiveness for weight loss by measuring changes in body weight, body mass index (BMI), lipid profiles, blood sugar levels, and serum levels of leptin (a hormone that regulates fat storage and appetite), especially when gymnema is combined

CAUTION Although few adverse effects have been reported, people with diabetes or other blood sugar regulation issues should consult with their health-care practitioner before using gymnema. Since it is so effective at lowering blood sugar, the combined effect of the herb and drugs for lowering blood sugar may cause hypoglycemia.

Fructose: An Overused Sweetener

Fructose is a natural sugar that occurs in fruits and vegetables. However, when it is extracted, made into an isolated component, and used as a sweetener, it acts quite differently in the body than when eaten as part of a whole fruit. In a whole fruit, the fructose that makes the fruit taste sweet is attached to other substances, such as fiber and protein. This causes the fructose to be absorbed into the bloodstream slowly. However, when isolated fructose is used, as a white powder or high-fructose corn syrup, it is absorbed quickly and has a different effect on the body than other sugars, which may lead to harmful consequences.

When glucose is consumed, it signals the body to release insulin, which then alerts the cells to absorb the glucose. Glucose also influences other hormones, increasing leptin levels (which regulates fat storage and appetite), and decreasing ghrelin levels (a stomach hormone that regulates appetite). This is why eating sweet food made with sugar usually decreases hunger. However, when fructose is consumed, it does not stimulate insulin or leptin, nor does it decrease ghrelin. Therefore, the body does not get a satiety signal. With-

out this signal, the body still craves more food, which leads to increased appetite and more weight gain.

In addition, isolated fructose raises uric acid, which plays a role in the development of metabolic syndrome.[55] Certain indicators of aging, such as lipid peroxidation (breakdown of cell membranes) and unhealthy changes in skin collagen have been linked to long-term fructose consumption to a higher degree than sucrose consumption.[56] Fructose can be converted by the body to triglycerides more readily than other sugars, thus it increases triglyceride levels (this is more apparent in men than women).[57] When the liver metabolizes fructose, it causes increased lipogenesis (fat production) and contributes to obesity.[58] Also, fructose interferes with the important mineral magnesium in the body, which may adversely effect bone and kidney health.[59] These negative effects of fructose vary depending on the amount consumed and the sensitivity of each individual.[60] It is unfortunate that fructose is so widely used, even in so-called health foods, and in meal replacement powders and other supplements that claim to be useful for weight control.

with chromium and hydroxycitric acid (a compound found in *Garcinia cambogia*).[61] Gymnema has other positive effects, including acting as an antimicrobial agent.[62] Typical doses range from 1 to 2 grams in traditional Ayurvedic medicine to 300 to 800 mg per day standardized for 25% gymnemic acids.

Bitter melon (*Momordica charantia*) is a prolific vine that produces a lanternlike orange flower and a very bitter fruit. The fruit is commonly used medicinally in all areas of the world where it grows. Science has uncovered a variety of constituents in bitter melon that have the effect of lowering blood sugar, including steroidal saponins and insulin-like peptides. The extract of bitter melon has been found to lower blood sugar[63] and has been studied for its antidiabetic effects.[64] Experiments on obese rats found that those fed dried bitter melon lost body fat more efficiently than those not fed bitter melon.[65] Human trials examining the use of bitter melon along with pharmaceutical drugs for lowering blood sugar, such as metformin (Glucophage), have found that the addition of bitter melon increases the drug's action in lowering blood sugar.[66]

Exercise

Exercise helps in every aspect of healthy weight management. Not only does it burn fat, elevate mood, increase energy, and improve motivation, it also helps to stabilize blood sugar levels.[67] Balancing your blood sugar level by exercising will also help reduce food cravings and addictive behaviors. Any program designed to restore healthy blood sugar levels should include daily sessions of light exercise, such as walking, swimming, or cycling. There is no way around it: Exercise is critical to your entire weight-loss program.

 For more on the **importance of exercise,** see chapter 2, Start Exercising, page 52.

six

Overcome a Sluggish Thyroid

In this chapter, we'll look at the relationship between the thyroid and weight gain. I'll discuss the symptoms and causes of hypothyroidism (low thyroid function) and tests used to diagnose an underactive thyroid. Finally, I'll offer effective alternative therapies for correcting this problem.

Many people who have trouble losing weight will often blame it on the function of their thyroid gland. On one level, this may be a convenient excuse for not having the motivation to make the changes in diet, exercise, and other aspects of lifestyle that are critical components of any healthy weight management program. However, in many instances, thyroid dysfunction actually is one among a variety factors that work together to impede weight loss. And in fact, studies indicate that a surprising number of people have some kind of abnormal function of the thyroid gland. The Colorado Thyroid

Disease Prevalence Study tested 25,862 people and found that over 9% of them had undiagnosed thyroid dysfunctions.[1] This suggests that as many as 13 million Americans may have this problem.

The thyroid gland is a butterfly-shaped organ that wraps around the windpipe right behind the Adam's apple. It is the largest of the body's endocrine glands and produces several different hormones that are extremely important to the function of a vast array of metabolic processes in the body, including brain development, mood, and weight regulation. The thyroid gland plays a key role in weight problems because it controls the body's overall metabolic rate. When it's not working properly, it may lead to an variety of health problems, including weight gain, arthritis, depression, cold hands and feet, dry skin, high cholesterol, chronic constipation, and hair loss. Symptoms caused by low thyroid function are so varied that they can easily be confused with those of other conditions. Beyond physical symptoms, this condition also leads to many mental and emotional problems.

Mental and emotional symptoms: Depression, poor memory, difficulty concentrating, mood swings, personality disorder, paranoia, irritability, inappropriate crying, excessive worry, insomnia, slow reaction time, mental sluggishness, and attention-deficit/hyperactivity disorder (ADHD).

Physical symptoms: Weight fluctuations, difficulty losing (or gaining) weight, edema, hypoglycemia, skin problems, chronic infections (respiratory, viral, or bacterial), chronic fatigue syndrome, lethargy, weakness, constipation, low body temperature, cold extremities, slow pulse, hair loss, headaches, infertility, rheumatic pain, muscle aches and weakness, burning or prickling sensations, anemia, labored breathing, brittle nails, poor vision, hearing impairment, menstrual disorders (excessive flow or cramps), heart disease, cancer, hypertension, high cholesterol, and multiple sclerosis.

Weight Gain and Your Thyroid

The thyroid is the body's metabolic thermostat, controlling body temperature, energy use, and, in children, the body's growth rate. It sends chemical messages via hormones to every cell in the body, maintaining a normal, resting body temperature of 98.6°F and regulating heart rate, the rate at which organs function, and the speed with which the body uses food. When the thyroid is dysfunctional or underactive, it sends out fewer hormones, causing metabolism to slow down. When metabolism slows, the body will store rather than burn calories, causing an accumulation of fat. Beyond that, slowed metabolism affects nearly every function in the body, causing weight problems in several other ways:

- Many people with low thyroid function have puffy, thick skin and retain fluid.
- Hypothyroidism leads to a sluggish digestive system, often resulting in a number of gastrointestinal problems, including constipation, gas and bloating, abdominal pain, and decreased absorption of nutrients. Decreased digestive efficiency may lead leaky gut syndrome, a condition in which undigested food particles enter the bloodstream, causing allergic reactions and depleting the immune system. Weight gain is one of the potential results of these digestive disturbances.
- Hypothyroidism is linked to pancreatitis, a decrease in insulin production by the pancreas. Insulin is the hormone that controls how the body processes sugars. When insulin imbalances occur, blood sugar is turned into fat rather than being burned off.
- Imbalances in the levels of thyroid hormones reduce the body's thermogenic, or fat-burning, capacity, leading to increased fat storage.
- Because low thyroid function causes fatigue and lack of stamina as well as muscle aches or weakness, people with this condition may find it difficult to exercise, a very important factor in weight problems.

Success Story: Tending the Thyroid Reverses Weight Gain

Adrienne, 46, ate a low-fat diet and exercised six times weekly. Nevertheless, her weight remained steady at 188 pounds—far too much for her height of 5 foot 3. Her feet were always sore, and she felt depleted in energy. When Adrienne underwent the routine TSH test for underactive thyroid, the results came back "normal." Around this time, a physician suggested she try Weight Watchers and put her on a conventional weight-loss drug, but the drug dropped her blood pressure to a

The Thyroid and Its Hormones

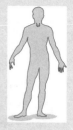

The thyroid has four principal hormones: T1, T2, T3, and T4. Thyroid hormones are stored in the thyroid and released to the body as needed. T1 (monoiodothyronine) and T2 (diiodothyronine) are not considered especially active. T3 (triiodothyronine) represents only about 7% of the thyroid hormone complement, but it's three to four times more biologically active than T4 (thyroxine), which is produced exclusively in the thyroid gland and accounts for almost 93% of the thyroid's hormones. Its chief function is to increase the speed of cell metabolism, or energy conversion.

Iodine and the amino acid tyrosine are essential to forming normal amounts of T4. When the body requires more T3, T4 can give up its iodine to form T3. About 80% of the body's T3 comes from converting T4, typically in the liver and kidneys. When T4 conversion runs smoothly—that is, when the necessary sequence chemical reactions takes place—normal body temperature and metabolic rates are maintained.

If the thyroid is functioning poorly, however, T4 breaks down to form reverse triiodothyronine, or rT3 (a different chemical version of T3). Stress, fasting, illness, or elevated cortisol (a hormone produced by the adrenal glands) can contribute to the occurrence of this faulty conversion. As rT3 levels increase, metabolism and body temperature decrease and various enzymes fail to function properly. In addition, as rT3 levels build, levels of T3 decrease, leading to low T3 syndrome and thyroid dysfunction.

Total blood levels of T3 and T4 consist of only 1% biologically active components (called the free levels), while 99% is the metabolically inactive portion bound to proteins. In a healthy person, total T4 levels as indicated in a blood test (or thyroid panel) are 4.5 to 12.5, but for someone with hypothyroidism, those values will be less than 4.5. For free T4, the normal range is 0.9 to 2.0; in hypothyroidism, it's less than 0.9. For free T3, normal is 80 to 220; in hypothyroidism, it's less than 80. TSH (see below) is normally 0.3 to 6.0; in hypothyroidism, it's greater than 6.0.

The formation and secretion of T3 and T4 are regulated by thyroid-stimulating hormone, or TSH (thyrotropin), secreted in the brain by the pituitary gland. TSH, in turn, is directed by another hormone called thyrotropin-releasing hormone (TRH), which is secreted in the brain by the hypothalamus gland. When TSH reaches the thyroid gland, it signals it to secrete more hormones (both T4 and T3). The hormones released by the thyroid not only speed up metabolism, but also send a feedback message to the brain, telling it to stop secreting TSH and TRH. TSH blood levels are conventionally taken as the best index for thyroid dysfunction, both hypothyroidism and hyperthyroidism (an overactive thyroid). When thyroid function is low, TSH levels normally go up.

Subclinical hypothyroidism, the early stage of the disease, is particularly difficult to diagnose because of the action of TSH. During this phase, the pituitary gland recognizes that the thyroid isn't producing enough hormones, so it releases more TSH. The extra TSH causes the thyroid to work overtime to secrete more T4 and T3. A weak thyroid is thus often propped up by high levels of TSH during the early stage of the disease, and this masks the symptoms of the condition. Without adequate treatment, the thyroid will continue to deteriorate.

dangerously low level of 78/57. Her body temperature was also subnormal, just 95°F to 96°F in the morning, and she felt very tired.

When she finally consulted a holistic physician, he ordered in-depth thyroid tests—T3, T4, and TSH—to more accurately pinpoint possible thyroid problems. While her T4 and TSH results were in the normal range, Adrienne's T3 was below normal (see "The Thyroid and Its Hormones," page 153). To support her thyroid, Adrienne's physician prescribed a combination of T4, T3, and Armour Thyroid (made from desiccated animal glands), which is especially effective when a patient's T3 level is lower than their T4.

The holistic physician also assessed Adrienne's vitamin and mineral levels, which had been completely ignored by conventional doctors. The analysis uncovered low levels of zinc, manganese, vitamin B_{12}, and chromium, and high copper levels. Adrienne began a program of nutrients that support the thyroid, along with an appropriate vitamin and mineral protocol. In addition, she visited a reflexologist once per week to increase circulation to her feet. Within three months, Adrienne reported a marked increase in energy, better mood, and no more aching feet. After six months, she had lost 50 pounds and felt like a new person.

Causes of Hypothyroidism

Thyroid problems may be due to a number of factors, including genetic predisposition, disease, environmental pollutants, dietary excesses or insufficiencies, certain drugs (such as lithium and phenylbutazone), stress, and yeast infections.

Thyroid Disease

Most people with thyroid problems that make weight loss difficult have mild to moderate disorders of thyroid function. There are also serious illnesses related to the thyroid: Goiter is an enlargement of the thyroid sometimes caused by iodine deficiency. Cretinism is a form of hypothyroidism that impairs both mental and physical development. Myxedema is severe hypothyroidism that can lead to coma and death. Hashimoto's thyroiditis is an autoimmune disease of the thyroid gland wherein the body releases antibodies that attack the thyroid gland as if it were a foreign invader. Characterized by an enlarged thyroid, other symptoms of Hashimoto's thyroiditis include deep fatigue, memory loss, and depression. This condition can also lead to psychological disturbance, including extreme anxiety, panic attacks, and overeating syndrome, which increases weight gain.

Toxic Environment

Thyroid problems have been on the rise due to the increasingly toxic environment in which we live. Exposure to radiation, fluoride (in water and toothpaste), mercury from silver amalgam dental fillings, pollutants in cigarette smoke (thyocyanide), and chlorinated compounds (found in wood and leather preservatives) are just a few of the many environmental causes of hypothyroidism. Radiation is probably the greatest environmental cause of hypothyroidism and other thyroid problems, including thyroid cancer.[2] PCBs (polychlorinated biphenyls), chlorinated pesticides, and heavy metals such as mercury (which comprises up to 50% of silver amalgam fillings) have been scientifically proven to disrupt endocrine function.[3] Experimental techniques have been developed to help determine the extent of accumulation of heavy metals, such as lead and cadmium, in thyroid tissue.[4] Even low exposure to environmental contaminants while in the womb can interfere with a person's thyroid status in later life.[5] Heavy metals also interfere with an enzyme critical in converting the less active form of thyroid hormone (T4) into the more potent form (T3).

Diet

Dietary factors that depress thyroid function include synthetic and genetically engineered hormones in meat, dairy products, poultry, and eggs, which block the release of thyroid hormones, and an imbalance (either a deficiency or excess) of the mineral iodine. Excess accumulation may occur due to an overabundance of iodine in commercial salt, baked goods (in dough conditioners), and dietary supplements.

Some vegetables that have a wide variety of health benefits, such as raw cruciferous vegetables (cabbage, broccoli, cauliflower, brussels sprouts, and the like) contain thyroid inhibitors called goitrogens, which may cause an enlargement of the thyroid gland and inhibit hormone synthesis.[6] However, lightly steaming the vegetables deactivates these thyroid-suppressing substances. Soy products, especially if not fermented, may also depress thyroid function, mostly in people who are already at risk for hypothyroidism.[7] Other dietary influences include vitamin deficiencies (particularly vitamins A and B), mineral deficiencies (zinc, copper, iron, and selenium), and excessive intake of polyunsaturated

After many years of clinical work, E. Denis Wilson, MD, of Longwood, Florida, author of *Wilson's Syndrome: The Miracle of Feeling Well*, identified the thyroid syndrome that bears his name. According to Dr. Wilson, the symptoms of Wilson's syndrome include all the symptoms of hypothyroidism plus the additional symptoms of migraines, aggravated premenstrual syndrome (PMS), panic attacks, night sweats, ringing in the ears, mood swings, itchiness, allergies, and asthma.

Emotional or physical stress reduces the rate of conversion of T4 to T3, which, according to Dr. Wilson, is a natural survival mechanism that helps conserve energy. After the stressful period passes, the body should resume converting T4 to T3. However, for reasons that are still unclear, the body sometimes fails to do this.

In addition to the problem of conversion, cell membranes within the body may stop responding to T3. Each cell has an area on its surface, a receptor site, where T3 attaches. When the chemical shape of these areas is altered, T3 cannot attach itself and the metabolism of the cell consequently slows. Diets high in low-quality animal fats, particularly from red meat and chicken, will damage these receptor sites and interfere with the uptake of T3, thus slowing metabolism.

fats (abundant in soybean, safflower, and corn oils).

Medications

A long list of medications can interfere with thyroid function. These include prednisone, sulfa drugs, antidiabetic agents, birth control pills, estrogen replacement therapy (ERT), lithium (in up to 33% of users), certain heart drugs, interferon, methimazole, propylthiouracil (PTU), and others. Check with your physician and pharmacist for a list of possible adverse effects and interactions of any medications that you are taking.

Stress

The action of thyroid hormones in the body is also uniquely affected by the stress hormones adrenaline and cortisol. They interfere with the body's ability to convert the thyroid hormone T4 into the more potent T3. As T3 levels decrease, the body produces even more adrenaline and cortisol to try and speed up metabolism, which further inhibits the conversion. Wilson's syndrome is a stress-related condition where the body has difficulty converting T4 to T3 (see "Wilson's Syndrome," left).

Yeast Infections

Hypothyroidism is associated with the spread of *Candida albicans* (a yeast-like fungus normally confined to the lower bowels, skin, and vagina) in the body. As it spreads, candida takes on an aggressive form that affects not only the thyroid, but many other body systems. Holistic health-care practitioners often note a significant overlap between the hypothyroidism and yeast infections.

Candida infections can cause serious damage to the intestinal tract by permeating the lining of the intestines and breaking down the barrier between the inside of the digestive tract and the bloodstream. The damaged lining allows undigested food to pass into the bloodstream, an ailment known as leaky gut syndrome. The immune system then produces antibodies to attack these food particles as though they were allergens and may ultimately become confused and begin to attack the body's own tissues. This reaction of the body against itself, called an autoimmune response, can seriously damage the thyroid gland. The most severe form of this autoimmune reaction can cause Hashimoto's thyroiditis. This condition can lead to a variety of symptoms, including depression and weight gain.

Detecting Hypothyroidism

Despite its high incidence, hypothyroidism has remained a hidden disease. Many cases of hypothyroidism remain undetected and untreated because the conventional tests used by mainstream physicians are inadequate. Fortunately, there are test procedures available that can more accurately assess the functioning of the thyroid. While most of these tests require the assistance of a health-care professional, you can perform the basal temperature yourself (see page 158).

Standard Thyroid Tests

The most common conventional test for assessing thyroid function are total T4, T3 uptake, free thyroxine index, and TSH level. However, these tests may show normal levels despite a weakened thyroid. If these tests indicate normal levels but the person's symptom picture suggests low thyroid, many holistic practitioners will take testing a step further and measure the patient's free T3 and free T4; these tests are more sensitive than the standard tests. They'll also take a thyroid sonogram, which shows if the thyroid is swollen, and have the patient measure their resting body temperature, or basal body temperature.

To further complicate the interpretation of thyroid tests, morbidly obese individuals often have higher-than-normal levels of T3, T4, and TSH even if they actually have hypothyroidism. This may occur due to an imbalance in the set point of their thyroid regulation mechanisms.[8] Elevated levels of TSH are considered an indication of low thyroid function, since the pituitary gland oversecretes TSH in an attempt to increase hormone secretion by the thyroid gland. In conventional medicine, the normal range of TSH is considered 0.3–3.0. Holistic physicians, on the other hand, often note that even with a reading as low as 1.5, patients can have many of the symptoms associated with low thyroid function.

The Thyroid Gold Standard Test

A more sophisticated test, the TRH (thyrotropin-releasing hormone) stimulation test, is considered by some practitioners to be the gold standard for accurately detecting an underactive thyroid. As mentioned above, TRH is a hormone released by the hypothalamus that energizes the pituitary gland to release TSH. The TRH stimulation test is inexpensive and is performed by most laboratories. The physician measures the patient's TSH level using a simple blood test, gives an injection of TRH, then draws blood again 25 minutes later and remeasures TSH. If the first TSH level is normal and the second TSH level is high—above 10—it indicates that the patient's thyroid is underactive, and that the pituitary gland is compensating by releasing more TSH. A TSH reading of 20 strongly points to hypothyroidism.

Routine tests diagnose hypothyroidism by documenting its effects (such as low body temperature), while the TRH test uncovers the physiological causes behind an under-functioning thyroid. A stressed pituitary gland, worn down by a weak thyroid, will overreact to TRH, while a healthy one will not. It is one of the best ways to accurately assess thyroid function. The TRH test was once widely used by American physicians, but was then replaced by the quicker, easier, although less reliable TSH test.

Basal Temperature Test

Broda O. Barnes, MD, Ph.D., a pioneer in thyroid research and author of *Hypothyroidism: The Unsuspected Illness,* was the first to use basal temperature (resting body temperature), as an indicator of thyroid function. Based on more than four decades of research, Dr. Barnes found that consistently low basal temperature is a dependable indicator of problems with thyroid function. His test involves taking underarm temperatures on consecutive mornings. In clinical practice, I've found a much easier method to do this test. All you need is a basal thermometer (available in most drugstores) and several small disposable Styrofoam cups with lids. Immediately upon awakening, urinate in the cup, place the basal thermometer through the hole in the top of the cup, and submerge it in the urine. Wait about 3 minutes, then record the temperature. Repeat the test every day for one month. At the end of the month, calculate your average daily temperature. An average temperature of less than 97.8°F usually indicates an underactive thyroid, although it can indicate low adrenal function as well. Do not use any heat sources in your bed, such as electric blankets, heating pads, or hot water bottles, as these may interfere with an accurate reading. Women who are menstruating are likely to have an elevated temperature and should begin recording their temperature after the third day of their cycle.

Alternative Medicine Therapies for a Healthy Thyroid

Conventional medicine's approach to an underactive thyroid is limited to drug therapy. The usual prescription is levothyroxine (brand names Synthroid, Levoxyl, and Levothroid). This is T4. While some patients get a lot of relief from hypothyroid symptoms after initial treatment, others do not. In many cases, this is because the body must be able to convert T4 to T3 in order to use the hormone efficiently. Research shows that specific symptoms, including those affecting mood and neuropsychological function, show a much greater level of improvement if T3 (triiodothyronine) is supplemented along with T4.[9] Many holistic physicians will prescribe Armour Thyroid, which is a naturally derived hormone supplement that is a mixture of T3 and T4. This product is derived from pork sources and is not acceptable to vegetarians and other people who prefer not to ingest pork products. Cytomel, another form of T3, isn't derived from animal sources and may also be used along with T4.

Alternative Medicine Therapies for Thyroid Support

- Lifestyle Suggestions
- Dietary Recommendations
- Nutritional Supplements
- Herbal Remedies
- Thyroid Glandular Therapy

Alternative medicine practitioners take a much more comprehensive view of treating thyroid problems. Generally, they begin by strengthening intestinal health and digestion. Proper nutrition combined with regular exercise can help restore a weakened thyroid, and lead to weight loss as well. To help spark proper thyroid function a combination of specific foods, nutrients, exercises, and therapies is needed. Thyroid glandular therapy and thyroid hormone therapy are two additional options available to return the thyroid to normal functioning. These may be used in addition to conventional therapies.

Lifestyle Suggestions

Yoga, reflexology, and castor oil packs can provide a much-needed boost to other therapies.

Yoga: Specific yoga postures can help activate a sluggish thyroid. The shoulder stand is an inverted posture that puts gentle pressure on the thyroid gland and stimulates circulation to the area. The fish is a counterpose to the shoulder stand that stretches the thyroid area and further enhances energy flow to the area. Both of these postures need to be learned as part of a yoga instruction program.

Reflexology: Reflexology is the application of pressure to areas of the feet, hands, and earlobes to influence and heal internal organs. Pressure at precise points releases blockages that inhibit energy flow and cause pain and disease. This pressure is thought to affect internal organs and glands by stimulating reflex points of the body. Typically, practitioners use their thumbs to press on the various areas of the feet, known as zones, that correspond to organs or other parts of the body. Reflexology helps to detoxify organs, such as the kidneys and liver, and stimulate sluggish glands, including the thyroid and adrenals.

 For instructions on how to apply a **castor oil pack,** see chapter 1, Detoxification, page 40.

Castor oil pack: Applying a castor oil pack directly over the thyroid gland area can help to stimulate thyroid activity. Repeat this procedure for 45 minutes 3 times per week.

Dietary Recommendations

Goitrogens are substances found in certain foods that reduce the release of thyroid hormone and interfere in the conversion of T4 to T3. Foods containing goitrogens include walnuts, sorghum, cassava, almonds, peanuts, soy flour, millet, and apples. These foods should be eaten only in moderation by anyone suffering from hypothyroidism. Mustard greens, kale, cabbage, spinach, brussels sprouts, cauliflower, broccoli, and turnips, when eaten raw, also have a mild antithyroid effect.

Some foods stimulate thyroid hormone production and increase the conversion of T4 to T3. Examples include sea vegetables (bladderwrack, laminaria, kelp, and dulse), garlic, radishes, watercress, seafood, egg yolks, wheat germ, brewer's yeast, and mushrooms. Fruits and fruit juices (especially tropical varieties), watermelon, and coconut oil are also thyroid-stimulating. A two- to four-week diet of only raw foods, with heavy emphasis on raw greens, sea vegetables, nuts, seeds, sprouted beans and seeds, and freshly extracted juices, is an effective way to improve thyroid function, and you can watch the pounds melt away at the same time!

Here are some general dietary recommendations for supporting the thyroid:

- Eat adequate amounts of protein. Organic beef or poultry, certain kinds of fish (such as halibut and whitefish), organic eggs, and organic raw milk products (such as kefir, yogurt, and cottage cheese) are all good choices.

- Avoid iodized salt. Use organic sea salt or purified seawater with no added iodine.

- Include coconut oil in your diet. Probably the most healthful type of saturated fat other than raw butter, coconut oil stimulates thyroid function.

Nutritional Supplements

A number of nutrients can play a critical role in revitalizing the thyroid.

Vitamin A: People with hypothyroidism do not effectively convert beta-carotene — the natural form of vitamin A found in yellow and green fruits and vegetables — to a biologically usable form of vitamin A.[10] Vitamin A is necessary for the production of thyroxine and is required by the thyroid to absorb iodine. Most vitamin A supplements are sold in the beta-carotene form. As a typical recommendation, patients with impaired thyroid function should take 10,000 to 20,000 IU of pure vitamin A, rather than beta-carotene, daily. Unless closely supervised by a physician, intake of vitamin A should never exceed 20,000 IU per day.

Iodine: The interplay between iodine intake and thyroid function is extremely complex. For example, both iodine deficiency and iodine excess are linked to autoimmune thyroid disease.[11] While iodine deficiency causes goiter, hypothyroidism, myxedema, or cretinism, iodine excess can lead to either overactivity or underactivity of the thyroid gland. Iodine excess appears to be of greater concern than deficiency in today's environment.[12] Taking additional natural sources of iodine may help an underactive thyroid, if it is due to iodine deficiency. The best food supplements for iodine are sea vegetables, such as kelp and bladderwrack. Lobster, shrimp, crab, and saltwater fish such as haddock, cod, halibut, and herring are also good sources of iodine. The recommended daily allowance for iodine is 100 mcg for women and 120 mcg for men. Since too much iodine can suppress the formation of T3, iodized table salt should be avoided; it can imbalance the relative concentrations of sodium and potassium in the body, which in turn can result in serious disorders, such as heart disease, high blood pressure, and obesity. Better choices include Celtic Sea Salt and granular kelp, which you can sprinkle on food.

Zinc: The trace metal zinc is essential for the activity of many enzymes and plays an important role in regulating several hormones involved in healthy weight maintenance, such as insulin, leptin, and thyroid hormones.[13] Zinc helps in the conversion of T4 to T3 and increases the sensitivity of cell membranes to these hormones. In the ZENITH study, which investigated the effect of zinc on various health parameters,[14] zinc supplementation was found to be an effective way to raise the level of zinc available for metabolic processes in the body,[15] such as supporting thyroid function and increasing metabolic rate, which helps weight loss.[16] A typical dose is 25 mg per day along with 3 mg of copper, because zinc tends to deplete copper reserves. With medical supervision, the dosage of zinc can be increased; however, dosages should be increased with caution, as too much zinc can interfere with immune system function.

Selenium: Selenium also plays an important role in the conversion of T4 to T3. Selenium supplements must be used with caution because there is an interaction between selenium and iodine that can further impair thyroid function.[17] However, if iodine is deficient, selenium supplementation can help to normalize T4 levels.[18] Due to these complicating factors, it is best to consult with a health-care practitioner trained in the correct use of supplements before using selenium.

Iron: Iron deficiency has been linked to low thyroid function.[19] This may be due to low iron intake, which causes anemia, which in turn is linked to hypothyroidism.[20] The recommended amount of iron supplementation is 18 mg per day. Higher doses may be needed with more severe deficiencies, which should be determined by testing iron levels. Supplements made from ferrous sulfate cause constipation and other side effects.[21] Ferrous fumarate and ferrous gluconate are better forms.[22]

Tyrosine: The amino acid tyrosine is an important building block of both T4 and T3 hormones. Tyrosine is found in soybeans, beef, chicken, fish, carob, bean sprouts, oats, spinach, sesame seeds, and butternut squash. L-tyrosine can also be taken as a nutritional supplement. The typical recommended dose is 250 to 500 mg per day, taken between meals.

Herbal Remedies

Herbs have traditionally been used to help balance thyroid function. Science has validated their thyroid supporting actions.

Guggulipid, an Ayurvedic herb that has been used in India for over 2,500 years, is helpful for supporting the thyroid. It is derived from the resin of a small myrrh tree native to Asia and is traditionally used for a number of health conditions, including rheumatoid arthritis and high cholesterol. Studies have shown that guggulipid stimulates thyroid function.[23] Guggulipid is often

Other Weight-Loss Hormones:

Thyroid hormones are well known to be actively involved in metabolism and weight regulation. However, there are many other hormones that play a role in weight gain and loss. Research is uncovering the fact that fat cells themselves release hormones that influence insulin release as well as appetite. Here are some of the more notable players:

Leptin: Produced by fat cells, especially those located around the abdomen, leptin's normal function is to signal the brain to decrease appetite. When you lose fat due to dieting, the amount of leptin released also decreases, which can increase the appetite and induce rebound weight gain. This is yet another in the long list of reasons why slow and steady weight loss is more effective in the long run.

Ghrelin: This hormone secreted by the gastrointestinal tract increases appetite. Ghrelin levels rise when the stomach is empty and also while dieting by severely restricting calories. Obese individuals have higher-than-normal ghrelin levels, and these increase even further during dieting. Ghrelin can be regulated by eating frequent high-protein meals. In addition, sleep deprivation elevates ghrelin levels, so getting enough sleep can help weight-loss efforts.[24]

Adiponectin: Produced by fat cells, adiponectin improves insulin sensitivity, lowers triglyceride levels, helps to avoid hardening of the arteries, and acts as an anti-inflammatory agent. Current research is reviewing the role of adiponectin as a treatment for diabetes, atherosclerosis, and obesity.[25]

available as an extract standardized to 2.5% to 5% guggulsterones. A common recommended dose is 75 to 100 mg per day in divided doses.

Coleus forskohlii, a member of the mint family, is another Ayurvedic herb that has been used to help stimulate the thyroid. Research has shown that its primary active ingredient, forskolin, increases the production of thyroid hormones and stimulates their release.[26] Extracts of the *Coleus forskohlii* plant are often standardized to 18% forskolin. The usual recommend dose is 50 to 100 mg two times per day.

Thyroid Glandular Therapy

Natural health-care practitioners will often suggest the use of desiccated thyroid glandular extract rather than synthetic hormones. Thyroid glandular is usually derived from calves or pigs and contains both T3 and T4 hormones. Whole glandular derivatives provide protein precursors to both thyroid hormones in a natural proportion of T4 to T3, and at times this works well to re-educate the body to effectively produce these hormones. Typical doses range from ¼ grain to 1 grain per day, taken with food. Glandular extracts should be used under medical supervision.

seven

Break Food Allergies and Addictions

Do you find certain foods irresistible? Are you often a victim of uncontrollable bingeing? If so, you may be suffering from a food allergy. Although largely ignored by mainstream medical practitioners, food allergies and addictions affect millions of Americans, causing a variety of symptoms, including weight gain. Alternative medicine offers testing procedures that can determine if you suffer from such an allergy, an important step in finally breaking your addiction. For many, pinpointing hidden food allergies has been the key to finally realizing permanent weight loss and a healthier life. This chapter will introduce you to methods of determining what foods you might be allergic to. It will also describe techniques and alternative medicine therapies to help you overcome food allergies.

IN THIS CHAPTER

- Success Story: Food Allergy Awareness Relieves Weight Gain
- The Allergy Connection to Weight Gain
- Causes of Food Allergies and Addictions
- Success Story: Overcoming a Carbohydrate Addiction
- Diagnosing Food Allergies
- Alternative Medicine Therapies for Food Allergies
- Success Story: Reprogramming Hunger with Acupuncture

Success Story: Food Allergy Awareness Relieves Weight Gain

Angela, age 40, suffered from bloating, cramps, and intestinal discomfort after every meal. She was also chronically overweight and afflicted with sinus and ear infections, muscle and joint pain, mood swings, and hyperactivity. Angela was eventually diagnosed with ulcerative colitis and esophageal reflux, in which stomach acids leak upward into the esophagus, producing an intense sensation of heartburn. In addition to physical symptoms, she reported emotional disturbance, describing herself as irritable, argumentative, and overbearing, adding that most of the time she "didn't feel good inside." Angela consulted with a wide array of physicians, but none of the drug therapies they offered helped, and in fact, they seemed to worsen several of her conditions.

She finally decided to conduct her own research into her problem. She discovered a lot of information about food allergies, which sounded like a possible cause of her health issues. After learning that some food allergies are hidden, or delayed, making them difficult to track down, she decided to try a vegetarian, dairy-free diet, to see if that would help. After three months, Angela had gained 12 pounds and was excessively bloated all the time, and none of her symptoms had improved. The diet was a dismal failure.

Finally, Angela heard about a physician who specialized in food allergy testing. On her first visit, she was relieved to finally meet someone who was open to the possibility of her health issues being triggered by food allergies. In addition, this physician outlined a plan of action to determine what foods triggered Angela's symptoms. The doctor explained that the vegetarian diet might have worked very well for someone else, but that she was probably highly sensitive to the very grains that her new diet had emphasized: wheat, rye, oats, and barley. He explained that these grains contain gluten, a highly allergenic protein now linked with at least 100 medical conditions.[1] The physician ordered a test that helps determines both immediate (IgE) allergic reactions and delayed (IgG) allergic reactions. He explained that conventional doctors usually only test for the former, but that the delayed reaction is most often related to the kinds of symptoms that Angela was experiencing.

The test revealed that Angela was sensitive to 17 foods, including bananas, chile peppers, clams, eggs, oysters, green peppers, pineapple, scallops, spinach, sugar cane, wheat, yeast (baker's and brewer's), and green, kidney, and yellow wax beans. Angela also had an overgrowth of *Candida albicans*, a yeastlike fungus that often overgrows in the intestines as a result of a diet high in sugar and foods made with yeast. Angela immediately altered her eating pattern by removing all of her allergenic foods and anything that contained yeast, including buttermilk, cereals, cheeses, mushrooms, olives, wine, soy sauce, and pickles. She started practicing food rotation—not consuming the same foods or drinks two days in a row.

Angela experienced excellent results from these dietary changes. Over the next few months, she lost 22 pounds without any restriction of calories, her bowel stopped bleeding, and her remaining symptoms cleared up. Not only did Angela's physical symptoms resolve, but her state of mind improved as well—she no longer felt tense, hyperactive, and argumentative.

The Allergy Connection to Weight Gain

An allergy is the immune system's abnormal reaction to a substance that is harmless to most people. The immune system usually responds only to dangerous invaders, such as bacteria or viruses, and ignores normal substances, such as foods. People develop allergies when the immune system has become weakened or compromised and can no longer distinguish between harmful and harmless substances. In response to these otherwise normal substances, the immune system releases chemicals, such as histamines, resulting in many of the symptoms associated with allergies (see "A Primer on Allergies," page 170).

Allergies are a contributing factor in a number of health problems, including depression, hyperactivity, learning disabilities, gastrointestinal problems, diabetes, arthritis, and obesity. Unsuspected food allergies are also one of the major reasons overweight people fail to lose weight, especially in situations where cutting calories and exercising have yielded only minimal results. In addition to weight gain, food allergy symptoms include stomach pains, joint pain, insomnia, mood swings, and apathy. Food allergies specifically lead to weight gain in several ways:

- By slowing the metabolism
- By stimulating overproduction of insulin
- By causing food addictions and the related problems of bingeing, bloating, and cravings

Slowing the Metabolism

Metabolism is the biological process by which energy is extracted from food. Basal (or base) metabolism refers to the number of calories used by the body at complete rest to maintain basic functions such as breathing and circulation. Basal metabolism is controlled by the thyroid gland, which, when functioning properly, keeps the body at a normal temperature of 98.6°F. When the thyroid is underactive (known as hypothyroidism) it sends out fewer hormones, causing basal metabolism to slow down and fewer calories to be burned. Food allergies are one of the root causes of hypothyroidism, because the overactivated immune system can damage the thyroid. Hypothyroidism causes a number of problems, including general feelings of sluggishness and increases in body weight.

 For a complete discussion of the **thyroid,** see chapter 6, Overcome a Sluggish Thyroid, page 150.

Insulin Imbalance

High levels of the hormone insulin can lead to hypoglycemia, a condition that can cause significant weight gain. Insulin is the body's chief regulator of sugar (glucose); it also controls appetite, affecting your choice of when and how much you eat. The physiological mechanism that regulates insulin can be thrown off balance by food allergies, as the immune system becomes stressed and overburdened by the constant response to allergenic foods. This causes too much insulin to enter the blood, precipitating insulin resistance, a condition in which the body's cells no longer respond to insulin. As a result, insulin cannot get glucose into the cells and instead converts more and more sugar into fat.

 For more on **hypoglycemia** and **insulin and weight gain,** see chapter 5, Strengthen Your Sugar Controls, page 121.

Food Addictions

Although overweight individuals are often accused of laziness or lack of willpower, the truth is that, for some, the failure to control eating habits is due to a food addiction brought on by an allergy. Food addictions, like all addictions, can be a difficult challenge to overcome. Moreover, like alcoholics, most food addicts often do not even recognize that they have a problem.

When the person stops consuming a food to which their body is addicted, such as coffee or chocolate, they experience unpleasant withdrawal symptoms. Eating more of this addictive substance can alleviate the situation by suppressing the withdrawal symptoms. This becomes an unhealthy cycle of addiction, craving, and fulfillment that eventually leads to serious health problems, including obesity. Similar to the withdrawal from other substance addictions, withdrawal from a food addiction only occurs when the person completely stops eating the food for an extended period of time.[2]

Causes of Food Allergies and Addictions

The tendency to develop allergies is due to a combination of genetic and environmental factors,[3] and poor food choices, stress, and lack of exercise can all increase a person's susceptibility to allergies. Indeed, as the pace of life and levels of stress increase and the quality of food declines, allergies become increasingly commonplace. Allergies are usually rooted in underlying problems, with their onset often linked to a weakened immune system, leaky gut syndrome, and a repetitive diet.

Weakened Immune System

The immune system is the body's first line of defense against harmful substances. Allergies are often caused by an overload of toxins, which continually stimulates the immune system. Over time, the body's normal feedback mechanisms, which usually turn the immune system off, malfunction. The system becomes dysregulated and attacks molecules that a normal system would recognize as harmless. Many different substances may initiate this deregulation, including junk foods, allergenic foods, pesticides and herbicides, pollutants, immunizations, steroids, birth control pills, antibiotics, and other pharmaceutical drugs. Once the immune system becomes dysregulated, it loses its ability to distinguish friend from foe. Instead of attacking invaders, it begins to attack food molecules that would be recognized as harmless by the immune system if it were functioning normally. When the immune system is triggered into attack mode, it releases a variety of chemicals that can have a negative impact on the body and even cause an increased craving for the offending allergen.

Leaky Gut Syndrome

As its name indicates, this illness occurs in the intestines, where most digestion and absorption of nutrients occurs. Leaky gut syndrome occurs when there is a breakdown in the lining of the intestines, creating tiny

A Primer on Allergies

An allergy is an adverse immune system reaction — sometimes mild, sometimes severe — to a substance that other people find harmless. Quite often, an allergen (a substance provoking an allergy symptom) is a protein that the body judges to be foreign and dangerous. The adverse reaction that follows is called an allergic response. Common manifestations of this allergic response include fatigue, headaches, sneezing, watery eyes, and stuffy sinuses following exposure to an allergen. Allergies fall into two categories, those caused by environmental factors and those caused by food. The most common source of environmental allergies is the pollen of plants, particularly trees, weeds, and grasses. The most common culprits in food allergies are yeast, wheat, corn, milk and other dairy products, egg whites, tomatoes, soy, shellfish, peanuts, chocolate, and food dyes and additives.

Common symptoms of a typical allergic reaction: Breathing congestion, tears, sneezing, coughing, itching, nosebleeds, puffy face, flushing of the cheeks, dark circles under the eyes, runny nose, swelling, hives, vomiting, stomachache, intestinal irritation or swelling, watery eyes, and inflamed, bloodshot, or scratchy eyes.

The cycle of food allergies: With food allergies, there is a strange paradox: often a person becomes addicted to a food that produces an allergic response. When a person stops eating an allergy-producing food to which their body is addicted, there is a three-day period in which they experience unpleasant withdrawal symptoms, such as fatigue; eating more of the addictive substance can suppress these withdrawal symptoms. Allergy experts call this suppression of symptoms masking, because it disguises the true allergic symptoms. This becomes an unhealthy cycle of addiction, food craving, and masking that eventually leads to serious health problems.

What happens in an allergic response: The typical allergic reactions people have to foods, dust, pollen, and other substances are the body's way of fending off the intrusion of toxins that disrupt the body's equilibrium. Allergens enter the body through breathing or absorption through the skin, by eating or drinking foods, or by injection, such as insect bites or vaccinations. Because the body judges the substances to be dangerous to its health, the immune system identifies them as antigens. Antigens trigger an allergic inflammatory response. The mobilized immune system then releases specific forms of protein called antibodies

fissures that allow partially digested food particles to seep out into the bloodstream. The immune system reacts to the particles of partially digested food that leak through the gut as if they were foreign material, which sets off an allergic reaction.

One of the leading causes of a leaky gut syndrome is a harmful overgrowth of the yeastlike fungus *Candida albicans.* When an overgrowth occurs, this microorganism grows mycelia, rootlike structures that attach to the intestinal lining and literally poke tiny holes through the cell membranes, causing increased permeability through the tight junctures that are normally in place between the cells of the intestinal lining. Candida overgrowth may be caused by the use of antibiotics, to deactivate the allergenic antigens, setting in motion a complex series of events involving many biochemicals. These chemicals then produce the inflammation or other symptoms typical of an allergy response. The antibody most commonly involved in the allergic response to pollens and other environmental allergens is IgE, one of five immunoglobulins (SEE QUICK DEFINITION) involved in the immune system's defense response to foreign substances. Mast cells, which produce the allergic response, next come into play; they tend to be concentrated in the skin, nose, and lung linings, gastrointestinal tract, and reproductive organs. When the IgE antibody senses an allergen, it triggers the mast cells to release histamine and other chemicals and the allergic response flares into action. The IgE molecules also attach themselves, like a key fitting a lock, to the allergens.

Immediate versus delayed allergic reactions: The most common allergic reactions occur immediately after exposure to a certain substance (peanuts, pollen, bee stings, or cats). These reactions are typically caused by IgE immunoglobulins, resulting in a runny nose, watery eyes, itching, and skin rashes; more severe reactions include constriction of the bronchial tubes and difficulty breath-

 QUICK DEFINITION An **immunoglobulin** is one of a class of five specially designed antibody proteins produced in the spleen, bone marrow, or lymph tissue and involved in the immune system's defense response to foreign substances. The main types of immunoglobulins, grouped according to their concentration in the blood, are IgG (80%), IgA (10% to 15%), IgM (5% to 10%), IgD (less than 0.1%), and IgE (less than 0.01%).

ing. In delayed allergic reactions, symptoms may manifest up to 72 hours after exposure to a triggering substance. These can commonly appear as seemingly unrelated conditions, such as lethargy, attention-deficit disorder, fatigue, hyperactivity, acne, itchy skin, mood swings, insomnia, and inflammation. Many of these reactions are caused by IgG immunoglobulins. Up to 100 different medical conditions — from arthritis, asthma, and autism to insomnia, psoriasis, and diabetes — have been clinically associated with IgG food allergy reactions. Many people display few or no immediate sensitivity reactions (produced by IgE), but instead show moderate to severe delayed reactions (produced by IgG).

eating animal products that are not organic (since they often have antibiotic residues), or a diet high in simple carbohydrates and sugar (which also leads to weight gain). Other causes of leaky gut syndrome include alcohol consumption, excessive stress, exposure to radiation, premature birth, and vitamin, mineral, amino acid and/or essential fatty acid deficiencies.

Repetitive Diet

Food allergies are also caused by a repetitive and monotonous diet, generally limited to 30 foods or less. Food intolerance can develop when the same food, such as bread, is eaten over and over again. The immune system becomes overexposed to the molecules of this particular food, begins to recognize it as an invader, and initiates an attack against it. The cells and chemicals involved in this attack then begin to destroy the body's own tissues. In the gastrointestinal tract, the immune system normally responds only to pathogens and toxins while remaining unresponsive to food. However, it can go out of control when bombarded with a repetitive diet. This overreaction is linked to the development of gut permeability and food allergies.

Success Story:
Overcoming a Carbohydrate Addiction

Robert, age 51, was 5 foot 11 and weighed 258 pounds. He was constantly hungry and ate almost continually. He was tired all the time, had intermittent chest pains, and suffered from indigestion and high blood pressure. He visited a nutritionist to discuss his problem, and she determined that Robert had all the signs of carbohydrate addiction.

When a person who isn't addicted eats carbohydrates, their body produces a number of neurotransmitters, such as serotonin, that make them feel satisfied. The carbohydrate addict, however, has a dysregulated "reward circuit" that does not appropriately turn off.[4] This may be due to a deficiency in neurotransmitters, an imbalance in sugar regulation, psychological factors, or a combination of all of these. When these factors are present, it sets the stage for a carbohydrate addiction: the more carbohydrates a person eats, the more they crave them. Robert had been eating high amounts of carbohydrates for years, starting with his morning bagel, and was putting on about 20 pounds per year because of his addiction.

To control Roberts's cravings, he was put on a food plan based on proteins, vegetables, and a small amount of healthy fats like flaxseed and olive oils for breakfast and lunch. He then ate complex carbohydrates such as brown rice with dinner. Breakfast could include proteins like eggs, chicken, or ham. For lunch, he could eat vegetables like green beans or broccoli, salad with chicken or shrimp, or a hamburger without the bun. There were less restrictions for dinner, and carbohydrates such as pasta could be included occasionally. (Limiting carbohydrates to only the evening meal keeps insulin production in control, which reduces food cravings. It also helps with weight loss because the body tends to burn stored fat as fuel when there are fewer insulin bursts throughout the day.) The nutritionist also recommended a supplement program to complement his new diet. She suggested that he take an amino acid combination along with carnitine, coenzyme Q10, and lipoic acid in the midmorning and midafternoon to boost his protein intake and level his blood sugar, both of which would help decrease carbohydrate cravings. He was also instructed to take pancreatic enzymes with each meal to help with heartburn.

At the end of one week, Robert had lost 5 pounds. This gave him motivation to stick with the program and even add a half hour of exercise daily. After two months, Robert had lost 21 pounds, his heartburn had disappeared, and his blood pressure was almost normal. He was amazed at how much his energy level had increased. And at last he could easily make it from meal to meal without being hungry. He had won the appetite battle.

Diagnosing Food Allergies

Diagnosing food allergies can be challenging, because reactions are often varied and inconsistent, and they may take several days to develop after eating an allergy-causing food. How much of an allergenic food you eat, how often you eat it, and how it is cooked may also be factors in whether or not you have a reaction. In addition, multiple foods are often involved, and finally, symptoms may be masked by regular consumption of the foods.

Despite the complexity surrounding the detection of food allergies, mainstream medical practitioners generally take a highly simplified approach to the problem. Most rely on procedures that are minimally accurate at detecting food allergies: scratch tests, prick tests, and patch tests. These are most useful for identifying reactions caused by pollen or dust, or an immediate food allergy, such as swelling that occurs very soon after eating shellfish or peanuts. Another common test procedure is the radioallergosorbent test (RAST). This blood test is useful for diagnosing allergies to pollens, dust, molds, bee venom, and other allergens, but is not accurate in detecting food allergies, especially those involving delayed reactions. Most alternative medicine practitioners rarely use these tests, instead relying on self-evaluation techniques, the elimination diet, and other tests for identifying allergens, such as applied kinesiology, electrodermal screening, the IgG ELISA test, blood typing, and skin testing. Regardless of which type of test you use, it is best to consult a nutritional counselor or other health-care practitioner to help guide you through the process.

Do You Suffer from Food Allergies?

The following questionnaire, developed by London naturopath Leon Chaitow, ND, DO, can help you determine if you have a food allergy. If you answer no or never to any question, give yourself a score of zero for that particular question; the other scores are provided with each question.

- Do you suffer from unnatural fatigue? (Score 1 if occasionally, 2 if regularly — three times a week or more.)

- Do you sometimes experience weight fluctuations of 4 or more pounds in a single day, accompanied by puffiness of the face, ankles, or fingers? (Score 1 if infrequently, 2 if frequently — more than once a month.)

- Do you have hot flashes (apart from menopause) or find yourself sweating for no obvious reason? (Score 1 if infrequently, 2 if several times a week or more.)

- Does your pulse race or your heart pound strongly for no obvious reason? (Score 1 if infrequently, 2 if several times a week or more.)

- Do you have a history of food intolerance, causing any symptoms at all? (Score 2 if your answer is yes.)

- Do you crave bread, sugary foods, milk, chocolate, coffee, or tea? (Score 2 if your answer is yes.)

- Do you suffer from migraines or severe headaches, irritable bowel syndrome, eczema, depression, asthma, or muscle aches? (Score 2 if your answer is yes.)

If your score is five or higher, there is a strong likelihood that hidden food allergies are part of your symptom picture.

The Elimination Diet

The elimination diet allows you to study your reaction to different foods without undergoing laboratory tests. It takes some time and dedication, but it will give you an excellent idea of which foods you react to and how different foods make you feel. Here's how you do it:

1. Eliminate the possible allergenic foods for 10 to 14 days.

2. Carefully observe any changes in symptoms.

3. Test the eliminated foods by bringing them back into the diet, one by one, and noting any return of symptoms.

Test foods that are likely allergens, which probably fall into one of these categories:

- Foods you eat often, especially those you eat daily, such as wheat and dairy
- Foods you crave
- Foods that you notice any reaction to, such as feeling tired or light-headed after eating them

It is important to eliminate all of the suspected foods on your list, as multiple allergies are quite common. If all are not eliminated, it could skew your results. Also, read the ingredients on any packaged foods very carefully to ensure you do not inadvertently consume whatever it is you are trying to eliminate (for example, sugar or the flavor enhancer monosodium glutamate). Remember that delayed food allergies can take as long as 72 hours to exhibit symptoms. If you experience symptoms such as irritability, fatigue, headaches, and intense cravings during the elimination period, you may be going through withdrawal, which is indicative of both food allergies and food addictions.

Although the elimination diet is accurate, it is time-consuming and requires a level of discipline that overweight people often find difficult. The following techniques are faster and more convenient, and are done by many holistic health-care practitioners.

Common Allergenic Foods

Here's a list of a few of the more common foods that provoke allergies:

- Wheat
- Yeast
- Corn
- Sugar
- Eggs
- Soybeans
- Citrus fruits
- Strawberries
- Chocolate
- Shellfish
- Coffee
- Tomatoes
- Potatoes
- Spices
- Beef and pork
- Nuts
- Milk and other dairy products
- Food additives, such as nitrates, sulfites, and monosodium glutamate (MSG)

Food Allergy Timetable

When experiencing the symptoms below, notice if they began within the given time after eating a particular food. If so, they may be due to food allergies:[5]

Delayed Food Allergy Symptoms	
Symptom	Elapsed Time
Indigestion or heartburn	30 minutes
Headache	Within 1 hour
Asthma or runny nose	Within 1 hour
Bloated stomach or diarrhea	3 to 4 hours
Rashes or hives	6 to 12 hours
Weight gain by fluid retention	12 to 15 hours
Fits, convulsions, or mental disturbance	12 to 24 hours
Mouth ulcers, joint or muscle pain, or backache	48 to 96 hours

Applied Kinesiology

First developed by Detroit chiropractor George Goodheart, applied kinesiology is the study of the relationship between muscle dysfunction (evidenced by weakness) and related organ or gland dysfunction. Applied kinesiology employs a simple strength resistance test on a specific indicator muscle related to the organ or part of the body that is being tested. If the muscle tests strong (maintaining its resistance), it indicates health. If it tests weak, it can mean infection or dysfunction. To isolate the allergy-inducing substances, the person who is being tested provides small samples of foods in their regular diet. While holding one food sample in their hand, pressure is applied to a specific muscle. If the muscle can resist the pressure, then the tested food does not cause allergic reactions in the person. But if the muscle cannot withstand the applied pressure, then the tested food is suspected of causing an allergic response. The process is repeated until the most common foods in the diet have been tested. This technique is so easy and noninvasive that people can learn it and test themselves at home. Their results aren't always precise, but it gives them a feeling of control over their food allergies.

Nambudripad Allergy Elimination Technique

Another method that uses kinesiology to detect food allergies is the Nambudripad Allergy Elimination Technique (NAET). Developed by Devi Nambudripad, DC, it also treats and eliminates allergies using acupuncture or acupressure and chiropractic. After determining which substances are allergens through muscle testing, the patient again holds the offending substance while the NAET practitioner uses acupuncture or acupressure to reprogram the way the body responds to the substance, thereby removing the allergic charge.

Electrodermal Screening

Electrodermal screening is a form of computerized information gathering based on physics, not chemistry. A blunt, noninvasive electric probe is placed at specific points on the patient's hands, face, or feet, corresponding to acupuncture points at the beginning or end of energy meridians. Minute electrical discharges from these points provide information about the condition of the body's organs and systems, useful for the physician in evaluation and developing a treatment plan. It's widely used by holistic practitioners in Europe and the United States to screen for a wide range of allergens, including food and environmental substances. It also helps determine what remedies to use to properly neutralize allergic reactions and can be used to monitor the success of prescribed remedies.

IgG ELISA Test

Most allergy tests only measure the presence of the antibody IgE, or immunoglobulin E. IgE allergies cause immediate reactions that patients can usually recognize soon after eating the offending food. However, some allergies are more difficult to identify because they result in delayed reactions that occur as much as 48 to 72 hours after ingestion of the offending food. Delayed food allergies involve another type of antibody, IgG. The IgG ELISA (enzyme-linked immunoabsorbent assay) test, which can detect delayed food allergies, involves computer analysis of a blood sample for the presence of IgG antibodies in response to over 100 foods.

Skin Testing

There are two types of skin tests used to determine allergies to molds, dusts, pollen, and other environmental factors. Serial endpoint titration (SET) is far more accurate than the commonly used scratch test. During a SET test, a diluted form of a potential food allergen is injected just under the skin. The body immediately reacts to the introduction of this foreign substance by forming a wheal about 4 millimeters in diameter. After 10 minutes another measurement is taken. The wheal will grow according to the severity of the immune reaction. A 5-millimeter-diameter wheal indicates no allergic reaction, while a 7-millimeter wheal (or larger) indicates an allergic response. If the test shows a positive result, the process is then repeated with increasingly diluted forms of the same allergen to evaluate the degree of sensitivity. After the offending foods or environmental allergens are determined, a formula is created specifically for the patient. Each allergic substance is combined in a vial in the exact titration needed to help neutralize the allergic effect. The patient still needs to avoid those foods to which they are highly allergic, but doing home injections of the formula helps rebuild the immune system and lessen the overall allergic response.

Alternative Medicine Therapies for Food Allergies

Decreasing your allergic response to foods will not only help you feel better, it will aid you with weight loss. The first step in treating a food allergy is to remove problem foods from your diet. In addition, a number of nutrients and herbs are helpful for treating allergies and supporting the digestive system. Overcoming a food allergy or food addiction can be a formidable challenge, despite a carefully planned menu and nutritional supplements. Acupuncture, flower essence therapy, and aromatherapy, three alternative medicine therapies used to help treat addictive behaviors, can give you the extra support you need to curb your desire for sugar or other addictive foods.

Alternative Medicine Therapies for Food Allergies

- Dietary Changes
- Supplements and Herbs
- Acupuncture
- Flower Essence Therapy
- Aromatherapy

Dietary Changes

Once you have identified the foods you are allergic to, the next step is to eliminate them from your diet. Initially, you should completely refrain from eating all allergenic foods for 60 to 90 days. When a person eliminates an allergenic food, it can cause withdrawal reactions similar to those experienced by alcoholics when they stop drinking. The withdrawal phase usually lasts 3 to 5 days. During that time, it is common to experience tiredness, cravings, mood swings, irritability, feeling of loss and distress, and other symptoms. After this period, you can begin to slowly reintroduce the allergenic foods, one at a time, into your diet. Once the withdrawal phase has passed, the cravings also abate, and the person is free of dependence on foods that had been problematic—free of both the physiological and psychological desire to consume it so frequently, and in such great quantities. But even after food allergies have been overcome, it's best to practice food rotation, wherein foods are varied on a daily basis, to avoid developing new allergies.

Many people have discovered that identifying and treating food allergies was the key to solving their weight problems. However, it is important to understand that the desire to lose weight is rarely the source of the kind of motivation needed to beat a food addiction and break a food allergy. To overcome an allergy, people often need to completely overhaul their eating patterns. Depending on how many foods a person is sensitive to, the process can be a very demanding and daunting task. It means saying no to popular foods, party foods, and comfort foods. However, focusing on embracing health rather than just losing pounds supports a total commitment to healthy living, including maintaining a healthy weight.

Supplements and Herbs

A combination of quercetin and bromelain is one of the most effective supplements for combating a food allergy. Quercetin is a bioflavonoid derived from plants such as blueberries, cranberries, cherries, onions, and tomatoes. It enhances the body's ability to use vitamin C, increasing its absorption by the liver, kidneys, and adrenal glands. Bromelain, a digestive enzyme derived from pineapple, enhances the absorption of quercetin. Taken together, quercetin and bromelain strengthen the membranes of the body's cells so that they are less likely to be damaged in the presence of an allergen. This, in turn, lessens the allergic response and reduces the symptoms of the allergy. The typical recommended dosage is 250 mg of quercetin and 125 mg of bromelain, taken three times daily, 20 minutes before each meal.

The reaction of the digestive system to offending foods can be reduced by using the appropriate enzyme supplements: proteases digest proteins, lipases digest fats, amylases digest carbohydrates, lactases digest dairy products, and disaccharidases digest sugars. Supplementing with beta-

Helpful Hints for Breaking a Food Addiction

Breaking a food addiction is never easy. Nevertheless, there are a few basic measures to follow that can help you make it through the cravings and withdrawal:

- Have plenty of nonallergenic foods on hand at all times, including when you're away from home.

- Drink at least six to eight glasses of pure water every day, as adequate water intake is essential for good health; use springwater, distilled water, or filtered tap water.

- Don't go it alone. You may need extra help to break an addiction, so consider the support of a trained counselor.

- Maintain good nutrition because malnourishment only increases cravings. Try working with a nutritional expert to determine your unique nutritional needs.

- Engage in light exercise on a regular basis. A brisk walk twice a day is all it takes to obtain some health benefit.

ine hydrochloric acid, the primary acid in the stomach, may also help digestive function. As digestion improves, allergic reactions to food should be minimized or eliminated.

Herbs can also help to counteract the effects of an allergy. Curcumin, an extract from the spice plant turmeric (*Curcuma longa*), decreases the symptoms of an allergic reaction. Another allergy-relieving herb is cayenne (*Capsicum annuum*), or red pepper. This herb is a systemic stimulant, meaning it invigorates the function of the whole body, and it's especially helpful for digestive function.

Other nutrients and supplements are useful for supporting overall digestion, which will help with any food allergy. These include the amino acid glutamine, vitamin E, chlorophyll, and aloe vera. Herbs for digestive support include slippery elm, marshmallow root, cat's claw, and pau d'arco. Probiotics introduce healthy flora into the digestive system, which helps to improve digestion and decrease allergic reactions. Beneficial bacteria, such as *Lactobacillus acidophilus*, *Lactobacillus bulgaricus*, and *Bifidobacterium bifidum*, are the key players in this process. Probiotic supplements are available at most health food stores.

Acupuncture

Acupuncture is a proven means of combating cravings and controlling weight,[6] and has been used extensively in treating many kinds of addictions, such as smoking, alcoholism, and drug addictions.[7] Needles are placed mainly on points on the ear to influence two parts of the brain located in the hypothalamus: the feeding center, which is responsible for the feeling of hunger, and the satiety center, which tells you when you've eaten enough.

Success Story:
Reprogramming Hunger with Acupuncture

Ramond, 34, stood 5 foot 7 and weighed 249 pounds. He worked long days as a traveling sales representative and, due to the stress of his job, he tended to eat erratically, relying on fast foods and late-night snacks. His food choices were high in calories, fats, and salt, all of which contribute to weight gain. While he had tried different diets, herbs, and weight-loss drugs, nothing had yielded permanent weight loss. His body mass index (BMI) was 37 (20 to 25 is a healthy level). Ramond spoke to a friend who suggested that he try acupuncture. He figured he had nothing to lose but some weight, so he made an appointment with a licensed acupuncturist.

The acupuncturist advised Ramond that strictly dietary approaches to weight loss tend to fail over time because they are too restrictive and leave people feeling deprived, with no joy in their life regarding food. He explained that acupuncture helps to reduce the appetite, raise the body's metabolic rate, and enhance digestion so that more nutrients are extracted and absorbed from what is eaten. He also explained that the placement of acupuncture needles can activate the parasympathetic nervous system, which controls appetite, metabolism, and digestion, and that the goal is to decrease nervous tension, which frequently triggers the desire to overeat.

The needles are placed mainly on points on the ear, plus some points along the spine and abdomen, to influence two parts of the brain located in the hypothalamus: the feeding center, which is responsible for the feeling of hunger, and the satiety center, which tells you when you've eaten enough. Acupuncture can reset the operation of these two centers so you feel less hunger and feel more satisfied after eating less food. The clinician also placed an acupuncture "earring" (a tiny silver pellet) in Ramond's ear so that merely by pressing on it he could activate the treatment point to reduce his food cravings whenever he felt the need.

In addition to the acupuncture treatments, Ramond made a commitment to modify his diet. He ate 10% to 30% less at each meal, and learned new ways of cooking and choosing more healthful foods on the go. This minimized feelings of deprivation and eased his transition to a healthier diet. For example, Ramond substituted baked Atlantic salmon with shiitake mushroom pesto instead of unhealthy fried foods and he used whole-grain toast with almond butter with natural fruit jam as a late night snack instead of apple pie with ice cream.

After three months of acupuncture and improved diet, Ramond lost 37 pounds and his BMI to dropped to 31.5. What pleased him the most was that he achieved the lasting (and ongoing) weight reduction without the feeling of sacrifice so typical of other weight-reduction programs.

Flower Essence Therapy

Flower essence therapy helps control addictive behaviors by treating underlying emotional, psychological, and spiritual issues. The approach was pioneered by British physician Edward Bach in the 1930s, when he introduced the Bach flower remedies, based on English plants. Flower essences are made by floating blossoms in springwater, then letting them sit in the sun for a few hours. The blossoms are removed, leaving the essence of the flower, which is then diluted to a dosage level.

 For more information on **flower essences**, see chapter 4, Heal Your Emotional Appetite, page 115.

Drops of the essences are either placed under the tongue, ingested in a tonic, or diluted in a bath. Although you can administer a flower essence treatment yourself, a trained practitioner can help tailor a treatment program specific to your psychological needs.

Aromatherapy

Another way to control appetite is through aromatherapy. Rather than water-based flower essences, aromatherapy relies on oils extracted from the leaves, flowers, or roots of plants. The small size of the molecules in these oils allows them to penetrate bodily tissues via the skin or the olfactory nerves, affecting central nervous system activity. Aromatherapy can be performed at home, using either a diffuser, which spreads microparticles of the oils into the air, or floral waters, which can be sprayed. One formula that has been used to help suppress the appetite is 15 drops of bergamot oil and 10 drops of fennel oil. To make a spray, add both of the oils to a 4-ounce spray bottle of water.[8]

Inhalants are essential oils that you can breathe directly from the bottle. As the soothing aromas travel through your respiratory system, they trigger a positive reaction in the brain. You might feel the difference —elevated mood, lower stress level, or reduced appetite—in as little as a few seconds. To make an inhalant, just place your choice of essential oils in a small glass bottle with an airtight cover. Then blend the oils by gently turning the container upside down or rolling it between your hands. After a few minutes, the oils are well blended and your inhalant is ready for use. If you would like to use your inhalant throughout the day, try placing a few drops of the blend on a tissue or handkerchief, then carry the scented item with you so you can enjoy an aromatherapy break anytime.

Part III
Customize Your Weight-Loss Program

Copyright 2003 by Randy Glasbergen. www.glasbergen.com

GLASBERGEN

"What fits your busy schedule better, exercising one hour a day or being dead 24 hours a day?"

eight

Individualize Your Diet

If you have already incorporated the recommendations in this book that apply to your situation, great! In that case, you're well on your way and can use this section to help you fine-tune your path toward optimum health, wellness, and weight management. If you have skipped to this section looking for the perfect quickie weight-loss diet, then you may be disappointed!

The Diet Debate

Diet fads proliferate throughout the media and popular culture. Anyone seeking the "perfect" diet can easily be overwhelmed by the plethora of options and strong opinions, sometimes in support of diametrically opposite approaches. Much of the debate among weight-loss experts focuses on what proportion of protein, carbohydrate, and fat should be included in a diet. Some claim a high-carbohydrate, low-fat, mostly vegetarian diet is best, while others argue that carbohydrates need to be balanced by a fair amount of protein and fat. Other diets propose that eating mostly protein and almost no carbohydrates is the fastest way to a trim figure. So who should you believe?

IN THIS CHAPTER

- The Diet Debate
- Different Body Types, Different Diets
- Sizing Up the Popular Diets

Recognizing that individuals have different nutritional requirements, alternative medicine practitioners don't promote the use of any specific diet for all patients. The key is to match an appropriate diet to each person's physiology. In addition, individual needs are not static; they change according to conditions such as illness, stress, exposure to environmental toxins, and other factors that vary the person's need for different nutrients. All of these variables must be taken into account in making the right dietary decisions. The first step in tailoring a diet to fit your individual needs is to look more closely at your body type.

Different Body Types, Different Diets

Just like fingerprints, each person has a unique metabolism, which affects how food is converted into energy. Many alternative medicine practitioners use body-typing systems to gain insight into a person's unique nutritional needs, allowing development of a diet plan appropriate to that person. The concept that people can be categorized into different body types is not a new one. Such systems for understanding people's physiological functioning and unique needs have been around for millenia.

Traditional Chinese Medicine

One of the most ancient systems of healing is traditional Chinese medicine (TCM), which originated over 5,000 years ago. TCM is a comprehensive system of medical practice that heals the body according to the principles of nature and balance. A Chinese medicine physician considers the flow of vital energy (qi) in a patient through close examination of the patient's pulse, tongue, body odor, voice tone and strength, and general demeanor, among other elements. Underlying imbalances and disharmony in the body are described in terminology analogous to the natural world (heat, cold, dryness, or dampness). TCM employs a body-typing paradigm called the five element theory, which holds that each individual expresses the energy of the elements of fire, wood, air, water, and metal in different measures and that an interplay of yin (passive, watery, stationary, dark, calming) and yang (active, fiery, moving, bright, energizing) energies influences each person's health.

Ayurvedic Medicine

Another venerable healing tradition is Ayurveda, the 5,000-year-old traditional medicine of India. Ayurveda describes three metabolic and

Optimum Foods for Ayurvedic Body Types

Foods That Balance *Kapha*

Fruit	
Lemon	
Lime	
Grapefruit	
Cranberries	
Apple	
Dried fruits	

Vegetables	
Chiles	Asparagus
Broccoli	Lettuce
Cabbage	Cilantro
Celery	Watercress
Carrot	Mustard greens
Green beans	Alfalfa
Peas (fresh)	Sunflower sprouts
Beet	Chard
	Bell pepper
	Cauliflower
	Parsley
	Spinach

Grains
Barley
Quinoa
Corn
Millet

continued on next page

constitutional body types (*doshas*) in association with the basic elements of nature—*vata* (air and ether, rooted in the intestines), *pitta* (fire and water, rooted in the stomach), and *kapha* (water and earth, rooted in the lungs). Ayurvedic physicians use these categories (which also have psychological aspects) as the basis for prescribing individualized programs of herbs, diet, massage, breathing, meditation, exercise, and detoxification techniques.[1]

For more details on each of these body types, see the descriptions of Sheldon's somatotypes below, which include not just physical characteristics, but also personality traits and potential health issues. *Kapha* corresponds to endomorph; *pitta* to mesomorph; and *vata* to ectomorph. In brief, the *kapha* type is soft and round, the *pitta* type is muscular, and the *vata* type is thin and delicate. See the following chart for food recommendations for each of these types.

Optimum Foods for Ayurvedic Body Types, *continued*

Foods That Balance Kapha, *continued*

Rye

Buckwheat

Basmati rice (moderate)

Beans

Adzuki

Soy

Lima

Lentils

Tofu

Mung

Kidney

Peanuts (raw)

Split peas

Nuts and seeds

Sunflower seeds

Pumpkin seeds

Oils

Mustard oil

Canola oil

Sunflower oil

Safflower oil

Corn oil

Dairy

Goat's milk

Lassi (a yogurt beverage)

Sweeteners

Raw honey

Animal Products

Chicken (white meat)

Turkey (white meat)

Beverages

Soy milk (warm)

Goat's milk (boiled)

Fruit juices (pineapple, pomegranate, cranberry, grapefruit, lemon, lime)

Vegetable juices (celery and other green vegetables)

Teas (alfalfa, dandelion, hibiscus, raspberry)

Condiments

Ginger (dried)

Fenugreek

Basil

Black pepper

Horseradish

Cloves

Cinnamon

Foods That Balance *Pitta*

Fruit

- Apple
- Pear
- Pomegranate
- Pineapple
- Cranberries
- Persimmon
- Melons
- Prunes
- Dates
- Figs
- Grapes
- Mango
- Plum
- Raspberries

Vegetables

- Cauliflower
- Cilantro
- Alfalfa sprouts
- Sunflower sprouts
- Celery
- Broccoli
- Cabbage
- Brussels sprouts
- Asparagus
- Lettuce
- Beans (fresh or dried)
- Peas (fresh or dried)
- Cucumber
- Okra
- Parsley
- Bell pepper
- Corn (fresh)
- Squash

Grains

- Whole wheat
- Basmati rice
- Long-grain rice
- Oats
- Granola
- Couscous
- Quinoa
- Blue corn
- Millet

Beans

- Adzuki
- Tofu
- Lima
- Kidney
- Soy
- Split pea
- Chickpeas
- Nuts and seeds
- Coconut
- Sunflower seeds

Oils

- Ghee (clarified butter)
- Sunflower
- Butter (unsalted)

continued on next page

Optimum Foods for Ayurvedic Body Types, *continued*

Soy oil

Dairy

Ghee (clarified butter)

Milk (boiled and cooled)

Yogurt

Lassi (a yogurt beverage)

Cottage cheese (unsalted)

Sweeteners

Cane sugar

Maple syrup

Molasses (in moderation)

Animal products

Egg whites

Chicken (white meat)

Turkey (white meat)

Fish (freshwater)

Beverages

Aloe vera

Fruit juices (using the fruits above)

Carob

Vegetable juices (using the vegetables above)

Milk (boiled and cooled)

Teas (alfalfa, barley, burdock, chamomile, chicory, chrysanthemum, dandelion, hibiscus, jasmine, lavender, lemon grass, nettle, mint, raspberry, red clover, rose, saffron, sarsaparilla)

Condiments

Coriander

Mint

Fennel

Turmeric (in moderation)

Rock salt (in moderation)

Foods That Balance *Vata*

Fruit

: Lemon
: Lime
: Grapefruit
: Cherries
: Grapes
: Strawberries
: Raspberries
: Berries
: Pineapple
: Papaya
: Mango
: Apple (baked)
: Pear (baked)
: Kiwi
: Melons (sweet)
: Dried fruits (soaked prunes, raisins, dates, figs)
: Oranges
: Peach
: Plum
: Apricot
: Pomegranate
: Persimmon

Vegetables

: Sweet potato
: Carrot
: Beet
: Cilantro
: Parsley

: Sea Vegetables
: Avocado (in moderation)
: Corn (fresh)
: Green beans (well-cooked)
: Peas (fresh)
: Zucchini
: Squash
: Artichoke
: Mustard greens
: Watercress
: Bell pepper
: Okra
: Fenugreek greens
: Leeks (cooked)
: Olives (black and green)
: Parsnip
: Pumpkin
: Rutabaga

Grains

: Wheat
: Basmati rice
: Oats
: Couscous
: Pasta (whole-grain)
: Bread (whole-grain, yeast-free, and toasted)

Beans

: Mung
: Tofu

continued on next page

Individualize Your Diet   191

Optimum Foods for Ayurvedic Body Types, *continued*

Foods That Balance Vata, continued

Nuts and seeds

- Almonds (raw, soaked, and peeled)
- Sesame seeds (or tahini)
- Walnuts
- Pecans
- Pine nuts

Oils

- Sesame oil
- Ghee (clarified butter)
- Almond oil
- Olive oil

Dairy

- Milk (organic and boiled)
- Yogurt
- Lassi (a yogurt beverage)
- Ghee (clarified butter)
- Cottage cheese
- Buttermilk (homemade)
- Sour cream
- Kefir
- Cream
- Cheese (in moderation)

Sweeteners

- Natural sugar cane
- Maple syrup
- Raw sugar
- Raw honey
- Fruit sugar (in moderation)
- Jaggery (unrefined sugar from palm sap)

Animal products

- Fish
- Eggs
- Chicken (white meat)
- Turkey (white meat)

Beverages

- Milk
- Lassi (a yogurt beverage)
- Buttermilk
- Fruit juices (using the fruits above)
- Vegetable juices (using the vegetables above)

- Water (with lime or lemon)
- Herbal teas

Condiments

- Cardamom
- Cinnamon
- Fennel
- Mint
- Coriander
- Turmeric
- Basil
- Rock salt

Adapted from *The Ayurveda Encyclopedia* by Swami Sada Shiva Tirtha (copyright 1998, reprinted with permission).

Type	Endomorph (kapha)	Mesomorph (pitta)	Ectomorph (vata)
Physical characteristics	Endomorphs have a round body shape with poorly defined muscular development and soft tone. They tend to have a large abdomen and enjoy eating, often making poor food choices.	Mesomorphs have a rectangular shaped, muscular body with good tone, especially if they exercise. They have a mature appearance at a younger age than other body types. They have thick skin and good posture.	Ectomorphs are small framed, with a thin, delicate build. They have light musculature and may have stooped shoulders and a flat chest. They tend to have a large brain and appear young for their age.
Character traits	Endomorphs are usually sociable, relaxed, and even tempered. They are usually in a good mood. They enjoy creature comforts and need a lot of affection.	Mesomorphs are bold and assertive, seek power, and move themselves into dominant positions. They are willing to go out on a limb and try something adventurous. They crave competition and physical activity, and they are indifferent to the opinions of others.	Ectomorphs are often artistic and intellectually oriented with restrained emotions. They can be inhibited and introverted with a preference for privacy.
Possible health issues	Endomorphs often develop health issues associated with overeating, including high cholesterol, obesity, allergies, chronic congestion and sinus problems.	Mesomorphs tend to have strong constitutions, but may develop conditions associated with too much acid, such as profuse sweating, acne, hemorrhoids, ulcers and stomach ailments.	Ectomorphs can suffer from stress-related syndromes such as anxiety, insomnia and bowel irregularities including constipation. Woman may experience premenstrual syndrome.

Sheldon's Somatotypes

There are also modern systems that categorize people according to body types. In 1940, Dr. William Sheldon (1898–1977), an American psychologist, proposed three somatotypes, or body types—endomorph,

Are You a Candidate for Metabolic Typing?

Consulting a dietitian or other health-care practitioner regarding your diet is always a good idea, but there are basic warning signals that your diet may be working against you (and your metabolic type), causing you to go further out of balance and gain weight:

1. Appetite: Are you always hungry no matter how frequently or how much you eat?

2. Digestion: After you eat, do you experience any bloating, gas, or indigestion? Do you find it difficult to digest certain foods, such as dairy, meats, or wheat products?

3. Energy levels: Are you excessively tired a few hours after eating? Do you have difficulty performing tasks that require concentration and alertness?

4. Cravings: Do you crave certain foods such as salty snacks, sweets, caffeine, or fat?

5. Regularity: Do you experience any constipation?

6. Sleep: Do you find it difficult to fall asleep? Do you wake up still feeling tired after sleeping 7 hours or more?

7. Sense of well-being: Do you experience mood swings or mild depression?

If you answer "yes" to three or more of these questions, you may want to consider metabolic typing to help you choose the right foods for your particular biochemistry and to restore a healthy balance in your life.

mesomorph, and ectomorph—based on the three tissue layers: endoderm, mesoderm, and ectoderm. These categories have an amazingly close correspondence to the Ayurvedic types. In Sheldon's system, each body type is associated not just with physical characteristics, but also with personality characteristics.

Blood Type Diet

In the system of eating referred to as the blood type diet, designed by James D'Adamo and expounded upon by his son Peter D'Adamo, ND, each blood type is assigned a specific diet. Observations of more than 3,000 patients led to the conclusion that the four basic blood groups —O, A, B, and AB (plus six additional subtypes)—have different physiological and nutritional needs. As with many diets, there are varied opinions. Many people who try this diet find that they feel very well, are able to lose weight, have less congestion and sinus trouble, and experience improved bowel function and balanced blood sugar. Others, however, question if there is sufficient scientific research to back up the claims of this dietary regimen.

Metabolic Typing

One of the most detailed body-typing systems is metabolic typing, which is based on research done by George Watson, Ph.D., William Donald Kelley, DDS, and Francis Pottenger, MD. They believed that each individual has a particular metabolic type that determines how quickly—or slowly—the body burns calories and stores fat. Metabolic type is determined by a series of diagnostic tests that reveal which physiological systems tend to drive the body. Determining a person's metabolic type allows them to use specific foods and supplements that are most likely to support their unique biochemistry.

Tests Used to Determine Metabolic Type

Metabolic typing relies on a series of medical tests. When an experienced health practitioner analyzes these tests in a comprehensive manner, they can accurately identify your metabolic type and recommend a diet and exercise program specific to you.

- Blood pH: The first step in figuring out a person's metabolic type is determining the acid/alkaline state, or pH, of their blood. Ideal blood pH is slightly alkaline at 7.46. A blood pH with a higher number is considered alkaline, and below 7.46 is acid. Body type can predispose you to being more acidic or more alkaline. When you are too acid or too alkaline, your body doesn't absorb nutrients as well, which can lead to an array of problems, including weight gain, fatigue, allergies, high blood pressure, and other chronic illnesses.

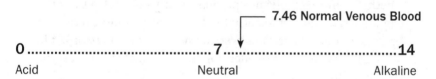

7.46 Normal Venous Blood

0 .... 7 14
Acid   Neutral   Alkaline

- Blood typing: Blood is classified into four blood types or groups according to the presence of type A and type B antigens on the surface of red blood cells. These antigens, also called agglutinogens, pertain to the blood cells' ability to agglutinate, or clump together. In the United States, 43% of the population has type O blood (containing neither A nor B); 40% are type A; 12% are type B; and 5% are type AB.[2] Blood type is considered relevant to metabolic typing because agglutination also occurs in the body in response to a type of protein called lectins (SEE QUICK DEFINITION, page 196). Found in 30% of the foods we eat, lectins have characteristics similar to blood antigens and are thus some-

QUICK DEFINITION

Lectins are protein fragments of incompletely digested foods that bind with specific sugar receptors on the surface of all cells of the body. They tend to stick like Velcro to the lining of the gastrointestinal tract, where they irritate the tissues and can destroy cell membranes. Most dietary lectins come from the indigestible fractions of plant products, often deriving from beans, grains, soy, and wheat. Lectins can lead to food allergies and toxic reactions at the mucosal membranes in the intestines. In particular, soybean and wheat lectins can produce an increase in permeability in the cells they bind to, often leading to cell death. Further, lectins can cause atrophying of the intestinal villi (the fingerlike projections that afford the intestines their absorptive surface area).

times recognized as an enemy by the immune system, which may lead to allergic reactions.

■ Glucose metabolism: During a glucose tolerance test, you drink a preparation rich in sugars after fasting overnight. Saliva and urine samples are then measured to determine how quickly or slowly the body is burning off, or oxidizing, the sugars. The person's sense of well-being, hunger, and energy are noted prior to taking the drink and at intervals over the next few hours. Different patterns of response indicate different metabolic types.

■ Oxidative or autonomic: As an adjunct to the glucose metabolism test, blood pressure, heart rate, pulse, and respiratory rate are measured both before and after the glucose test is administered. Changes in the readings will reflect whether your metabolism is predominantly controlled by your oxidative rate (how efficiently food is converted into energy) or by your autonomic nervous system (SEE QUICK DEFINITION). This information can aid in the development of a diet that is best for your metabolic type.

■ Basal body temperature: Also known as resting body temperature, this provides a clue as to whether your metabolism, essentially the internal "furnace" that burns the calories you consume, is operating efficiently. For instructions on measuring your basal temperature at home, see page 158.

■ Food diary: The diary provides a detailed list of all the foods consumed over a three-day period — not just meals, but all the snacks and foods eaten on the run, which people sometimes forget they consume if they don't keep a food diary.

■ Hair analysis: Hair analysis reveals what minerals a person may be lacking. Much like the rings on a tree, hair provides a nutrient his-

tory. This information reveals what supplementation may
be needed to restore health.

- Photos of the body: Photos are used to record what parts of
  the person's body tend to store fat.

- Electroacupuncture test: This
  test is administered to determine
  if any organs, such as the liver,
  thyroid, or spleen, are underactive
  or overstimulated.

- General health: Finally, the
  practitioner will ask the person
  to complete n extensive survey
  with questions regarding what
  they eat, what snacks they crave,
  sleeping habits, and general outlook on life. This reveals general
  tendencies and any obvious imbalances, such as intense cravings for
  salty snacks or interrupted sleep.

 The **autonomic nervous system** (ANS) is like your body's automatic pilot. It maintains functions that keep you alive, such as breathing, heart rate, and digestion, without your being aware of it or participating in its activities. The ANS has two divisions: the sympathetic, which expends body energy and prepares us physically when we perceive a threat or challenge by increasing heart rate, blood pressure, and muscle tension, and the parasympathetic, which conserves body energy by slowing heart rate and increases intestinal and gland activity.

Taken together, these tests give an overview of the person's general
health and whether any of their body systems are creating imbalances
that affect their metabolism.

The Five Metabolic Types

With all of this information, an experienced practitioner can determine
the person's metabolic type as one of the following:

Fast burners: Also known as fast oxidizers, these people have a tendency
to burn off their carbohydrates too quickly for their energy needs. At
the same time, they are poor at converting fats to fuel that can be used
by the body. They have acid blood and do best on a whole foods diet
including whole grains, quite a bit of animal protein, and full-fat dairy
foods. Wheat is to be avoided as it is too acid-forming.

Slow burners: Also known as slow oxidizers, these people are alkaline
and do well eating a diet limiting high-fat animal proteins. Low-fat

dairy foods and whole grains are allowed, but wheat should be favored as it is acid-forming.

Energizers: Considered to be sympathetic dominant, these people tend to have acid blood and their bodies are dominated by the thyroid, pituitary, and adrenal glands. They do well on a low-protein, relatively low-fat diet.

Conservers: Considered to be parasympathetic dominant, these people do well on a diet that includes full-fat dairy foods and more animal protein. This type is characterized by increased activity in the liver, intestines, and, pancreas.

Balanced: A small number of people are blessed with balanced, well-functioning endocrine systems. They maintain a healthy weight and eat intuitively, selecting foods that provide them with a steady supply of energy that discourages overeating.

Although wide-ranging in their origins and principles, all these systems share a belief that everyone has a distinct physiological "fingerprint" that cannot be ignored. Finding out your body type may be helpful, but it also may be complicated, and this might give you yet another reason to put off the commitment to healthy eating and exercise. No matter what your body type, these are key to feeling great and maintaining a healthy weight. Use the information about body typing to your advantage. If it helps you get motivated, learn about the system that seems to make the most sense to you. If it makes you feel even more discouraged and overwhelmed, just skip it and use a simple and direct approach instead.

Sizing Up the Popular Diets

Walk into any bookstore and you will find hundreds of books on dieting. The most popular diets have many enthusiastic fans who have initially shed pounds following their program, but more often than not, those same people are not successful at maintaining a healthy weight in the long term. If you look at the overall plan of most popular weight-loss programs, they fall into one of the following categories.

High-Carbohydrate, Low-Fat

According to this diet plan, your fat intake should not exceed 10% of total caloric intake. The majority of calories (70%) should come from carbohydrates and only 20% from proteins. This kind of diet is usually mostly vegetarian, since meat contains high levels of fat and cholesterol. It advocates eating small portions and grazing throughout the day. Studies have found that this kind of diet can be very effective at lowering LDL (bad) cholesterol, and decreasing the risk of heart disease, diabetes, and obesity,[3] especially if emphasis is placed on including nutrient-dense plant-based foods.[4] It's important to focus on the *kind* of carbohydrates that are eaten on this diet. You should choose nutrient-dense, high-fiber vegetables and fruits, *not* processed foods high in sugar. A further modification is to include carbohydrates with a low glycemic index to avoid the release of too much insulin.[5]

However, many people find that they do not feel full or satisfied on this type of program, and they find it hard to follow as a long-term lifestyle. In addition, eating too many carbohydrates (especially processed foods and refined carbohydrates) can lead to insulin imbalance, which ultimately leads to more fat storage by the body. Also, limiting fats for extended periods of time, especially healthy fats, interferes with hormone production and other metabolic processes.

High-Protein, Low-Carbohydrate

The high-protein, low-carb approach is the exact opposite of low-fat, high-carb diets. In this approach, protein is the mainstay of every meal, with high-fat meat and animal products taking center stage, while carbohydrates are completely eliminated for a short time and then slowly reintroduced in limited amounts. Although there are concerns that this raises cholesterol, studies have shown that this approach leads to rapid weight loss, as well as improvements in risk factors for coronary heart disease. High-protein, low-carb diets result in a greater decrease in LDL (bad) cholesterol and triglycerides, and a greater increase in HDL (good) cholesterol, than high-carb, low-fat diets.[6] Metabolic syndrome markers, including high fasting glucose and insulin levels, high plasma triglycerides, low HDL, and high blood pressure, are all normalized quite effectively by following a high-protein, low-carb diet.[7]

High-fat diets are successful because most people find they feel full and satisfied after eating fat, which helps to suppress appetite and cravings. However, there are dangers associated with this diet, especially if it is used for more than a few months. Eating a high-protein, high-fat, low-carbohydrate diet can put the body into a state of ketosis, forcing it to burn stored fat for fuel instead of using carbohydrates from daily consumption. This can put added stress on the liver and kidneys and may cause serious kidney problems if adhered to for long periods of time. Ketosis can also cause some unpleasant side effects, such as headaches and mental fatigue. High-fat diets may be too high in saturated fats, and too low in fiber and several important nutrients, including calcium, vitamin C, vitamin A, folate, and thiamin, which can lead to other health problems.

Mediterranean Diet

The Mediterranean diet refers to a style of eating that is common in countries found around the Mediterranean Sea, such as Turkey, Italy, and Spain. Of course, there are great differences in traditional diets between the many countries in this area, but they have some aspects in common:

- Whole grains, vegetables, beans, nuts, and seeds are emphasized as the mainstay in most meals.
- Consumption of monounsaturated fats, particularly olive oil, is high.
- Red meat is almost never eaten, and fish, poultry, eggs, and dairy products are used as flavor accents, not as the main course.
- Wine is used in moderate amounts.

This eating style is one of the best ways to maintain a healthy weight. It has been proven to be beneficial for heart health and provides protection against other diseases, such as cancer.[8] It supplies a high level of antioxidants and helps the body produce detoxification enzymes, which can help you process the toxins created during weight loss. This kind of diet formed the basis for the Lyon Diet Heart Study, which proved the health benefits of this eating style over an extended period of time (four years). The American Heart Association features the Mediterranean-style diet as a scientifically proven eating program to sustain cardiovascular health.[9] The Mediterranean diet has been scientifically proven to be very effective for weight loss in both short-term and long-term follow-ups. In fact it has been found to be at least as effective as any diet or drug therapy for weight loss, while providing an incredibly rich nutrient base with no known negative effects.[10] That's an impressive track record for such delicious food! The high fat content due to the use of olive oil increases satiation (feeling full), while the emphasis on vegetables ensures the consumption of lots of nutrients while keeping down the calorie count.

The Jump-Start Eating Plan

The eating plan outlined below restricts carbohydrates while focusing on protein and vegetables. Most individuals will experience immediate weight loss after following this eating plan for just one week. You can continue it for up to four weeks and then gradually introduce a wider variety of healthy foods. At the end of this book you'll find an appendix with recipes you can use on this plan that are based on a wide range of delicious whole foods. Before we get into the specifics, here are some general guidelines for the Jump-Start Eating Plan:

- Choose organic and free-range food sources whenever possible.
- Eat only what is on the plan. However, you can add two to three bowls of Detoxifying Vegetable Soup (page 7) daily if you wish.
- Repeat week 1 for the second, third, and fourth weeks.
- Eat normal portions. Eat enough to be satisfied, but do not overeat.
- A protein shake can be used for any breakfast or lunch.
- Meats should be baked, steamed, or grilled, but not fried.
- Salad dressings may only include lemon, olive oil, flaxseed oil, and herbs and spices; no commercial salad dressings.
- Snacks may consist of green peppers, celery, radishes, cucumber, green apples, blueberries, or 10 almonds per day.
- The only beverages allowed are water, coffee, and tea (herbal or green, with no sugar or artificial sweetener).
- No alcohol.
- No artificial sweeteners.
- If you must use a sweetener, choose stevia or organic brown rice syrup.

The Jump-Start Eating Plan

Monday

Breakfast
- 1 hard-boiled egg and 1 to 2 egg whites
- ½ grapefruit
- Coffee or tea without sugar or artificial sweetener

Lunch
- Salad (lettuce, tomatoes, and cucumber)
- Turkey or chicken breast, skinned

Dinner
- Fish, lobster, or shrimp
- Green beans, asparagus, or cauliflower
- 1 slice of low-carb whole-grain bread

Tuesday

Breakfast
- Omelet: 2 eggs
  with low-fat ham, low-fat cheese, and green pepper
- Coffee or tea without sugar or artificial sweetener

Lunch
- Salad (lettuce, celery, and olives)
- Tuna salad (light mayo)

Dinner
- Lamb, veal, or lean pork, trimmed of fat
- Salad (lettuce, tomato, and radishes)
- Broccoli or cauliflower
- 1 slice of low-carb whole-grain bread

Wednesday

Breakfast

- Canadian bacon or turkey sausage, trimmed of fat
- 1 slice of low-carb whole-grain bread
- Coffee or tea without sugar or artificial sweetener

Lunch

- Salad: lettuce, tomato, and cucumber
- Low-fat ham
- Low-fat cheese

Dinner

- Fish, lobster, or shrimp
- Green beans, spinach, or asparagus
- Apple as dessert

Thursday

Breakfast

- Scrambled eggs
- Turkey sausage
- ½ grapefruit
- Coffee or tea without sugar or artificial sweetener

Lunch

- Salad (lettuce, tomato, green peppers, and olives)
- Tuna or salmon salad (light mayo)

Dinner

- Chicken, skinned (white meat only)
- Carrots, green beans, or spinach
- 1 slice of low-carb whole-grain bread

Friday

Breakfast
- ½ cup oat bran with a small amount of skim milk
- Apple or pear

Lunch
- Raw vegetables: carrots, broccoli, bell peppers, or celery
- Turkey, chicken, or low-fat ham

Dinner
- Lean ground sirloin
- Salad (lettuce, tomato, and celery)
- 1 slice low-carb whole-grain bread

Saturday

Breakfast
- Omelet: 2 eggs
  low-fat cheese,
  green peppers
  turkey or Canadian bacon
- Coffee or tea without sugar or artificial sweetener

Lunch
- Raw vegetables: carrots, broccoli, bell peppers, or celery
- Grilled chicken or turkey

Dinner
- Filet mignon or lean steak, trimmed of fat
- Broccoli, cauliflower, asparagus, green beans

Sunday

Breakfast

- ½ grapefruit
- 1 slice of low-carb whole-grain bread
- Coffee or tea without sugar or artificial sweetener

Lunch

- Salad: lettuce, tomato, cucumber, bell pepper, and radishes
- Tuna or salmon salad with light mayo

Dinner

- Filet mignon or lean steak, trimmed of fat
- Broccoli, cauliflower, asparagus, or green beans

nine

Supplements for Weight Loss

People who have decided they want to lose weight will often turn to this chapter first, hoping that there is a one-pill way to achieve weight loss. But this chapter is placed near the end of the book for a good reason. Don't even consider using the information here without first addressing diet, psychological factors, and exercise. Only then is using supplements a reasonable adjunct therapy that will help you fine-tune your overall health and wellness program.

Strange as it sounds, if you have trouble losing weight, you may not be eating enough food. A good weight-loss plan must be based on a well-rounded diet, as a deficiency in one or more essential nutrients may be interfering with your weight-loss goals. These nutrients are often referred to as micronutrients because they are required in much smaller quantities than the macronutrients: proteins, carbohydrates, and fats. A deficiency in any of the micronutrients can cause an imbalance that increases appetite and slows metabolism, both of which lead to fat storage. For example, a deficiency in the nutrient choline (a vitamin B complex cofactor) is known to cause an insatiable appetite.

IN THIS CHAPTER

- Overconsumption and Undernutrition
- Detecting a Nutritional Deficiency
- Success Story: Addressing Nutrient Deficiencies Leads to Weight Loss
- Getting the Nutrients You Need for Weight Loss
- Brown Fat — The Body's Calorie-Burning Furnace
- Supplements to Increase Fat Burning

A healthy diet is the best way to obtain the nutrients needed for weight loss, but a supplement program tailored to your specific nutritional needs can also be valuable. Ideally, you should work with a health-care practitioner or nutritionist to develop a program of nutritional supplementation individualized for you. Whatever approach you take, this chapter will give you much-needed background. I'll discuss the most common nutrient deficiencies associated with weight gain, along with food sources, supplements, and dosage recommendations for each. I'll also discuss herbs that are useful for weight loss, as well as supplements that can provide a boost to your body's fat-burning capacity.

Overconsumption and Undernutrition

Many leading health professionals approach the problem of weight loss by assessing micronutrient deficiencies. They understand that the growing problem of obesity in the United States is due to a nutrient-poor diet. Many Americans do not get enough nutrients in their diet to meet the recommended daily allowance (RDA) for vitamin A, vitamin C, B complex vitamins, and the essential minerals calcium, magnesium, and iron.[1] This is particularly troubling in light of the fact that many nutritional experts consider the RDA standards to be below what is needed for optimum health, even though they may reduce the risk for deficiency diseases.

To understand why we have become so malnourished, it is necessary to look more closely at how our diet has changed. In the early 1900s, most people's diet consisted mostly of whole, unprocessed foods. Things have gone downhill quite rapidly since the late 1970s, with Americans typically eating far fewer nutrient-rich foods, such as whole grains, unrefined cereals, fruits, and vegetables; 150% more refined sugars; and 500% more sweetened beverages, such as soda.[2]

The startling increase in sugar consumption has been matched by a

Total Nutrition in a Box?

Some boxed cereal manufacturers claim that you can obtain all the nutrients you need for an entire day by eating one bowl of their product. Researchers at Tufts University took issue with these claims and demonstrated that the nutrients added to boxed cereals (which are sprayed onto the surface of the flakes) are not efficiently absorbed by the body. For example, the researchers showed that only 2% of the supplemental iron added to cereal is effectively absorbed by the body. Zinc is even more problematic, as its absorption is inhibited by the presence of fiber in the cereal and the calcium in milk — so much so that virtually no zinc will be absorbed from this food source.

corresponding rise in consumption of harmful fats, such as trans fats. Today, two-thirds of the average American diet consists entirely of high-calorie sugars and fats. The result is that we are eating more but getting less of what we need to stay healthy. While the decline in the American diet can be attributed, in part, to the popularity of junk foods, even some so-called healthy food choices fail to deliver adequate quantities of nutrients. For example, canned vegetable soup, considered by most to be a healthy choice, generally contains few nutrients. Although the ingredients used in these foods may be high in vitamins, enzymes, and other nutrients, high-heat processing often destroys their value.

While some manufacturers try to compensate for the destruction of nutrients in their products by artificially adding some of the nutrients back in, this method rarely is able to restore the nutritive value available in the raw, unprocessed food.

Food quality has also been affected by changes in agricultural practices. Over the past century, commercial farmers have adopted intensive cropping methods that rely on large quantities of synthetic chemical fertilizers. The fertilizers return only a fraction of the vital minerals that growing plants remove from the soil. Consequently, the mineral content of American soils, along with the nutritive value of plants, has steadily declined. Since 1948, levels of the essential minerals iron, manganese, and copper have declined significantly in a variety of crops. The iron content of lettuce, for example, has dropped from an average of 52 mg per 100 grams in 1948 to a mere 0.5 mg today.[3]

Detecting a Nutritional Deficiency

Which nutrients you need to supplement and how much you need to take, beyond what you get in your diet, depends on your individual biochemical needs. It can take years of personal research and experimentation to put together a good dietary and supplement program. To eliminate a lot of the guesswork and frustration, consult a qualified health professional trained in the intricacies of nutritional biochemistry, who can help you assess your needs and develop an effective, individualized program. The following tests can be used to analyze your nutrient status, pinpoint specific deficiencies, and provide a basis for recommending supplement dosages that best suit your needs. (Refer to Resources for information on laboratories that perform these tests.)

Blood tests: Many mainstream physicians assess nutritional status using blood tests. These tests measure nutrient concentrations only in the blood serum, the liquid fraction of blood, and not in the blood cells (the globular or nonliquid fraction of blood). The cells are generally separated out and discarded. Unfortunately, a good deal of information about an individual's nutritional status is thrown out along with these cells. Whole blood analysis, which examines both the serum and the blood cells, is not commonly done since most mainstream physicians are looking at blood primarily to diagnose a disease and serum testing is generally adequate for that purpose. As most mainstream physicians are oriented toward using drugs to treat symptoms, they have no interest in nutritional status and are thus not inclined to order the proper tests. Additional restrictions due to regulations of HMOs may deter physicians from ordering appropriate in-depth testing.

Hair analysis: This methodology measures the body's levels of various minerals, including calcium, iron, magnesium, potassium, and zinc, among others. As the hair is considered a storage organ, it provides a biochemical record of nutritional status over a period of several months. Hair analysis can also uncover high levels of toxic metals, such as mercury and aluminum. Hair analysis does not assess vitamin deficiency, however, so other testing procedures are needed to augment the findings of a hair analysis.

Individualized Optimal Nutrition (ION) Panel: This test uses blood and urine samples to measure levels 150 biochemical components. Specifically, it checks for nutritional status in categories including vitamins, minerals, amino acids, fatty and organic acids, lipid peroxides, general blood chemistry (cholesterol, thyroid hormone, glucose), and antioxidants.

Functional Intracellular Analysis (FIA): Another accurate and comprehensive technique, the FIA measures how micronutrients are naturally functioning within the activities of living white blood cells rather than simply measuring micronutrient levels in the blood. This nutritional assay must be ordered by a health-care professional, but the lab will refer individuals to nutritionally oriented practitioners in their area.

Success Story: Addressing Nutrient Deficiencies Leads to Weight Loss

Julia, 51, weighed 302 pounds and suffered from severe fatigue. She claimed that her shortness of breath was sometimes so severe that she could not walk and breathe at the same time. In addition, she complained of night sweats, disturbed sleep, loss of concentration, colds, fevers, sore throats, and constant hunger. Although she tried to control her eating habits, she frequently binged, practically inhaling food as though she couldn't get enough.

Julia decided to seek treatment from a nutritional medicine specialist. After taking Julia's complete history and having her undergo a comprehensive nutritional analysis, he discovered that Julia was seriously deficient in vitamin B_{12} and the mineral chromium, and had a slight manganese deficiency. These deficiencies had severely impaired Julia's metabolism, making it difficult for her to burn fat. Julia was started on vitamin B_{12} shots, along with oral supplements of chromium and manganese. Within three days, she stopped having hunger pangs. She also began feeling full after eating an ordinary meal and felt satisfied between meals.

Julia was instructed to eliminate all white flour and sugar from her diet and continue on a regimen of supplements that included vitamins A, C, and E, iron, beta-carotene, lysine, and garlic. Since Julia had also tested positive for candida, her doctor also prescribed antifungal agents for two months, including caprylic acid and acidophilus. After several weeks, Julia began to respond. Her energy returned and her hunger subsided. In six months, she lost 63 pounds. After a year, she had lost slightly over 100 pounds and felt like she had a new lease on life. She was able to walk longer distances without experiencing shortness of breath, and needless to say, she felt much healthier and happier.

Getting the Nutrients You Need for Weight Loss

The best way to get the nutrients your body needs to lose weight is by eating healthy food. Instead of fretting about calories, start focusing on whether the food you are eating is wholesome and rich in essential nutrients. The place to start is with a whole foods diet. Stop eating processed, refined foods, fried foods, and anything adulterated with artificial sweeteners and other additives. Instead fill your diet with healthy and delicious alternatives. Giving up unhealthful foods doesn't entail deprivation. It means choosing from a wide variety of vegetables, fruits, and grains; raw seeds and nuts and their butters; beans; fermented milk products, such as yogurt and kefir; and fish, poultry, and bean products like tofu.

Yet even a whole foods diet may not succeed in satisfying all of your nutritional requirements. The declining nutrient content of plants makes it difficult to obtain an adequate intake of many essential nutrients. In addition, exposure to environmental toxins, such as exhaust fumes, industrial chemicals and wastes, and agricultural pesticides, puts a heavy demand on the body's detoxification systems, which tends to deplete nutrient reserves even further. Moreover, if you restrict your calorie intake to 1,500 to 2,000 calories per day, you are unlikely to consume even the fairly minimal recommended dietary allowance (RDA) of most essential vitamins and minerals. All of these factors make nutritional supplementation essential to maintaining good health and controlling body weight.

Essential and Accessory Micronutrients

Essential nutrients are those nutrients the body cannot manufacture on its own and must derive from food (or supplements). Absolutely necessary for human life, these nutrients include at least 13 vitamins and 15 minerals. Essential vitamins are broken up into two groups, fat-soluble and water-soluble. The fat-soluble essential vitamins include vitamins A, D, E, and K. The water-soluble essential vitamins are C (ascorbic acid), B_1 (thiamin), B_2 (riboflavin), B_3 (niacin), B_5 (pantothenic acid), B_6 (pyridoxine), B_{12}, folic acid, and biotin. The essential minerals include calcium, magnesium, phosphorus, iron, zinc, copper, manganese, iodine, chromium, potassium, sodium, and a number of trace elements. The nutrients listed above form necessary elements of body tissues, fluids, and other organs and play an active role in the body's regulatory functions.

In addition to the essential nutrients, there are "accessory nutrients," cofactors that work in harmony with the essential nutrients to aid in the breakdown and conversion of food into cellular energy and help support all of the body's physical and mental functions. Some of the key accessory nutrients include the vitamin B complex cofactors choline and inositol, coenzyme Q10 (which acts like a spark plug for cellular energy), and lipoic acid. Other accessory nutrients that have demonstrated preventative functions include the B complex cofactor PABA (para-aminobenzoic acid) and bioflavonoids (substances that enhance the beneficial effects of vitamin C).

Vitamins and minerals that work to control body weight can be separated into two general categories: energy nutrients, which are principally involved in the conversion of food to energy; and protector nutrients, which help defend the cells against damaging toxins from drugs, alcohol, radiation, environmental pollutants, or the body's own enzyme processes. Examples of protector nutrients are vitamins C and E, beta-carotene, and the minerals zinc, copper, manganese, and selenium, which play a critical role as antioxidants in preventing the effects of damaging free radicals. Both categories are vital to the management of body weight. Without enough energy nutrients, calories cannot be burned in the body's cells and instead are stored as fat. And when protector nutrients are scarce, cells are damaged by free radicals and other harmful substances, resulting in impaired metabolism and weight gain. These nutrients often work synergistically, each enhancing the other's function.

Let's take a look at the key micronutrients that can support healthy weight maintenance. In addition to vitamins and minerals, the sections below will discuss amino acids, green foods, and fiber. I'll explain how each substance works in your body and provide information on the best dietary sources of each, as well as supplement forms and standard daily dosages.

Vitamins

A good quality multivitamin formula is helpful for general dietary support. In addition, a number of vitamins have been shown to be useful specifically for weight loss.

Vitamin A and Beta-Carotene

Vitamin A facilitates the efficient absorption of nutrients by strengthening the lining of the digestive tract. Along with vitamins C and E, it strengthens the immune system and thus makes the body more resistant to infection from parasites and yeast overgrowth, two common causes of weight gain. Vitamin A is also necessary for the production of thyroxine, a thyroid hormone, and helps the thyroid to absorb iodine, a key nutrient. The healthy functioning of the thyroid is essential to maintaining effective metabolism and preventing the accumulation of body fat. The body obtains vitamin A from food sources or manufactures it through the conversion of carotenes (alpha, beta, and gamma). Because high levels of vitamin A can be toxic, it is usually safer to supplement with carotenes, which the body will convert into sufficient amounts of vitamin A.

Beta-carotene is not only a precursor to vitamin A, it also has additional antioxidant properties not found in vitamin A. For most people, beta-carotene is the preferred source of vitamin A, most vitamin A supplements found in health food stores are actually beta-carotene. The only exception is people with an impaired thyroid, because they cannot effectively convert beta-carotene to its biologically usable form.

 Prolonged intake of excessive doses of vitamins A, D, B3, and possibly B6 may produce toxic effects. In addition, anyone currently under medical care, taking medications, or with a history of health problems should always consult a health-care professional (preferably one knowledgeable about nutrition) before making any changes in diet or using supplements.

Food sources of vitamin A: Fish oil (such as cod liver oil), liver, chile peppers, carrots, dried apricots, sweet potatoes, and leafy greens.

Vitamin A supplements: Those with impaired thyroid function typically should take 10,000 IU to 20,000 IU of vitamin A daily in a form that is already converted from beta-carotene.

Precautions: Very high levels of vitamin A can cause headaches and irritability and can be toxic; high levels should be avoided during pregnancy.[4]

Typical recommended dosage: Unless closely supervised by a physician, your intake of pure vitamin A should at no time exceed 25,000 IU per day.

Food sources of carotenes: All yellow and green vegetables, including carrots, beet greens, spinach, and broccoli.

Supplements: Most multivitamins contain beta-carotene.

Typical recommended dose: 10,000 to 30,000 IU.

Vitamin B Complex

The B vitamins (collectively known as B complex) nutritionally support the brain, eyes, intestines, liver, muscles, and skin. They act as a team to help maintain healthy energy metabolism, which is crucial for burning off calories and avoiding weight gain. Stress levels, diet, and lifestyle can deplete the body's store of B vitamins.

Vitamin B₁ (Thiamin) and Vitamin B₂ (Riboflavin)

Vitamins B_1 and B_2 primarily serve in the maintenance of mucous membranes, formation of red blood cells, and metabolism of carbohydrates. Deficiencies of vitamin B_1 may lead to blood sugar imbalances.

Food sources: Brewer's yeast is an excellent source of both of these vitamins.

Supplements: B1 and B2 are commonly found in B complex supplements.

Typical recommended dosage: 25 mg to 100 mg daily.

Vitamin B3 (Niacin)

Niacin is necessary for transport of oxygen in the blood, and formation of fatty acids and nucleic acids. It is also vital to the actions of more than 150 enzymes in the body, and without these enzymatic reactions, the body's energy production would quickly shut down. Low levels of B_3 can cause muscle weakness, fatigue, skin sores, irritability, and depression. Eating a diet high in refined sugar or prolonged use of antibiotics deplete B_3 reserves in the body.

Food sources: Meat, chicken, fish, peanuts, wheat germ, brewer's yeast, and whole grains, particularly rice.

Supplements: Niacin, the natural form of vitamin B_3, is available in supplement form. When taken in dosages of over 100 mg, niacin can cause a very distinctive flushing, tingling, and redness that begins in the lower part of the body and moves up to the face, hands, and head.[5] Niacinamide causes no flushing and is the form found in many supplements. However, there is some evidence that this form is less effective for lowering blood lipids.[6]

Typical recommended dosage: 50 mg.

Precautions: Liver enzymes may be affected by taking high levels of B_3 or niacinamide. Another form of B_3, inositol hexaniacinate, has shown no toxicity and may be the best choice for this supplement.

Vitamin B5 (Pantothenic Acid)

Vitamin B_5 is vital for the synthesis of hormones and support of the adrenal glands. A deficiency can cause fatigue, insomnia, and depression.[7] B_5 is also involved in lipid metabolism. Even a mild deficiency of pantothenic acid can raise triglyceride levels.[8] Pantothenic acid can be a useful weight-reducing agent, in part by helping to decrease hunger.[9]

Food sources: Liver, meat, chicken, whole grains, and legumes. Eating a variety of foods can ensure adequate levels of vitamin B5.

Supplements: Pantothenic acid is the usual source, although at times pantothine, which is a byproduct of pantothenic acid, is used instead.

Typical recommended dosage: 10 mg to 2,000 mg.

Vitamin B6 (Pyridoxine)

Vitamin B_6 strongly influences the immune and nervous systems. It aids in fat and protein metabolism and the conversion of the amino acid tryptophan to the brain neurotransmitter serotonin, which helps to control appetite. B_6 is also essential in the production of prostaglandins, which influence a variety of biological processes, including strengthening the immune system and controlling inflammation. A prostaglandin imbalance may cause some people to develop food sensitivities and allergies, leading to food addictions and other reactions that frequently cause weight gain. Deficiencies are rare, but suboptimum levels of B_6 can occur as a result of eating a diet high in fats and low in fruits and vegetables. Supplementation with B_6 has helped kidney transplant patients avoid obesity.[10]

Food sources: Brewer's yeast, whole grains, legumes, nuts, and seeds.

Supplements: There are two forms of B6, pyridoxine hydrochloride and pyridoxal-5-phosphate (the most active form).

Typical recommended dosage: 50 mg.

Precautions: High levels of pyridoxine (over 250 mg per day) can cause toxic side effects.[11]

Vitamin B₁₂ (Cobalamin, Methylcobalamin)

Vitamin B_{12} is virtually absent in vegetable food sources, which means vegans are likely to be deficient in this vitamin. B_{12} is essential for normal formation of red blood cells and maintenance of the nervous system and mucous membrane linings. These linings are important for the proper absorption of nutrients and to prevent parasites and other pathogens from entering the body.

Food sources: Meat, most fish (especially trout, mackerel, and herring), egg yolks, and yogurt.

Supplements: B_{12} can be taken in sublingual or nasal spray forms, or via injection.

Typical recommended dosage: 10 to 500 mcg daily.

Choline

Choline is a B vitamin that helps the body break down fats and transport them in and out of cells. It is particularly important in helping to clear the liver of fats by keeping cholesterol from solidifying in the gallbladder.

Food sources: Choline is found in lecithin (used as a thickener in some foods) and is also present in high amounts in egg yolks, meat, milk, whole grains, and soybeans. Lecithin granules, which can be sprinkled on salads, cereals, and casseroles, are a good source. Lecithin is also present in the herb chickweed (*Stellaria media*).

Supplements: Choline is available in lecithin capsules or as phosphatidylcholine.

Typical recommended dosage: 100 to 200 mg per day, or 1 to 2 tablespoons of lecithin granules per day.

Folic Acid (Folacin, Folate)

Folic acid is important for red blood cell formation, breakdown and utilization of proteins, and proper cell division, which is especially important in the early stages of pregnancy (folic acid prevents spina bifida and neural tube defects). It is also useful for anemia, atherosclerosis, fatigue, immune weakness, infection, and osteoporosis.

Food sources: Green leafy vegetables such as spinach and kale, asparagus, broccoli, lima beans, green peas, sweet potatoes, bean sprouts, whole wheat, cantaloupe, strawberries, and brewer's yeast.

Supplements: The folic acid content in foods can be depleted by cooking, so supplementation may be necessary.

Typical recommended dosage: 400 mcg daily.

Inositol

Inositol is important for the eyes, intestines, and bone marrow. It assists in metabolizing fats in the blood and liver and lowers cholesterol. Inositol helps control arteriosclerosis (hardening of the arteries) and hypertension.

Food sources: Whole grains, citrus fruits, brewer's yeast, liver, cabbage, and some nuts. Caffeinated beverages can deplete the body of inositol.

Supplements: Inositol is best taken in combination with other B vitamins.

Typical recommended dosage: 500 mg daily.

Para-Aminobenzoic Acid (PABA)

PABA is important for the skin, hair pigment (color), and blood cell formation. PABA aids in the metabolism and assimilation of amino acids (proteins) and is essential for the growth of "friendly" intestinal bacteria and supports their production of vitamin B_{12}.

Food sources: Brewer's yeast, wheat germ, whole grains, and eggs.

Supplements: PABA should be taken in a time-released form.

Typical recommended dosage: 50 to 100 mg, three times daily.

Vitamin C (Ascorbic Acid)

Vitamin C is an important antioxidant and also helps to keep the adrenal glands and the thyroid healthy and functioning. Vitamin C is particularly important when the body is under stress, as stress severely impacts the adrenal glands.[12] Damage to the adrenals can, in turn, cause shortages of protective hormones, such as DHEA, leading to diminished energy and overeating, as the body attempts to compensate for low energy levels. This may deprive the body of essential nutrients, which can prompt urgent food cravings. A vitamin C deficiency can also cause capillaries in the thyroid to bleed, and normal cells in the gland to multiply abnormally, a condition called hyperplasia. Blood plasma vitamin C levels are lower in people with high waist-to-hip ratios, one of the indicators of obesity, probably due to poor dietary patterns and high levels of oxidative stress.[13]

Food sources: Most fruits and vegetables, including oranges, grapefruit, kiwis, lemons, avocado, parsley, leafy greens, kale, collard, and broccoli. Red chile peppers have over seven times more vitamin C than oranges.

Supplements: Esterified vitamin C, may be absorbed more efficiently because it is retained for a longer period of time by body tissues. Because it isn't acidic, esterified vitamin C is also less likely to cause gastrointestinal distress.[14]

Typical recommended dosage: 100 to 200 mg.[15] Many holistic practitioners recommend higher doses of 1,000 to 2,000 mg per day.

Vitamin E (Alpha-Tocopherol)

Vitamin E is one of the primary agents used to protect cell membranes against the damage caused by environmental pollutants. Since chemical exposure can lead to a toxic liver, lymph, or colon—three conditions that contribute to weight gain—vitamin E should be an important component of any weight-loss program. A study of teenage boys found that those who were overweight (more than 30% over their ideal weight) had half the blood levels of vitamin E as teenage boys of normal weight.[16] A vitamin E deficiency can also reduce iodine absorption by the thyroid. When the thyroid lacks iodine, it secretes fewer hormones, resulting in hypothyroidism and a sluggish metabolism.

Food sources: Cold-pressed polyunsaturated vegetable oils (such as sunflower and safflower), leafy green vegetables, avocados, nuts, seeds, and whole grains.

Supplements: Vitamin E is actually a group of compounds called tocopherols. When purchasing supplements of vitamin E, avoid products that contain vitamin E in the "dl" form — this means that it is a petroleum-based synthetic form of the vitamin. The natural form of vitamin E will be designated only with the letter "d." The best form will be called natural mixed tocopherols and will include alpha-, beta-, and gamma-tocopherols.

Typical recommended dosage: 30 IU daily; for those suffering from hypothyroidism, 800 to 1,200 IU per day.

Minerals

A combination mineral formula is generally recommended for dietary support, and several minerals have specific actions helpful for weight loss.

Calcium

Calcium consumption has been found to have specific weight-loss benefits. Population studies have found that people who consume more calcium tend to be thinner than people who have low calcium consumption.[17] People who are overweight have been shown to experience increased weight loss if they include calcium-rich foods as part of a healthy diet.[18] Most studies have concluded that the calcium found in dairy products appears to be more effective to aid weight loss than calcium taken as a supplement.[19] Calcium supports healthy weight through several mechanisms, including reducing the accumulation of body fat and increasing thermogenic activity, which breaks down fat cells.[20]

Antioxidants

An antioxidant is a natural biochemical substance that protects living cells from the damaging effects of free radicals. Free radicals cause oxidation, the same chemical process that causes metal to rust and apples to turn brown. In the body, if left uncontrolled, free radicals cause cell membranes to erode and die, leading to a variety of degenerative conditions. Produced as a by-product of cellular activities, free radicals are typically neutralized and rendered harmless by antioxidants. But when environmental and other toxins (such as poor diet, pollution, stress, or cigarettes) introduce an increased burden of free radicals, the body's reserve of antioxidants is quickly exhausted. Nutrients and biochemicals that act as antioxidants fall into many different categories:

- Amino acids: cysteine, glutathione, methionine

- Bioflavonoids: anthocyanins (found in fruit, especially grapes, cranberries, and bilberries), citrus bioflavonoids, oligomeric proanthocyanidins (found in pine bark or grape seed extract)

- Carotene: alpha- and beta-carotene (found in red, yellow, and dark green fruits and vegetables), lycopene (found in red fruits and vegetables, such as red grapefruit and tomatoes)

- Spices: cayenne pepper, garlic, turmeric

- Herbs: astragalus, bilberry, green tea, ginkgo, milk thistle, sage

- Minerals: copper, manganese, selenium, zinc

- Vitamins: A, B1, C, and E

- Enzymes: catalase, glutathione peroxidase, superoxide dismutase

- Hormones: melatonin

- Miscellaneous: coenzyme Q10, lipoic acid, NADH (nicotinamide adenine dinucleotide)

Food sources: Dairy is calcium rich, but some forms of dairy are healthier than others. Good choices include organic unsweetened yogurt, organic feta cheese, and organic cottage cheese. Kale and almonds are good nondairy sources of calcium.

Supplements: To maintain bone health, 1000 to 1500 mg per day of calcium (including food sources and supplements) is recommended (varies with age, weight, sex, etc.). It is often difficult to get this amount through diet alone; supplementation is often called for. This can be confusing, due to the many forms of calcium on the market, the differences in dosage levels, absorption rates, delivery forms (i.e., tablets, vs. liquids), cost, etc. Calcium citrate is absorbed better than tricalcium phosphate, calcium lactate, and calcium carbonate, (the kind of calcium in antacid tablets). Calcium citrate does not tend to cause gastric distress, and has a pleasant taste.

Typical recommended dosage: between 1000 to 1500 mg per day.

Chromium

Chromium is a mineral essential for regulating the production of the hormone insulin, which is responsible for stabilizing blood sugar levels and preventing the conversion of blood sugar into fat. Although the body requires only small amounts of this important mineral, Americans are more likely to be deficient in chromium than any other micronutrient. Chromium is found in the outer bran portion of grains, but much of it is lost in the processing of white flour (the staple ingredient in most refined bread and pasta products) and white rice. The chromium that we do obtain from food sources can be depleted in our bodies by various factors, including a high-carbohydrate diet, infections, repeated pregnancies, air pollution, exposure to radiation, and physical and emotional stress. The urinary excretion of chromium can increase as much as fiftyfold under stress.[21] Chromium has been shown to help add lean muscle tissue and reduce body fat.[22] Regular chromium supplementation can be useful for both general health and weight management.

Food sources: An excellent source of chromium is brewer's yeast (available in powder form or in tablets). Other good choices are wheat germ, beef, chicken, liver, whole grains, potatoes, eggs, apples, bananas, and spinach.

Supplements: Chromium and other minerals are better absorbed in the body when bound into a "transporter" molecule, called a chelate.[23] Chromium polynicotinate is a chelated variety that is chemically bound to niacin, a B complex vitamin. According to some researchers, this form of chromium is superior to either chromium chloride or chromium picolinate.

Typical recommended dosage: 200 mcg per day.

Iodine

Along with the minerals copper, zinc, and selenium, iodine is part of the structure of thyroid hormones (especially thyroxine), which regulate how fast the body burns calories. As the metabolism of all the body's cells (except for brain cells) is influenced by thyroid hormones, iodine's effects are far-reaching. Iodine deficiency most typically results in hypothyroidism, which may subsequently cause weight gain and fatigue. For many people with hypothyroidism, simply adding more iodine-containing foods to the diet is often enough to restore thyroid function.

Food sources: Kelp and other sea vegetables, cod liver oil, fish (haddock, cod, halibut, and herring), and iodized salt. People using sea salt as a replacement for table salt should consider supplementing with kelp, a vegetable rich in elemental iodine. Certain foods, called goitrogens, prevent iodine absorption. These include soybeans, turnips, cabbage, and pine nuts, especially if eaten raw.

Supplements: Supplements often contain inorganic iodine (such as sodium iodide and potassium iodide), which is not as beneficial as elemental iodine.

Typical recommended dosage: 100 mcg for women and 120 mcg for men.

Precautions: Too much iodine can suppress the formation of the thyroid hormone T3.

Iron

Iron is essential to red blood cell synthesis, oxygen transport, and energy production. A diet low in iron causes anemia, which has also been found to cause hypothyroidism.[24] An iron deficiency can also decrease hydrochloric acid in the stomach, impairing digestion and contributing to further nutritional deficiencies. People who follow low-calorie diets are particularly vulnerable to developing iron deficiencies.[25]

Food sources: Kelp, organ meats, egg yolk, blackstrap molasses, lecithin, almonds, walnuts and brazil nuts, millet, and parsley.

Supplements: The heme form of iron, found in desiccated liver or liquid liver extract supplements, is most easily absorbed and has fewer side effects. Of the nonheme forms, ferrous fumerate and ferrous succinate are recommended.

Typical recommended dosage: To ensure the proper functioning of the thyroid, the recommended dose is 100 mcg per day.

Precautions: Ferrous sulfate, commonly used in conventional supplements, can cause the production of free radicals and should be avoided. Elevated levels of iron in the blood are associated with an increased risk for heart attacks and other cardiovascular problems, as well as low immunity.[26] Overdose in infants can cause serious reactions or be fatal, so be sure that all iron supplements are out of the reach of children. Women who are menopausal and those who experience a heavy menstrual flow should consult their physician to determine an appropriate level of supplementation.

Selenium

Selenium plays an important role in maintaining balance among the thyroid hormones.[27] It is an important constituent of the antioxidant enzyme glutathione peroxidase, which protects the body from free radical damage. Selenium also protects against the absorption of toxic heavy metals such as aluminum, mercury, and lead.[28]

Food sources: Wheat germ, Brazil nuts, bran, and Swiss chard.

Supplements: Avoid multimineral supplements that contain sodium selenite, an organic salt that is not well absorbed. Organic selenium from yeast or the chelated mineral (such as selenomethionine) are better sources.

Typical recommended dosage: 200 to 1,000 mcg per day; those with thyroid imbalance should limit supplementation to 200 mcg per day.

Precautions: Selenium toxicity is possible but rare. An overdose can cause hair loss, nail malformations, weakness, and slowed mental function.[29]

Zinc

Zinc helps in the conversion of the thyroid hormone T4 to the more-active T3 form, increases the sensitivity of cell membranes to these hormones, and serves as a building block of the hormone thyroxine. Vegetarians are often deficient in zinc because beans, legumes, and grains —staples of a vegetarian diet—are high in the substance phytate, which lowers absorption of zinc by the body.[30]

Food sources: Meat, whole grains, nuts, seeds, oysters, shellfish, and pumpkin seeds.

Supplements: Zinc sulfate, found in many multivitamin-multimineral preparations, is not easily absorbed by the body. Other forms of zinc that are more readily absorbed are zinc picolinate, zinc citrate, and zinc monomethionine.

Typical recommended dosage: 25 mg of zinc per day, along with 3 mg of copper (zinc tends to deplete copper reserves).

Precautions: With medical supervision, the dosage of zinc could be increased, if necessary. However, dosages should be increased with caution, as too much zinc can interfere with the functioning of the

A Guide to Taking Supplements

In addition to knowing which supplements to take, it is also important to know how and when to take them. It is best to develop an individualized supplement program by working with a health-care practitioner who is knowledgeable in the correct use of nutritional supplements, such as a licensed naturopathic physician. Jeffrey Bland, Ph.D., and Lindsey Berkson, D.C., offer some basic guidelines for the correct use of supplements:

- Most nutritional supplements should be taken with meals to promote increased absorption. Fat-soluble nutrients (such as vitamins A and E, beta-carotene, and essential fatty acids) should be taken during the day with the meal that contains the most fat.

- Amino acid supplements should be taken on an empty stomach one hour before or after a meal. Take them with fruit juice to help promote absorption. When taking an increased dosage of an isolated amino acid, be sure to supplement with an amino acid blend, for balance.

- When taking an increased dosage of an isolated B vitamin, be sure to supplement with B complex, again, for balance.

- If you become nauseated when you take supplements in capsule or tablet form, consider taking a liquid form, diluted in a beverage.

- If you are taking high doses, do not take all of your supplements at one time; divide them into smaller doses throughout the day.

 If you become nauseated or ill within an hour after taking supplements, take the supplements with food. If you still have an adverse response, discontinue use.

- Take digestive enzymes with meals to assist digestion. If you are taking pancreatic enzymes for other therapeutic reasons, be sure to take them on an empty stomach between meals.

- Do not take mineral supplements with high-fiber meals, as fiber can decrease absorption of minerals.

- When taking nutrients, be sure to drink adequate amounts of liquid to mix with digestive juices and prevent side effects.

immune system. Toxicity of zinc is rarely reported, however prolonged use of over 150 mg a day can cause anemia.

Amino Acids

Amino acids are the building blocks of proteins, which are constructed from chains of amino acids linked together. Proteins are, in turn, the building blocks of the body. Twenty-two amino acids are vital to the body's growth, development, and maintenance. Some are manufactured in the body, while others, called essential amino acids, must be obtained from the diet or nutritional supplements. Semi-essential amino acids are those that can be made by the body in amounts adequate to maintain basic protein requirements; however, during times of growth or stress additional amounts are required and must be obtained from foods or supplements.

Amino acid deficiency may be an underlying factor, often undetected, for many common disorders. Vegetarians and vegans (vegetarians who eat no eggs or dairy products) with a limited diet may have difficulty meeting dietary protein requirements and should take an amino acid complex supplement. However, a well-rounded vegetarian diet provides sufficient amino acids, so this is generally not a concern. Amino acid supplementation is also valuable to athletes, bodybuilders, people who routinely experience mental or physical stress, and dieters who are trying to prevent sugar or carbohydrate cravings. Let's take a look at the amino acids that are particularly useful for people trying to lose weight. The branched-chain amino acids (BCAAs)—isoleucine, leucine, and valine—are of particular interest for weight loss and body building, as they're important in formation of muscles and muscle metabolism. They're most effective for this purpose when taken together in balanced proportions.

- Isoleucine aids in production of energy, formation of hemoglobin (which carries oxygen in blood), and regulation of energy from blood sugars. Since it assists in the metabolism and formation of muscles, isoleucine is a useful supplement for bodybuilders.

- Leucine helps heal injured or weakened muscles, fractured or weakened bones, and skin conditions or injuries. Leucine can also be used as a nutritional support for postsurgery recovery. It reduces excessive blood sugar levels and is a good source of fuel during prolonged workouts or exercise.

- Valine can be used by the body to produce energy and is important for the formation, metabolism, and repair of muscle tissue. It has a natural stimulating effect.

- Lysine assists in the formation of antibodies, enzymes, and hormones. It helps develop bones by assisting in the metabolism of calcium from the intestinal tract. Lysine is also useful for building muscles and for recovering from surgery or muscular and sports injuries.

- Methionine is the one of the body's sources of organic sulfur (which must be constantly replaced) and is a potent antioxidant. It aids with detoxification, protects against radiation damage, and helps prevent excessive accumulation of fats in the liver and vascular system.

- Phenylalanine is a precursor of the neurotransmitters dopamine and norepinephrine, which regulate mood, promote alertness, and enhance memory and cognitive function. It is used for certain types of depression, headaches (especially migraine), menstrual cramps, and Parkinson's disease. It also helps with weight loss by acting as a natural appetite suppressant.

- Arginine is most needed during times of growth (childhood or pregnancy) and great stress. It stimulates the release of human growth hormone (HGH) and is important for muscle metabolism, increasing muscle mass while decreasing body fat. It also combats physical and mental fatigue and enhances immune function.

- Alanine promotes immunity and assists the body in metabolizing glucose, which serves as fuel for the brain, nervous system, and muscles. Hypoglycemia may be associated with low alanine levels. Alanine assists in the metabolism of organic acids in the body and is important for the formation of vitamin B5.

- Glutamic acid is a neurotransmitter important for brain metabolism. It assists in transporting potassium across the blood-brain barrier and in detoxifying ammonia in the brain. Important for the metabolism of other amino acids, fats, and sugars, glutamic acid is useful for balancing hypoglycemia (low blood sugar) and overcoming fatigue.

- Glutamine assists in improving mental alertness and memory. It can readily pass through the blood-brain barrier and be converted into glutamic acid (see above). It also increases levels of GABA (gamma-aminobutyric acid), a central nervous system neurotransmitter important for brain function and mental ability. It has been used to treat alcoholism and alcohol poisoning, mental illness, and degenerative brain conditions. Glutamine helps stop alcohol and sugar cravings and aids in the absorption of minerals into the tissues. Glutamine also assists in the formation of muscles.

- Glycine has a calming effect on the brain and is important for central nervous system function. It supports immune function, promotes the healing of wounds, and assists in the conversion of stored sugars into energy. Glycine is used as a sweetener and is also a building block for other amino acids.

- Ornithine stimulates the release of growth hormone. When taken with arginine and carnitine, it has the effect of increasing muscle mass while decreasing body fat. Ornithine is needed for a healthy liver, as it detoxifies ammonia from the liver and is involved in liver regeneration. It supports immune function and tissue repair and healing.

- Serine is a component of brain proteins and the fatty myelin sheaths that protect nerves. It is a source of stored energy for the liver and muscles and helps metabolize fats, oils, and fatty acids. It also is important for muscle growth and a healthy immune system.

- Taurine is the primary building block for other amino acids and is crucial for the proper assimilation of calcium, magnesium, potassium, and sodium. It is important in the formation of bile and is a component of white blood cells, skeletal and heart muscles, and the tissues of the central nervous system. Taurine supports normal brain function and has been used to help control hyperactivity, epilepsy, and nervous system imbalance caused by alcohol or drug abuse. It has also been used to treat atherosclerosis (fatty buildup in the arteries), heart disorders, high blood pressure, hypoglycemia, and seizures.

- Tyrosine is a building block of the neurotransmitters norepinephrine and dopamine, which help regulate mood, appetite, anxiety, and depression. It helps regulate the adrenal, pituitary, and thyroid glands and increases muscle growth while reducing body fat.

When buying amino acids, look for USP pharmaceutical grade, L-crystalline, free-form amino acids. *USP* means that the product meets the standards of purity and potency set by a reference book called *The United States Pharmacopeia*. The term *free-form* refers to the highest level of purity of the amino acid. The *L* refers to one of the two forms in which most amino acids come, designated D- and L- (as in D-lysine or L-lysine). The L-form amino acids are proper for human biochemistry, as proteins in the human body are made from this form. The exception is phenylalanine, which consists of a combination of the D- and L- forms (thus DL-phenylalanine is the preferred form of this amino acid).

Other Nutrients for Weight Loss

A number of other nutrients have proven to be helpful for supporting weight-loss programs, especially "green foods" and fiber.

"Green Foods"

Green foods are rich in vitamins, minerals, and chlorophyll, the green pigment found in most plants. Chlorophyll has long been used as a healing agent and is well-known for its antiaging and highly nutritive properties. It helps heal wounds of the skin and internal membranes, stimulates the growth of new cells, and hinders the growth of bacteria. Important to detoxifying, chlorophyll also promotes regularity and is excellent for detoxifying and healing the liver. Chlorella and spirulina are excellent sources of chlorophyll, and both are easily taken in supplement form. Sprouted barley grass and wheatgrass, available at most health food stores and usually consumed in the form of juice, are also good sources.

 Generally, it is not advisable to take individual amino acids for extended or indefinite periods as this can create an imbalance of other amino acids in the body and possibly cause other health conditions. If you use individual amino acids for any reason, follow this course of treatment with a complex of free-form amino acids to ensure balanced nutrition. Please consult a qualified health-care professional before beginning such therapies. Individual amino acids often come with warnings or precautions for women who are pregnant or for people with certain health conditions.

Chlorella, a freshwater single-celled green algae, is more popular than vitamin C in Japan. There are an estimated 5 million people taking this algae every day. Chlorella is approximately 60% protein, and contains all the essential amino acids, 20 different vitamins and minerals, and high levels of carotenoids and chlorophyll. It has very high levels of RNA and DNA, which support tissue repair and healing. An antioxidant, chlorella is well documented for its ability to remove heavy metals and pesticides.[31] Chlorella absorbs toxins from the intestines and promotes the growth of healthy intestinal flora, both important for weight loss.

Spirulina contains eight times more protein than tofu, five times more calcium than cow's milk (in a more easily absorbed form), and more of certain amino acids than any other plant food. It is highly nutritious and helps to restore energy and vitality in people who have been undernourished (even if they are overfed!).[32] Spirulina is useful for reversing adrenal and thyroid exhaustion and battling depression and mood swings. It is also excellent for weight control because it acts as an appetite suppressor and inhibits the uptake of dietary fat from the intestines.[33] It also contains higher levels of vitamin B_{12} than any other plant, making it an important supplement for vegans. Spirulina aids in detoxification by binding with heavy metals and helping to remove them from the body.[34]

Fiber

Fiber helps flush wastes from the body, works to reduce blood sugar levels,[35] and contributes to feelings of fullness. Fiber acts like a sponge, absorbing water as it goes through the stomach and small intestine, and arrives in the colon full of moisture. Diets low in fiber cause fecal material to become dry and difficult to expel, causing a buildup of toxins that can lead to weight gain.

There are two basic types of fiber, soluble and insoluble. Insoluble fiber, which doesn't dissolve in water, is found in wheat and corn bran, whole grains, nuts, legumes, and some vegetables. Insoluble fiber increases fecal size and weight and promotes regular bowel movements. However, it can also irritate the bowel, especially if it is already sensitive or inflamed. Too much grain fiber, especially wheat bran, may interfere with the absorption of calcium, magnesium, iron, and zinc. Soluble fiber, found in fruits, vegetables, oats and oat bran, barley, beans, and peas, is not irritating to the bowel. Eating foods containing soluble fiber stimulates bowel movements, decreases appetite, and thus leads to weight loss.[36]

An excellent source of fiber is powdered psyllium husk, the form of fiber most often used for intestinal cleansing due to its superior ability to absorb moisture, lubricate the intestines, and mop up contaminants. Other good forms of soluble fiber are flaxseed, guar gum, apple pectin, and glucomannan (discussed later in this chapter). Mixing fiber products with water or juice produce a gelatinous mass that, when taken before a meal, creates a feeling of fullness and thus reduces appetite. This mixture also assists in controlling blood sugar, decreasing the number of calories absorbed, and cleaning out the intestinal tract. Start by taking 4 to 5 grams of fiber per day and gradually increase intake as your body adjusts. When supplementing fiber, it's important to drink six to eight glasses of water per day to prevent constipation.

Brown Fat—The Body's Calorie-Burning Furnace

The nutrients discussed above support optimum overall health and wellness, and can aid in weight loss and maintaining a healthy weight. In addition, there are specific weight-loss agents that function though the process of thermogenesis (increasing fat burning). Although you're probably eager to learn about these supplements, it's important that you first have an understanding of brown fat, the body's energy burning furnace.

The body has two kinds of fat, yellow (or white) fat, and brown fat. Yellow fat serves as an insulator and a warehouse for unused or excess calories. This is the type of fat most people want to shed. Babies are born with up to 5% brown fat by body weight, which diminishes with age. Brown fat is located deep in the body, near the shoulder blades and extending down the back around the spine; it is also found adjacent to the heart (where it warms the blood), kidneys, and adrenal glands. These are areas of intense metabolic activity. Brown fat differs from yellow fat because it contains a high number of mitochondria, cellular components that generate energy through a process called oxidation. The mitochondria impart the brownish hue to this type of fat. Brown fat is metabolically active, burns calories, and is actively involved in weight loss.[37] Therefore, brown fat and yellow fat have opposite functions; brown fat is the furnace, and yellow fat is the fuel.[38]

This is a clue as to why certain people can eat seemingly whatever they want and not gain a pound, while others find losing weight difficult even if they restrict calories. Being overweight can actually shut down the mitochondria in brown fat, essentially turning it into yellow fat.[39]

Brown Fat and Your Set Point for Body Weight

One reason dieting often fails has to do with the body's natural set point. The set point is a constant weight that most adults maintain under normal conditions. The set point automatically controls your body weight the way a thermostat controls the temperature in your home.

When a person of normal weight begins to gain weight, their body responds by increasing calorie-burning activity, the way a furnace turns on when room temperature falls below a preset level. Similarly, when weight is lost, the body's calorie-burning furnaces slow down in an effort to prevent the body from dropping below a set weight. In this way, the body maintains its weight within a narrow range. One of the mechanisms for controlling set point is increasing or decreasing the calorie-burning activity in brown fat.

Scientists believe that the set point is what enabled our agrarian ancestors to cope with annual cycles of food abundance and scarcity. The problem for dieters is that the body can't distinguish between a famine and a crash diet. Consequently, the body may fight to retain weight when it senses a decrease in calories and quickly regain weight to return to its natural set point. One of the ways this occurs is through deactivation of brown fat.

Why You Lose Brown Fat

Unlike yellow fat, we do not gain brown fat by eating more food. In fact, we slowly lose brown fat as we grow older. It is also possible for brown fat to become inactive as a result of exposure to toxins in food, water, or air. Once brown fat has been deactivated, your body can no longer burn off excess calories as effectively, and instead, it will store it as yellow fat. Brown fat can be lost or deactivated due to the following factors:

- Essential fatty acid deficiencies: Nutritional deficiencies brought on by a poor diet can cause brown fat to become inactive. Among the most important nutrients for keeping thermogenic processes healthy in brown fat cells are essential fatty acids (EFAs). These substances are the primary fuels that stoke the body's thermogenic furnace. When they are in short supply, brown fat becomes inactive, which can make weight loss more difficult. This is one reason why crash diets can seriously impair thermogenic capacity.

- Behavioral factors: Excessive exercise and fasting can deplete stores of brown fat. A yo-yo pattern of weight loss and gain may also make it more difficult to burn off excess calories, since the body will tend to store them as body fat.

- Age and genetics: You are born with a certain amount of brown fat, and if this amount is inadequate, you may be prone to weight gain. In addition, as we age, brown fat decreases in both amount and activity. Diabetes and hypothyroidism also affect brown fat function.[40]

- Toxins and medications: When taken daily, various medications can have devastating effects on brown fat, eventually interfering in the ability of their mitochondria to produce energy. A healthy liver can readily filter out the toxins that accumulate from a few days of medication or from brief environmental exposure to toxins, but after a prolonged period of exposure the body is no longer able to clean out these damaging chemicals.

Mitochondria produce energy in the cells by generating ATP (adenosine triphosphate), the primary cellular fuel. Damaged mitochondria often lose their ability to use fats to make ATP. When this occurs, the body may draw upon lean body tissue to fuel metabolism, which can cause serious weakness and fatigue. People who have problems at this cellular level often have trouble exercising, making them more susceptible to weight gain.

Supplements to Increase Fat Burning

Fortunately, there are many natural remedies that can help to stimulate thermogenesis through a variety of mechanisms.[41] Of these, exercise is first and foremost. As emphasized throughout this book, without adequate exercise, you may find it difficult to lose weight and keep it off. In addition to getting enough exercise, you can use certain supplements to boost your body's fat-burning capabilities.

For more on **exercise and weight loss,** see chapter 2, Start Exercising, page 52.

Fighting Fat with Fats (Boosting Thermogenesis)

You may have a hard time accepting that supplementing your diet with fats can actually help you lose weight. Although it may seem to make sense that the fat you eat is deposited directly on your body, this isn't necessarily true. The health benefits of certain fats are so significant that *not* consuming them can actually sabotage weight-loss efforts and negatively impact your health.

Essential fatty acids: Many overweight people suffer from chronic deficiencies of essential fatty acids (EFAs). Gamma-linolenic acid (GLA), an omega-6 fatty acid, is of particular concern. Normally, the body can manufacture GLA from dietary sources of linoleic acid, another omega-6 fatty acid. Sources of linoleic acid include safflower, sunflower, corn, soybean, and flaxseed oils. However, a diet high in saturated fats combined with stress, alcohol, aging, or illness, can block this conversion, resulting in a GLA deficiency. Evening primrose oil, black currant oil, and borage oil are good sources of GLA. The typical recommended dosage for GLA is 500 mg daily.

Medium-chain triglycerides: Medium-chain triglycerides (MCTs) have been shown to promote weight loss. MCTs tend to accelerate metabolism while lowering blood levels of cholesterol. Good sources of MCTs are grapeseed and organic virgin coconut oils, available at most health food stores. These oils can be used on vegetables, in salad dressings, and for cooking. Consider adding 1 to 2 tablespoons to your diet daily. However, diabetics and those with liver disorders should approach the use of MCTs with caution, as the fat tends to be burned very rapidly in the liver. People with these conditions should avoid MCTs entirely or use them only under a doctor's supervision.

Herbs to Promote Fat Burning

Cayenne or red pepper (*Capsicum frutescens*), ginger, and cinnamon, long considered warming spices in traditional healing systems such as Chinese medicine and Ayurveda, have been credited with helping to break down fat. Cayenne helps digestion and increases feelings of fullness and satiety.[42] It has many other health benefits, too, such as helping to rid the body of candida and other harmful organisms.[43]

Ephedra also known as ma huang, has been used in traditional Chinese medicine for centuries to help with congestion, breathing, and low energy. Herbal formulas based on ephedra can help raise the metabolic rate and increase the amount of fat the body burns.[44] Ephedra's active ingredient is ephedrine, which prompts the release of norepinephrine, a brain chemical that increases metabolism. Several studies have shown that ephedra, particularly if used with herbs that contain caffeine, promotes weight loss, reduces body fat, and improves blood lipids.[45] Caffeine-containing herbs include cola nut (*Cola nitida*) and guarana (*Paullinia cupana*), and yerba maté (*Ilex paraguariensis*), which also contains caffeine. However, ephedra can produce significant side effects, including hand tremors, heart palpitations, insomnia, and headaches. There have been many reports of serious side effects due to the abuse and overuse of ephedra, including suspected deaths.[46] In their haste to lose weight, people often take too many stimulants, such as ephedra. Due to ephedra falling out of favor, many supplement manufacturers are using other herbs in weight-loss formulas, such as bitter orange (*Citrus aurantium*), which contains similar chemical compounds.[47]

Although this herb may also be effective for supporting weight loss, it actually has side effects similar to ephedra, such as increasing blood pressure and heart rate.[48] Because ephedra and bitter orange are stimulants and their prolonged use is considered controversial, it is best to have your dose tailored to your specific requirements. A trained practitioner will take into account your sensitivities and preexisting health conditions, such as impaired thyroid or adrenal function and cardiovascular conditions. With professional guidance, these supplements may be useful for increasing thermogenesis.

 Pregnant women, nursing mothers, people with certain health problems — high blood pressure, heart or thyroid disease, diabetes, and prostate enlargement — and people taking monoamine oxidase (MAO) inhibitors (an antidepressant) or any other prescription drug should seek advice from a health-care practitioner before taking any ephedrine-containing product, including ephedra. Thermogenic formulas that utilize aspirin should be obtained only from physicians and used in accordance with their recommendations; their use is not advisable for everyone and should be avoided by those who are sensitive to aspirin.

Garlic (**Allium sativum**) is probably the most well-recognized medicinal herb. It is used by traditional medicines worldwide and its applications are as varied as its geographical distribution. The chemistry and pharmacology of garlic has been extensively studied — over 1,000 research papers have been published in the past 25 years. Among its many virtues is that garlic may be useful in boosting thermogenesis. Two groups of animals were fed identical high-fat diets, with one group given additional garlic powder. After 28 days, the body weights of the group given garlic were significantly lower. Amounts of brown fat as well as levels of norepinephrine and mitochondrial protein were also greater in the garlic group — all indicators of increased metabolic and fat-burning activities.[49] Other studies have shown allicin, one of garlic's active ingredients, is useful in preventing weight gain in overfed rats.[50] The benefits of garlic can be gleaned from any garlic preparation: raw, dried, garlic oil, or a prepared commercial product.

Ginseng has an ancient history and has accumulated much folklore about its actions and uses. Common varieties are Oriental ginseng (*Panax ginseng*), American ginseng (*Panax quinquefolius*), and *Eleutherococcus senticosus*, which was previously called Siberian ginseng. In traditional Chinese medicine, ginseng is used as a general tonic to improve stamina during exercise, sharpen mental abilities, and relieve fatigue. Studies on ginseng prove that this ancient remedy is a useful antiobesity agent.

It decreases the release of free radicals generated by exercise,[51] and also reduces levels of appetite-stimulating compounds such as leptin.[52] Extracts of both ginseng root and ginseng berry help to stabilize blood sugar.[53]

Green tea (**Camellia sinensis**) can increase the metabolic rate and stimulate thermogenesis.[54] Green tea is rich in a variety of compounds, including theophylline, theobromine, caffeine, and polyphenols such as epigallocatechin gallate (EGCG). These active ingredients allow green tea to support weight loss by several different means. Green tea increases the body's use of energy,[55] and can inhibit the absorption of fat[56] and break down fat cells as they form.[57] Since green tea has other positive health benefits in addition to supporting weight loss, it's a great addition to a weight-loss program. Green tea does contain caffeine, so people sensitive to caffeine should use it in the earlier part of the day to avoid sleep problems. The tea plant tends to accumulate a high level of fluoride in its leaves. Younger leaves have the lowest fluoride content, and they also tend to make the best tea, so those who want to minimize fluoride intake should choose high-quality tea.[58] Consider drinking one or two cups of green tea per day.

Hoodia (**Hoodia gordonii**) is a succulent plant that grows in the Kalahari Desert. In 1937, a Dutch scientist who was studying the habits of local tribal people noticed that they used the hoodia plant and claimed it helped them avoid feelings of hunger while on long journeys. They picked the whole plant, peeled away the outer covering, and ate the inner part. In 1963, South Africa's Council for Scientific and Industrial Research studied the effects of hoodia and isolated several constituents believed to be responsible for weight loss. Hoodia does not act by increasing thermogenesis, but by decreasing appetite. Hoodia's active ingredients cause the body to release a compound that signals the satiety center in the hypothalamus that enough food has been consumed, and this in turn stunts the appetite. Animal studies have confirmed hoodia's appetite-controlling effects.[59] Hoodia is a slow-growing plant that takes five years to mature, which is one of the reasons that it is difficult to find good-quality hoodia in the commercial marketplace. Much of the hoodia sold is of poor quality and may not give the desired results. There are no safety studies on humans and it may not be safe for use along with prescription medications.

Hydroxycitric acid (HCA) is derived from the dried rind of the tamarind fruit *(Garcinia cambogia)*. It helps to clear fats from the liver, suppresses appetite, and slows the rate at which the body converts carbohydrates into fat.[60] HCA has been found to be more effective when taken in combination with the mineral chromium (either the polynicotinate or picolinate form). A typical therapeutic dose is 250 mg of HCA three times daily, along with 100 mcg of chromium, taken 30 to 60 minutes before each meal.

Yerba maté (Ilex paraguariensis) traditionally consumed as a tea in South America, is available in health food stores in the United States. It acts as a stimulant to boost thermogenesis. Yerba maté's stimulating effect comes primarily from a compound called mateine, a close relative of caffeine, plus small quantities of theophylline and theobromine. Both mateine and caffeine have stimulatory effects.

Nutraceuticals to Promote Fat Burning

There are several other natural substances that have been researched for their positive support for weight loss.

L-carnitine is made by the body by combining two amino acids: lysine and methionine. Involved with fat metabolism,[61] L-carnitine is often promoted as a weight-loss supplement, although some studies have failed to illustrate any actual benefit for weight loss.[62] Carnitine's most important use is in decreasing oxidative stress[63] while at the same time increasing fat burning when exercising.[64] A typical dose of carnitine supplements is 1,000 to 3,000 mg per day.

Conjugated linoleic acid (CLA) is derived from linoleic acid, an omega-6 essential fatty acid. CLA is found in animal foods, including beef, poultry, eggs, and dairy products; it's also produced by normal intestinal bacteria from linoleic acid. It has been touted as a supplement that can help burn fat, as well as improve athletic performance. Studies have yielded mixed results. High amount of CLA (4 grams per day) have been associated with decreased body fat in some studies,[65] while other studies have found that CLA supplementation had negligible effects.[66] CLA may be linked to adverse effects, including increased blood lipids and decreased insulin sensitivity.[67] Both of these factors may actually work against a healthy weight-control program. The conflicting evidence regarding CLA's usefulness may be due to the fact that research is uncovering different forms of CLA and noting that specific forms can have opposing actions. For example, one form of CLA increases atherosclerosis in mice, while another form doesn't.[68]

DHEA (dehydroepiandrosterone), the most abundant hormone in the body, is naturally produced by the human adrenal glands and gonads and functions as an antioxidant and hormone regulator. DHEA levels are naturally high in most people in their twenties and tend to decrease with age. DHEA levels should be tested before taking DHEA supplements, because headaches, irritability, insomnia, and fatigue have been reported with high DHEA doses. The chemical compound 3-acetyl-7-oxo-dehydroepiandrosterone (7-keto-DHEA), may be more useful to promote weight loss than DHEA, while being less likely to cause unwanted side effects. 7-keto DHEA has been shown to increase weight loss and reduce body fat in people who exercised for 45 minutes three times a week and ate an 1,800-calorie diet.[69] A suggested therapeutic dose is 100 mg per day.

Glucomannan is a water-soluble, fermentable fiber derived from an Asian plant called the elephant yam, or konjac root *(Amorphophallus konjac)*. It forms a thicker and more mucilaginous mass than other fibers, so it moves through the large intestines easily and is less irritating and more effective. Glucomannan can be helpful for weight reduction through several mechanisms, including increased feelings of satiety, lower levels of blood lipids, and better blood sugar balance.[70] Glucomannan binds to bile and removes it from the body, which lowers cholesterol by inducing the body to convert cholesterol to bile acids. Since glucomannan slows the emptying of stomach contents, it causes sugars to be absorbed more slowly, which helps to reduce blood sugar levels. By lowering cholesterol and controlling blood sugar, glucommanan also decreases risk factors for heart disease.[71] The amount that has shown success for inducing weight loss is 1 to 3 grams of powder or capsules taken with 8 to 12 ounces of water. Adverse effects include bloating and gas. If this occurs, it usually can be controlled by taking a smaller amount.

Pyruvate occurs naturally in many foods, such as cheese, red wine, and red apples, and is made by the body in the form of pyruvic acid. Studies exploring the use of pyruvate as a weight-loss supplement have shown mixed results. These studies on pyruvate have included dietary restrictions and exercise programs, which, of course, are required for healthy weight maintenance. Several studies indicate that high doses of pyruvate (10 to 40 grams) resulted in a reduction of body fat and increased weight loss,[72] but one study, which used a lower dose of 5 grams, found that pyruvate did not significantly affect body composition or exercise performance.[73] In addition, supplementing with pyruvate may decrease HDL (good cholesterol).[74] In some people it causes digestive disturbances, such as bloating and diarrhea. Another form of pyruvate, called methyl pyruvate, may be more effective for enhancing weight loss by helping to regulate blood sugar levels.[75]

ten

Take Charge of Your Life and Lifestyle

Although most of the case histories in this book involve visits to nutritionists and health-care practitioners, there is only one person who can really change your eating and exercise behavior, and that is *you!* This chapter includes tips that can make the changes easier, and it is followed by the Appendix, where you will find healthy, easy recipes that emphasize whole foods.

Age is not a limiting factor. Don't allow your age to stop you from starting on a path toward weight loss and fitness. Wherever you are today, start with a commitment to daily exercise and health eating. The following success stories introduce you to individuals who did just that, with long lasting positive benefits.

Success Story: 7 Decades of Health and Fitness

Sondra is a 78-year-old woman who knows how to enjoy life. When she was a young girl. Sondra was very overweight. She remembers her mother always having to go the special chubby girl department to buy her clothes. Sondra was constantly overeating. She had twin sisters who refused to eat, and her mother would get very upset. To avoid seeing her mother go into a rage, Sondra secretly removed all the food from both of the twin's plates, and gobbled it up while her mother's back was turned. Meanwhile, her twin sisters were getting skinnier and she kept getting fatter! As they all grew up, the situation improved. Once she hit puberty, the excess weight started to come off. Sondra got very involved in exercise, including figure skating, swimming, jumping rope, and walking. Now, since she is older she has become more conscious of focusing on diet, along with exercise to maintain her weight. She eats fruit and a rice cake in the morning, salads with sardines or other proteins for lunch, and steamed vegetables and protein for dinner. When Sondra stopped smoking at 69 years old, she put on a few pounds and had to make more of an effort to be aware of what she was eating to take off the extra pounds. Sondra continues to exercise daily, usually swimming at least two miles. In fact, her license plate says SWIM 2!

Success Story: Self-Motivation Is the Key

MyKey is a 59-year-old man who decided to take control of his weight. In 1980, MyKey, 5 foot 8, weighed in at 223 pounds. He felt a great deal of fatigue, was "dragging around," and was not happy with his sloppy appearance. At first, he attributed his steady weight gain to genetics, since most of the members of his family were obese. Then he started to pay attention to their traditional diet, which included a lot of bread, pasta, processed meats, and fried food, and was almost devoid of fresh food and vegetables.

MyKey says, "The motivation to change came from a combination of health and vanity issues. At that time, I took it upon myself to start to pay attention to what I was eating. I actually made my own nutrition book by cutting nutrition labels off of food products. I noticed that they clearly stated the calories in every food, and I decided to design a 2,200-calorie diet based on the food pyramid that was circulating in the 1980s. Although it is different than the one that is out now, it emphasized three vegetables, three fruits, and protein. I also included pasta and milk and other sources of calcium, and I paid attention to the grams of protein, fats, and carbohydrates that I consumed. I did not want to go on a "starvation diet"; I wanted to design a program that I could live with long-term. In addition, I started to take a multivitamin-multimineral supplement. I began to include exercise in my daily routine. I walked three miles a day and did sit-ups and push-ups. I started to really notice a change after six months. I was definitely more flexible and felt awake and energetic. At that point, my weight had dropped to 199 pounds. By now I was convinced that I had made the right choice and kept up the pace. After one year, my weight was at 175, and it has remained within a few pounds ever since. The payoff to maintaining a healthy lifestyle of diet and exercise is the enthusiasm you have for life when you feel good and have lots of energy."

MyKey's Weight-Loss Tips

- Many people have the know-how, but need the "do-how."
- Eat whatever you want one day a week; stick to the program the rest of the time.
- On holidays, eat before the party to avoid overeating.
- Always eat breakfast to rev up your metabolism in the morning.
- Most of us eat the same amount of food we ate in our twenties even though we traded in the tennis racket for the remote control a long time ago. Eat less and keep moving!
- Always leave a little food on your plate no matter how small the portion is.
- Eating after exercise helps ignite a very potent calorie burn.
- When you're away from home all day, always bring along a plastic bag full of ready-to-eat veggies, such as cucumbers, bell pepper, asparagus, and radishes, to munch on between meals.
- While losing weight, eat more protein; dieters usually consume too little.
- The brisker the walk, the better the benefits.
- Try having bigger meals during the day, and a smaller one at night.
- Take a critical look at everything you eat and decide where you can remove a little bit of fat. For instance, trim meat before cooking.
- Instead of loading up with butter, squeeze fresh lemon juice over your food.
- Never forget your sense of humor!

Health Q and A Session—From the Lighthearted Side!

Q: I've heard that cardiovascular exercise can prolong life. Is this true?

A: Your heart is only good for so many beats, and that's it. Don't waste them on exercise. Everything wears out eventually. Speeding up your heart will not make you live longer; that's like saying you can extend the life of your car by driving it faster. Want to live longer? Take a nap.

Q: Should I cut down on meat and eat more fruits and vegetables?
A: You must grasp logistical efficiencies. What does a cow eat? Hay and corn. And what are these? Vegetables. So a steak is nothing more than an efficient mechanism of delivering vegetables to your system. Need grain? Eat chicken. Beef is also a good source of field grass (green leafy vegetables).

Q: How can I calculate my body fat ratio?
A: Well, if you have a body and you have fat, your ratio is one to one. If you have two bodies, your ratio is two to one, and so on.

Q: Will sit-ups help prevent me from getting a little soft around the middle?
A: Definitely not! When you exercise a muscle, it gets bigger. You should only be doing sit-ups if you want a bigger stomach.

Q: Is chocolate bad for me?
A: Cocoa beans—another vegetable! It's the best feel-good food around.

Q: Is swimming good for your figure?
A: If swimming is good for your figure, explain whales to me.

Q: Is getting in shape important for my lifestyle?
A: Hey! "Round" is a shape!

Well, I hope this has cleared up any misconceptions you may have had about food and diets. And remember, Life should not be a journey to the grave with the intention of arriving safely in an attractive and well-preserved body. Rather, aim to skid in sideways — Chardonnay in one hand, chocolate in the other — body thoroughly used up, totally worn out, and screaming "Woo hoo! What a ride!"

Natural Nurse Diet

Regardless of the kind of diet and exercise program you feel will work best for you, you'll have the best success at losing weight and keeping it off if you follow these guidelines:

- Food is your ammunition. As you begin to integrate a healthy eating plan into your life, it is of utmost importance that you stock your refrigerator and pantry with an abundant variety of easily accessible healthy foods. This requires an investment of a few hours of preparation each week, but it's time well spent.

  Natural Nurse Tip: I cook and make vegetable juice every Sunday afternoon. Then I have "grab and go" containers of organic meals and vegetable juice that I put in a cooler in the car and take with me wherever I go.

- Eat a wide variety of foods daily. Include foods that have a wonderful array of the colors of the rainbow. If your diet is mostly white and brown, that means it is filled with meat and refined foods, which lead to weight gain. If your plate is filled with the colors of the rainbow, you are eating a lot of whole vegetables and fruits, and a wide variety of them, too.

  Natural Nurse Tip: Steam a wide variety of veggies; red cabbage, zucchini, broccoli, asparagus, kale, onions, tomatoes, carrots. Drizzle with olive oil and oregano. Put in on-the-go containers to use as snacks all week.

- Try a new fruit or vegetable at least once a week. Starting on your path toward healthy weight maintenance is more about experimentation and expansion than it is about denial and deprivation. Avoid eating the same foods every day. This is especially important if you have food allergies.

  Natural Nurse Tip: Put a whole avocado and a whole carrot along with a plastic knife in your lunch bag. Try a starfruit or kiwi if you have never eaten one before.

- Include protein with every meal—even with snacks; do not eat carbohydrates alone. This will increase your sense of fullness and help you avoid cravings.

  Natural Nurse Tip: Put organic almond butter or cashew butter on Granny Smith apple slices.

- Eat at least six to eight small, nutrient-dense meals per day. You should eat your largest meal before 4 p.m. For dinner, consider options like soup and salad, followed by fruit and herbal tea.

- Natural Nurse Tip: Make lunch the biggest meal of the day. Bring a healthy meal with you, or eat at a restaurant that offers whole food, such as fish and vegetables.

- No *paragraphs!* Some people have trouble understanding what "no paragraphs" means. Think about it: only processed food has paragraphs of ingredients listed! Eat only whole, natural foods, avoiding processed, canned, preserved, packaged, synthetic, and artificially colored foods.

- Natural Nurse Tip: The more whole food you have with you at all times, the less processed food you will reach for at home or on the road.

- Begin each day with lemon water. Squeeze half an organic lemon into a 12-ounce glass of water. Drinking lemon water first thing in the morning will give you a feeling of being refreshed and will also help you avoid filling up on junk food and refined carbohydrates, like bagels and doughnuts — definite no-no's for breakfast!

- Natural Nurse Tip: If the morning is very hectic, prepare the lemon in water the night before in a sealed jar, and take it with you on the road.

- Avoid drinking liquids with meals. Drinking along with meals dilutes the digestive juices in your stomach, making it more difficult for your body to assimilate the foods you have consumed. Avoid cold drinks, which interfere with the digestive enzymes from working optimally, thereby slowing digestion and transit time, which allows for more fat absorption and weight gain; soft drinks are the worst offenders.

- Natural Nurse Tip: Carry herbal teabags which aid digestion, such as peppermint and chamomile. If you MUST drink with your meal, you can always get a cup of cold or hot water and use your own herbal tea bag for a healthful drink.

- Avoid refined sugar and artificial sweeteners, including aspartame (Nutra-Sweet), sucralose, sorbitol and other chemical sweeteners. If you avoid sweets altogether as a rule and use them only occasionally as a treat (once a week or less), you will quickly notice that you lose that strong sugar craving.

🧑‍⚕️ Natural Nurse Tip: If you must use a sweetener, try stevia, an herb with a sweet taste, which does not cause a spike in blood sugar.

- Minimize salt intake and avoid commercial salt: Purchase gray Celtic Sea Salt, or use Bragg Liquid Aminos on your food. It has a salty taste, but it's high in variety of essential minerals, not just sodium.

- Eat a lot of your food raw. That includes a large salad every day, with lean organic meat, fish, or chicken cut into it, if you so desire.

🧑‍⚕️ Natural Nurse Tip: Include raw fruits, vegetables, and organic nuts (commercial nuts are often coated with hydrogenated oils) as healthy snacks.

- Don't eat fried foods! Also, don't overcook meat or eat blackened, charred meat; it's high in heterocyclic amines, which are linked to the development of cancer.

🧑‍⚕️ Natural Nurse Tip: Cook by steaming, boiling, or baking. Almost all foods can be steamed!

- Avoid processed and sugary foods, especially candy, jam, jelly, ketchup, white rice, pastas, breads made with refined flour, crackers, refined or processed cereals, and soft drinks. The fastest path to shedding pounds is to stop drinking all soft drinks and eating processed flour products and replace them with water and vegetables. Whenever possible, drink only purified water.

🧑‍⚕️ Natural Nurse Tip: Become an avid label reader. Many sugars and artifical ingredients are "hidden" in other ingredients.

- Avoid all trans fats such as margarine and hydrogenated oils, as well as dangerous fat substitutes, such as olestra. (For more information on olestra, see chapter 3, page 89.)

🧑‍⚕️ Natural Nurse Tip: Look for hydrogenated or partially hydrogenated oils in the ingredients. These are trans fats—even if the front of the label claims 0% trans fats!

- Schedule time for stress reduction and daily exercise. Failing to plan means planning to fail!

🧑‍⚕️ Natural Nurse Tip: Set aside an hour each week to plan your exercise schedule. Get a daily planner in which to pencil in the one hour per day that you will devote to exercise for the upcoming week. The time can be flexible—morning, lunchtime, evening—just as long as it is regular. Arrive five minutes early to work and sit in your car, cell phone turned off; use the time to practice deep breathing and visualization. Visualize a healthy, happy, and attractive you!

If you follow these guidelines, you'll watch your weight gradually drop to a healthier level, while experiencing added benefits, such as an increase in energy and self-esteem, happier mood, less constipation, easier breathing, and a better sex life, to name just a few!

Key Healthy Recipes

The recipes that follow could be your key to a healthy life. Instead of feeling deprived when you give up foods that pack on the pounds, consider these recipes as a new culinary adventure that also support your journey to permanent health and wellness, which includes weight control.

Breakfast Ideas

■ Apple Oatmeal

Diet Type: Vegan
Cooking Time: Under 15 minutes

    1 ½ cups water
    ¾ cup oatmeal
    ¼ teaspoon ground cinnamon
    ¼ teaspoon salt
    ½ cup vanilla soy milk
    ½ cup chopped dates
    ½ cup chopped almonds
    1 apple, grated

Bring the water to a boil. Add the oatmeal, cinnamon, and salt. Cover, lower the heat, and simmer until the liquid is absorbed (about 10 minutes). Stir in the soy milk, dates, almonds, and apple and serve hot.

Servings: 2

Author: Polly Pitchford, Full Spectrum Health

Nutrition Facts				
Serving Size: 1	Dietary Fiber 12 g	48%	Zinc	14%
Servings per Recipe: 2	Sugars 1 g		Pantothenic acid	6%
Amount per Serving	**Protein** 11 g		Niacin	16%
Calories: 417	Iron	20%	Riboflavin	18%
Calories from Fat: 130	Calcium	10%	Thiamin	20%
	Vitamin B$_{12}$	0%	Folate	5%
% Daily Value*	Vitamin B$_6$	10%	Potassium	21%
Total Fat 14 g　22%	Vitamin C	3%	Phosphorus	27%
Saturated Fat 1 g　6%	Vitamin D	0%	Magnesium	33%
Monounsaturated Fat 8 g	Vitamin E	32%		
Cholesterol 0 mg	Vitamin A	1%	* Percent Daily Values are based on a 2,000-calorie diet. Your daily values may be higher or lower depending on your calorie needs.	
Sodium 306 mg　13%	Selenium	29%		
Total Carbohydrate 70 g　23%	Manganese	85%		
	Copper	30%		

▪ Baked Breakfast Apples

Diet Type: Vegan and Sugar-free
Cooking Time: Under 30 minutes

2 medium apples, cut into bite-sized pieces
2 tablespoons chopped dates
½ teaspoon ground cinnamon
½ cup apple juice
¼ cup low-fat granola

Preheat the oven to 350°F. Combine the apples and dates in a small casserole. Sprinkle on the cinnamon, then pour the apple juice over. Bake, covered, for 25 to 30 minutes, or until the apples are slightly tender. Sprinkle with granola and serve warm.

Servings: 2

Author: Polly Pitchford, Full Spectrum Health

Nutrition Facts				
Serving Size: 1	Dietary Fiber 5 g	18%	Zinc	8%
Servings per Recipe: 2	Sugars 3 g		Pantothenic acid	2%
Amount per Serving	**Protein** 2 g		Niacin	9%
Calories: 191	Iron	8%	Riboflavin	12%
Calories from Fat: 13	Calcium	3%	Thiamin	13%
	Vitamin B$_{12}$	7%	Folate	7%
% Daily Value*	Vitamin B$_6$	10%	Potassium	10%
Total Fat 1 g　2%	Vitamin C	35%	Phosphorus	5%
Saturated Fat 0 g　1%	Vitamin E	0%	Magnesium	6%
Monounsaturated Fat 0 g	Vitamin D	4%		
Cholesterol 0 mg	Vitamin A	3%	* Percent Daily Values are based on a 2,000-calorie diet. Your daily values may be higher or lower depending on your calorie needs.	
Sodium 36 mg　2%	Selenium	6%		
Total Carbohydrate 47 g　16%	Manganese	30%		
	Copper	5%		

▪ Apricot Smoothie

Diet Type: Vegan

Cooking Time: Under 15 minutes

    1 cup apricot juice

    1 to 1 ½ cups frozen ripe, pitted apricots

    ¹/₈ teaspoon ground nutmeg

Place the juice, 1 cup of the frozen apricots, and the nutmeg in a blender and blend until smooth. Add the additional ½ cup apricots for a thicker consistency.

Servings: 1

Author: Polly Pitchford, Full Spectrum Health

Nutrition Facts					
Serving Size: 1	Dietary Fiber 5 g	21%	Zinc	5%	
Servings per Recipe: 1	Sugars 0 g		Pantothenic acid	7%	
Amount per Serving	**Protein** 4 g		Niacin	8%	
Calories: 229	Iron	9%	Riboflavin	6%	
Calories from Fat: 12	Calcium	4%	Thiamin	7%	
	Vitamin B₁₂	0%	Folate	8%	
% Daily Value*	Vitamin B₆	10%	Potassium	23%	
Total Fat 1 g 2%	Vitamin C	78%	Phosphorus	6%	
Saturated Fat 0 g 0%	Vitamin E	9%	Magnesium	7%	
Monounsaturated Fat 0 g	Vitamin D	0%			
Cholesterol 0 mg	Vitamin A	68%	* Percent Daily Values are based on a 2,000-calorie diet. Your daily values may be higher or lower depending on your calorie needs.		
Sodium 7 mg %	Selenium	1%			
Total Carbohydrate 55 g 18%	Manganese	10%			
	Copper	15%			

Dressings and Sauces

▪ Almond "Cheese" Sauce

Diet Type: Vegan

Cooking Time: Under 15 minutes

Serve this creamy sauce over steamed broccoli, cauliflower, grains, or potatoes.

    ½ cup grated almond cheese

    2 teaspoons unbleached white flour

    ½ cup plain rice milk

    Salt and pepper

Toss the grated cheese with the flour until coated. Gently heat the rice milk in a saucepan until hot but not bubbling. Gradually add cheese and stir constantly until thick. Season to taste with salt and pepper.

Servings: 4

Author: Polly Pitchford, Full Spectrum Health

Nutrition Facts					
Serving Size: 1	Dietary Fiber 0 g		Zinc		1%
Servings per Recipe: 4	Sugars 0 g		Pantothenic acid		1%
Amount per Serving	**Protein** 4 g		Niacin		4%
Calories: 78	Iron	5%	Riboflavin		24%
Calories from Fat: 19	Calcium	10%	Thiamin		7%
	Vitamin B$_{12}$	0%	Folate		6%
% Daily Value*	Vitamin B$_6$	5%	Potassium		1%
Total Fat 2 g — 3%	Vitamin C	1%	Phosphorus		5%
Saturated Fat 0 g — 0%	Vitamin E	3%	Magnesium		4%
Monounsaturated Fat 0 g	Vitamin D	0%	* Percent Daily Values are based on a 2,000-calorie diet. Your daily values may be higher or lower depending on your calorie needs.		
Cholesterol 0 mg	Vitamin A	1%			
Sodium 151 mg — 6%	Selenium	5%			
Total Carbohydrate 11 g — 4%	Manganese	5%			
	Copper	0%			

▪ Soybean Hummus

Diet Type: Vegan

Cooking Time: Under 15 minutes

    1 15-ounce can organic soybeans

    1 tablespoon tahini (sesame paste) or extra virgin olive oil

    ½ teaspoon salt

    1 large clove garlic, chopped

    2 tablespoons freshly squeezed lemon juice

Place all of the ingredients, including the liquid of the beans, in a blender or food processor. Blend until smooth, then adjust the seasonings to taste. Serve with baked corn chips, whole wheat pita bread, or raw vegetables.

Servings: 4

Author: Polly Pitchford, Full Spectrum Health

Nutrition Facts					
Serving Size: 1	Dietary Fiber 6 g	22%	Zinc		8%
Servings per Recipe: 4	Sugars 0 g		Pantothenic acid		2%
Amount per Serving	**Protein** 15 g		Niacin		3%
Calories: 174	Iron	32%	Riboflavin		18%
Calories from Fat: 87	Calcium	11%	Thiamin		13%
	Vitamin B$_{12}$	0%	Folate		13%
% Daily Value*	Vitamin B$_6$	10%	Potassium		13%
Total Fat 10 g — 15%	Vitamin C	6%	Phosphorus		24%
Saturated Fat 1 g — 7%	Vitamin E	9%	Magnesium		20%
Monounsaturated Fat 2 g	Vitamin D	0%	* Percent Daily Values are based on a 2,000-calorie diet. Your daily values may be higher or lower depending on your calorie needs.		
Cholesterol 0 mg	Vitamin A	0%			
Sodium 296 mg — 12%	Selenium	12%			
Total Carbohydrate 10 g — 3%	Manganese	40%			
	Copper	20%			

Basil Pignoli Dressing

Diet Type: Vegan

Cooking Time: Under 15 minutes

¼ cup pine nuts

1 large clove garlic, chopped

¼ cup fresh basil leaves, packed

½ cup brown rice vinegar

2 tablespoons extra virgin olive oil

2 tablespoons water

1 tablespoon honey

Blend all of the ingredients in a food processor or blender until smooth.

Servings: 4

Author: Polly Pitchford, Full Spectrum Health

Nutrition Facts		Dietary Fiber 0 g	%	Zinc	3%
Serving Size: 1		Sugars 0 g		Pantothenic acid	0%
Servings per Recipe: 4		**Protein** 2 g		Niacin	2%
Amount per Serving		Iron	7%	Riboflavin	0%
		Calcium	1%	Thiamin	7%
Calories: 130		Vitamin B₁₂	0%	Folate	2%
Calories from Fat: 100		Vitamin B₆	0%	Potassium	3%
	% Daily Value*	Vitamin C	1%	Phosphorus	5%
Total Fat 11 g	17%	Vitamin E	6%	Magnesium	7%
Saturated Fat 2 g	8%	Vitamin D	0%	* Percent Daily Values are based on
Monounsaturated Fat 0 g		Vitamin A	1%	a 2,000-calorie diet. Your daily val-
Cholesterol 0 mg		Selenium	3%	ues may be higher or lower depend-
Sodium 1 mg	0%	Manganese	25%	ing on your calorie needs.
Total Carbohydrate 8 g	3%	Copper	5%	

Corn on the Cob with Scallion Pesto

Diet Type: Vegan

Cooking Time: Under 15 minutes

4 ears of corn, shucked

4 scallions, chopped

¼ cup extra virgin olive oil

1 large clove garlic, chopped

¼ teaspoon salt-free seasoning

¹/₈ teaspoon freshly ground black pepper

Boil the corn on the cob in plenty of water for 10 minutes, then drain well. Meanwhile, make the pesto by blending the scallions, olive oil, garlic, and seasonings in a blender until smooth. Use a pastry brush or the back of a spoon to spread the pesto over the corn. Serve hot.

Servings: 4

Author: Polly Pitchford, Full Spectrum Health

Nutrition Facts					
Serving Size: 1	Dietary Fiber 2 g	10%	Zinc		3%
Servings per Recipe: 4	Sugars 0 g		Pantothenic acid		7%
Amount per Serving	**Protein** 3 g		Niacin		6%
Calories: 209	Iron	5%	Riboflavin		6%
Calories from Fat: 130	Calcium	1%	Thiamin		13%
	Vitamin B$_{12}$	0%	Folate		11%
% Daily Value*	Vitamin B$_6$	5%	Potassium		7%
Total Fat 14 g 22%	Vitamin C	9%	Phosphorus		9%
Saturated Fat 2 g 10%	Vitamin E	9%	Magnesium		7%
Monounsaturated Fat 10 g	Vitamin D	0%	* Percent Daily Values are based on		
Cholesterol 0 mg	Vitamin A	1%	a 2,000-calorie diet. Your daily val-		
Sodium 16 mg 1%	Selenium	1%	ues may be higher or lower depend-		
Total Carbohydrate 21 g 7%	Manganese	10%	ing on your calorie needs.		
	Copper	5%			

Salads

Eat at least one fresh salad a day. This incorporates raw foods and a variety of slimming and healthy vegetables and fruits packed full of energy-enhancing nutrients, with virtually no fat-building calories.

■ Antipasto Salad with Toasted Flaxseed Dressing

Diet Type: Vegetarian
Cooking Time: Under 15 minutes

Dressing

1 tablespoon olive oil
2 tablespoons flaxseeds
2 cloves garlic, minced
2 tablespoons white wine vinegar
2 tablespoons water
2 tablespoons chopped fresh herbs (parsley, oregano, basil, or a combination)
½ teaspoon dry mustard
¼ teaspoon salt
Freshly ground black pepper

Salad

6 cups washed, dried, and torn green leaf or romaine lettuce
1 4 ½-ounce can sliced pitted ripe olives
1 6-ounce jar marinated artichoke hearts
12 mushrooms, halved
12 cherry tomatoes, halved
2 tablespoons grated Parmesan cheese
Pickled pepperoncini peppers, thinly sliced red onion, or bell
    pepper rings, for garnish (optional)

Heat the olive oil and flaxseeds in a small saucepan over medium heat, until the seeds starts to darken and pop, about 1 ½ minutes. Add the garlic and sauté for 30 seconds, then remove from the heat. In a blender, combine the vinegar, water, herbs, dry mustard, salt, pepper to taste, and the toasted flax seed mixture. Also pour in the marinade from the artichoke hearts. Blend until the flaxseed is coarsely ground, about 1 minute. In a large bowl, toss the lettuce, olives, artichoke hearts, mushrooms, and tomatoes with the dressing and the Parmesan cheese. Divide salad onto 6 chilled plates. Garnish with the pepperoncini, onion, or bell pepper rings, if desired.

Servings: 6

Author: Flax Council of Canada

Nutrition Facts					
Serving Size: 1	Dietary Fiber 5 g	22%	Zinc		6%
	Sugars 0 g		Pantothenic acid		8%
Servings per Recipe: 6	**Protein** 5 g		Niacin		10%
Amount per Serving	Iron	16%	Riboflavin		12%
Calories: 114	Calcium	9%	Thiamin		7%
Calories from Fat: 62	Vitamin B₁₂	0%	Folate		18%
% Daily Value*	Vitamin B₆	10%	Potassium		12%
	Vitamin C	11%	Phosphorus		12%
Total Fat 7 g 11%	Vitamin E	8%	Magnesium		13%
Saturated Fat 1 g 6%	Vitamin D	7%			
Monounsaturated Fat 4 g	Vitamin A	4%	* Percent Daily Values are based on a 2,000-calorie diet. Your daily values may be higher or lower depending on your calorie needs.		
Cholesterol 1 mg	Selenium	9%			
Sodium 372 mg 16%	Manganese	20%			
Total Carbohydrate 11 g 4%	Copper	20%			

▪ Beets for Life Salad

Diet Type: Vegan

Cooking Time: Under 15 minutes

4 beets
1 Granny Smith apple

1 tablespoon Bragg Liquid Aminos
1 quarter-sized piece of ginger root
Freshly squeezed lemon juice (optional)

Wash the beets and scrub them under lukewarm water. Slice the beets into ¼-inch slices, then cut the slices into fourths. Do the same with the apple. Peel the ginger and mash, then add the liquid aminos and ginger to apple and beet mixture. For a little more zip, add some fresh lemon juice.

Servings: 4

Author: Jennifer Smira

Nutrition Facts				
Serving Size: 1	Dietary Fiber 3 g	13%	Zinc	2%
Servings per Recipe: 4	Sugars 0 g		Pantothenic acid	1%
Amount per Serving	**Protein** 2 g		Niacin	2%
Calories: 58	Iron	5%	Riboflavin	0%
Calories from Fat: 3	Calcium	2%	Thiamin	0%
	Vitamin B$_{12}$	0%	Folate	23%
% Daily Value*	Vitamin B$_6$	5%	Potassium	9%
Total Fat 0 g — 0%	Vitamin C	7%	Phosphorus	4%
Saturated Fat 0 g — 0%	Vitamin E	2%	Magnesium	5%
Monounsaturated Fat 0 g	Vitamin D	0%	
Cholesterol 0 mg	Vitamin A	0%	* Percent Daily Values are based on a 2,000-calorie diet. Your daily values may be higher or lower depending on your calorie needs.	
Sodium 274 mg — 11%	Selenium	1%		
Total Carbohydrate 13 g — 4%	Manganese	15%		
	Copper	5%		

▪ Avocado Salad with Black Olive Dressing

Diet Type: Vegan

Cooking Time: Under 15 minutes

    3 tablespoons orange juice
    2 tablespoons extra virgin olive oil
    ¼ cup pitted kalamata olives, coarsely chopped
    1 clove garlic, minced
    1 teaspoon honey
    Salt and black pepper
    1 firm, ripe avocado, pitted, peeled, and cut into thin wedges
    ½ red onion, sliced thin
    ½ head romaine lettuce, washed, dried, and sliced into thin strips

In a small bowl, whisk together the orange juice, olive oil, olives, garlic, and honey. Season with salt and pepper to taste. In another bowl, combine the avocado and onion. Pour the olive dressing over the avocado mixture and toss lightly. Serve on a bed of sliced romaine.

Servings: 2

Author: Polly Pitchford, Full Spectrum Health

Nutrition Facts						
Serving Size: 1	Dietary Fiber 4 g	16%	Zinc	3%
Servings per Recipe: 4	Sugars 0 g		Pantothenic acid	6%
Amount per Serving	**Protein** 2 g		Niacin	6%
Calories: 178	Iron	11%	Riboflavin	6%
Calories from Fat: 141	Calcium	4%	Thiamin	7%
% Daily Value*	Vitamin B₁₂	0%	Folate	28%
Total Fat 16 g 24%	Vitamin B₆	10%	Potassium	15%
Saturated Fat 2 g 11%	Vitamin C	27%	Phosphorus	5%
Monounsaturated Fat 11 g	Vitamin E	10%	Magnesium	7%
Cholesterol 0 mg	Vitamin D	0%		
Sodium 102 mg 4%	Vitamin A	18%		
Total Carbohydrate 10 g 3%	Selenium	1%		
	Manganese	25%		
	Copper	10%		

* Percent Daily Values are based on a 2,000-calorie diet. Your daily values may be higher or lower depending on your calorie needs.

▪ Curried Shrimp and Rice Salad

Diet Type: Low-fat

Cooking Time: Under 15 minutes

1 cup cooked shrimp, cut in half

2 cups cooked brown rice

½ cup cooked peas

½ cup minced red onion

¼ cup chopped parsley

¼ cup low-fat mayonnaise

½ cup nonfat plain yogurt

Freshly squeezed juice of $^1/_2$ lemon

2 teaspoons curry powder

$^1/_8$ teaspoon ground cinnamon

Combine the shrimp, rice, peas, onion, and parsley in a serving bowl. In a smaller bowl, whisk the mayonnaise, yogurt, lemon juice, curry powder, and cinnamon together until smooth. Combine the dressing with the rice mixture. Serve chilled.

Servings: 2

Dried Plum Waldorf Salad

Diet Type: Dairy-free

Cooking Time: Under 15 minutes

To toast walnuts, arrange them in an even layer on a baking sheet. Bake at 350°F for 8 to 10 minutes, or until lightly browned.

¾ cup reduced-fat mayonnaise

3 tablespoons freshly squeezed orange juice

3 cups chopped red apples

1 ½ cups cubed smoked turkey

1 cup chopped dried plums

¾ cup chopped celery

½ cup coarsely chopped walnuts, toasted

Red or green lettuce leaves (optional)

In medium bowl, combine the mayonnaise and orange juice. Add the apples, turkey, dried plums, celery, and walnuts and toss to coat. Serve chilled, on a bed of lettuce, if desired.

Servings: 6

Author: California Dried Plum Board

Nutrition Facts				
Serving Size: 1	Dietary Fiber 5 g	18%	Zinc	5%
Servings per Recipe: 6	Sugars 2 g		Pantothenic acid	5%
Amount per Serving	**Protein** 8 g		Niacin	16%
Calories: 307	Iron	9%	Riboflavin	6%
Calories from Fat: 143	Calcium	4%	Thiamin	7%
	Vitamin B₁₂	8%	Folate	6%
% Daily Value*	Vitamin B₆	15%	Potassium	15%
Total Fat 16 g — 24%	Vitamin C	24%	Phosphorus	14%
Saturated Fat 2 g — 11%	Vitamin E	10%	Magnesium	10%
Monounsaturated Fat 1 g	Vitamin D	0%	* Percent Daily Values are based on a 2,000-calorie diet. Your daily values may be higher or lower depending on your calorie needs.	
Cholesterol 21 mg	Vitamin A	7%		
Sodium 629 mg — 26%	Selenium	17%		
Total Carbohydrate 36 g — 12%	Manganese	20%		
	Copper	15%		

Healthy Turkey Salad Pocket

Diet Type: Low-fat

Cooking Time: Under 15 minutes

You can make a vegetarian version of this sandwich filling by substituting tofu for the turkey. Try baked tofu. It has a more appealing flavor and texture.

2 cups diced cooked turkey or chicken
¾ cup pitted dried plums, quartered
½ cup sliced celery
½ cup nonfat plain yogurt
¼ cup sliced green onion (about 1 green onion)
1 tablespoon sweet hot mustard
Salt and pepper
3 whole wheat pita breads, halved
6 lettuce leaves

In a medium bowl, combine the turkey, dried plums, celery, yogurt, green onion, and mustard and stir until thoroughly mixed. Season to taste with salt and pepper. To serve, place 1 lettuce leaf in each pita half and spoon in ½ cup of the turkey mixture. Keeps well in a covered container in the refrigerator for up to 3 days.

Servings: 6

Author: California Dried Plum Board

Nutrition Facts		Dietary Fiber 4 g	18%	Zinc	12%
Serving Size: 1		Sugars 0 g		Pantothenic acid	9%
Servings per Recipe: 6		**Protein** 19 g		Niacin	24%
Amount per Serving		Iron	17%	Riboflavin	12%
		Calcium	8%	Thiamin	13%
Calories: 219		Vitamin B₁₂	5%	Folate	8%
Calories from Fat: 15		Vitamin B₆	20%	Potassium	14%
	% Daily Value*	Vitamin C	4%	Phosphorus	22%
Total Fat 2 g	3%	Vitamin E	4%	Magnesium	13%
Saturated Fat 0 g	0%	Vitamin D	0%	* Percent Daily Values are based on
Monounsaturated Fat 0 g		Vitamin A	6%	a 2,000-calorie diet. Your daily val-
Cholesterol 40 mg		Selenium	57%	ues may be higher or lower depend-
Sodium 348 mg	14%	Manganese	35%	ing on your calorie needs.
Total Carbohydrate 34 g	11%	Copper	10%	

■ Mediterranean Vegetable and Walnut Salad

Diet Type: Vegan

Cooking Time: Under 15 minutes

½ cup chopped walnuts
½ cup reduced-fat balsamic vinaigrette
1 tablespoon minced, pitted ripe olives
1 15-ounce can chickpeas (with no added salt)
1 red bell pepper, seeded and thinly sliced
1 large carrot, peeled and cut into matchsticks
1 small red onion, thinly sliced

4 cups spinach
4 cups arugula leaves

Heat the walnuts in a dry skillet over medium-high heat for 1 to 2 minutes, until slightly toasted. In a small bowl, whisk together the vinaigrette and olives. In a medium bowl, combine the chickpeas, bell pepper, carrot, and onion; add 3 tablespoons of the vinaigrette and toss to coat. In a large bowl, toss the spinach and arugula with the remaining vinaigrette. Divide the greens equally among 6 salad plates, top with the chickpea mixture, and sprinkle with the walnuts.

Servings: 6

Author: Walnut Marketing Board

Nutrition Facts					
Serving Size: 1	Dietary Fiber 7 g	28%	Zinc		11%
	Sugars 1 g		Pantothenic acid		5%
Servings per Recipe: 6	**Protein** 8 g		Niacin		4%
Amount per Serving	Iron	18%	Riboflavin		6%
Calories: 224	Calcium	10%	Thiamin		7%
Calories from Fat: 99	Vitamin B$_{12}$	0%	Folate		34%
% Daily Value*	Vitamin B$_6$	35%	Potassium		14%
Total Fat 11 g 17%	Vitamin C	57%	Phosphorus		16%
Saturated Fat 1 g 6%	Vitamin E	5%	Magnesium		18%
Monounsaturated Fat 1 g	Vitamin D	0%	* Percent Daily Values are based on a 2,000-calorie diet. Your daily values may be higher or lower depending on your calorie needs.		
Cholesterol 0 mg	Vitamin A	62%			
Sodium 488 mg 20%	Selenium	7%			
Total Carbohydrate 30 g 10%	Manganese	60%			
	Copper	20%			

Soups

▣ Cold Avocado Cucumber Soup

Diet Type: Vegan

Cooking Time: Under 15 minutes

    2 ripe avocados, peeled and coarsely chopped
    1 cucumber, peeled, seeded, and coarsely chopped
    ¾ cup low-fat soy milk
    2 tablespoons cilantro leaves
    2 green onions, coarsely chopped
    1 tablespoon freshly squeezed lemon juice
    Salt and pepper
    2 cups vegetable broth

In a blender or food processor, blend the avocados, cucumber, soy milk, cilantro, and green onion until smooth. Add the lemon juice and season with salt and pepper to taste. Add as much vegetable broth as you want to thin the soup to the desired consistency. Serve chilled.

Servings: 4

Author: Polly Pitchford, Full Spectrum Health

Nutrition Facts					
Serving Size: 1	Dietary Fiber 6 g	23%	Zinc	3%	
Servings per Recipe: 4	Sugars 2 g		Pantothenic acid	10%	
Amount per Serving	**Protein** 4 g		Niacin	10%	
Calories: 206	Iron	11%	Riboflavin	6%	
Calories from Fat: 142	Calcium	5%	Thiamin	7%	
% Daily Value*	Vitamin B$_{12}$	0%	Folate	20%	
Total Fat 16 g 24%	Vitamin B$_6$	15%	Potassium	21%	
Saturated Fat 2 g 11%	Vitamin C	15%	Phosphorus	7%	
Monounsaturated Fat 10 g	Vitamin E	6%	Magnesium	13%	
Cholesterol 0 mg	Vitamin D	4%			
Sodium 260 mg 11%	Vitamin A	17%	* Percent Daily Values are based on a 2,000-calorie diet. Your daily values may be higher or lower depending on your calorie needs.		
Total Carbohydrate 16 g 5%	Selenium	0%			
	Manganese	15%			
	Copper	15%			

▪ Curried Split Pea Soup

Diet Type: Low-fat

Cooking Time: 30 minutes to 1 hour

    4 cups water or broth
    2 cups yellow split peas
    1 medium onion, chopped
    1 bay leaf
    1 tablespoon curry powder
    Salt

Combine the broth, split peas, onion, and bay leaf in a soup pot and bring to a boil. Turn heat to low, add the curry powder, and simmer for 40 minutes, or until the pe as are tender. Season with salt to taste and simmer a few minutes more.

Servings: 6

Author: Polly Pitchford, Full Spectrum Health

Nutrition Facts				
Serving Size: 1	Dietary Fiber 17 g	70%	Zinc	14%
Servings per Recipe: 6	Sugars 0 g		Pantothenic acid	12%
Amount per Serving	**Protein** 16 g		Niacin	10%
Calories: 235	Iron	22%	Riboflavin	6%
Calories from Fat: 8	Calcium	5%	Thiamin	33%
	Vitamin B$_{12}$	0%	Folate	46%
% Daily Value*	Vitamin B$_6$	5%	Potassium	20%
Total Fat 1 g 1%	Vitamin C	3%	Phosphorus	25%
Saturated Fat 0 g 0%	Vitamin E	1%	Magnesium	20%
Monounsaturated Fat 0 g	Vitamin D	0%	* Percent Daily Values are based on a 2,000-calorie diet. Your daily values may be higher or lower depending on your calorie needs.	
Cholesterol 0 mg	Vitamin A	1%		
Sodium 403 mg 17%	Selenium	2%		
Total Carbohydrate 42 g 14%	Manganese	50%		
	Copper	30%		

Desserts

■ Dried Fruit Balls

Diet Type: Sugar-free

Cooking Time: Under 15 minutes

   1 cup pitted dates

   ¼ cup walnuts

   ¼ cup rolled oats (not instant)

   ¼ cup cocoa or carob powder

Place all of the ingredients in a food processor and blend until thoroughly combined. The mixture should look like a lumpy paste. With slightly wet hands, roll the paste into walnut-sized balls. Place on wax paper on a tray or plate and freeze until firm. Store in baggies in the refrigerator for up to 2 weeks.

Servings: 6

Author: Polly Pitchford, Full Spectrum Health

Nutrition Facts				
Serving Size: 1	Dietary Fiber 16 g	4%	Zinc	3%
Servings per Recipe: 6	Sugars 0 g		Pantothenic acid	3%
Amount per Serving	**Protein** 2 g		Niacin	4%
Calories: 128	Iron	7%	Riboflavin	0%
Calories from Fat: 36	Calcium	2%	Thiamin	7%
	Vitamin B$_{12}$	0%	Folate	3%
% Daily Value*	Vitamin B$_6$	5%	Potassium	8%
Total Fat 4 g 6%	Vitamin C	0%	Phosphorus	6%
Saturated Fat 1 g 4%	Vitamin E	1%	Magnesium	10%
Monounsaturated Fat 1 g	Vitamin D	0%	* Percent Daily Values are based on a 2,000-calorie diet. Your daily values may be higher or lower depending on your calorie needs.	
Cholesterol 0 mg	Vitamin A	0%		
Sodium 2 mg 0%	Selenium	4%		
Total Carbohydrate 26 g 8%	Manganese	25%		
	Copper	15%		

■ High-Protein Pudding

Diet Type: Vegetarian

Cooking Time: Under 15 minutes

The amount of protein powder needed may vary slightly because of the different consistencies of different brands of silken tofu. The amount of honey or maple syrup you choose to use will also affect the amount of protein powder needed. Silken tofu has a smoother texture and less beany taste than regular tofu. It works well in desserts, smoothies, and other sweet recipes. Look for it on grocery shelves as well as in the refrigerated section, since at least one brand (Mori-Nu) need not be refrigerated until after it is opened.

1 12.3-ounce package silken tofu

3 tablespoons or 1 scoop protein powder

2 tablespoons coffee substitute powder

2 tablespoons unsweetened carob powder or cocoa powder

Dash of vanilla

Pinch each of ground cinnamon, nutmeg, and cloves

¼ to ½ cup honey or maple syrup

Place all of the ingredients in a blender and whirl until smooth. Refrigerate for at least 1 hour. Serve as is or with a topping of granola. Variation: Add a ripe banana or other fruit.

Servings: 2

Author: Ellen Sue Spicer of Hands On Nutrition

Nutrition Facts					
Serving Size: 1	Dietary Fiber 4 g	16%	Zinc	21%
	Sugars 35 g		Pantothenic acid	4%
Servings per Recipe: 2	**Protein** 25 g		Niacin	9%
Amount per Serving	Iron	18%	Riboflavin	0%
Calories: 334	Calcium	13%	Thiamin	13%
Calories from Fat: 40	Vitamin B₁₂	2%	Folate	5%
% Daily Value*	Vitamin B₆	5%	Potassium	22%
	Vitamin C	0%	Phosphorus	20%
Total Fat 4 g — 7%	Vitamin E	2%	Magnesium	20%
Saturated Fat 1 g — 4%	Vitamin D	0%	
Monounsaturated Fat 1 g	Vitamin A	0%	* Percent Daily Values are based on a 2,000-calorie diet. Your daily values may be higher or lower depending on your calorie needs.
Cholesterol 0 mg	Selenium	43%	
Sodium 228 mg — 12%	Manganese	90%	
Total Carbohydrate 52 g — 17%	Copper	20%	

Recipes Courtesy of Sprouts Farmers Market

www.sprouts.com

Quick Definitions

Amino Acids

Amino acids are the building blocks of the 40,000 different proteins of the body, including enzymes, hormones, and the brain's chemical messengers, called neutrotransmitters. Eight amino acids cannot be made by the body and must be obtained through diet; others are produced in the body but not always in sufficient amounts. The amino acids that occur most commonly in the body are alanine, arginine, asparagine, aspartic acid, caritine, citrulline, cysteine, cystine, GABA, glutamic acid, glutamine, glycine, histidine, isoleucine, leucine, lysine, methionine, ornithine, phenylalanine, proline, serine, taurine, threonine, tryptophan, tyrosine, and valine.

Antibody

An **antibody** is a protein molecule made from amino acids by white blood cells in the lymph tissue and set in motion against a specific foreign protein, or antigen, by the immune system. Antibodies, also referred to as immunoglobulins, may be found in the blood, lymph, saliva, and gastrointestinal and urinary tracts, usually within three days after the first encounter with an antigen. The antibody binds tightly with the antigen as a preliminary step in removing it from the system or destroying it.

Antioxidant

An **antioxidant** is a natural biochemical substance that protects living cells against damage from harmful free radicals. Antioxidants work against the process of oxidation—the robbing of electrons from molecules. Oxidation can lead to cellular aging, degeneration, arthritis, heart disease, cancer, and other illnesses. Antioxidants react with free radicals and neutralize them before they can damage the body. Antioxidant nutrients include vitamins A, C, and E, beta carotene, selenium, coenzyme Q10, pycnogenol (found in grapeseed extract), L-glutathione, superoxide dismutase, and bioflavonoids. Plant antioxidants include ginkgo biloba and garlic.

Autonomic Nervous System

The **autonomic nervous system** (ANS) is like your body's automatic pilot. It maintains functions that keep you alive, such as breathing, heart rate, and digestion, without your being aware of it or participating in its activities. The ANS has two divisions: the sympathetic, which expends body energy and prepares us physically when we perceive a threat or challenge by increasing heart rate, blood pressure, and muscle tension, and the parasympathetic, which conserves body energy by slowing heart rate and increases intestinal and gland activity.

Basal Metabolism

Basal metabolism refers to the number of calories used by the body at complete rest to maintain basic life processes, such as breathing and circulation. Basal metabolism, which is controlled by the thyroid gland (the largest endocrine gland, located near the front of the throat where it wraps around the windpipe right behind the Adam's apple), keeps the body at a normal, healthy resting temperature of 98.6°F. Using hormones, the thyroid sends chemical messages to every cell in the body, controlling body temperature, heart rate, and muscle movements. When the thyroid is dysfunctional or underactive—a condition called hypothyroidism—it sends out fewer hormones, causing basal metabolism to slow down. This slowing causes a number of problems, including general feelings of sluggishness and increases in body weight.

Bioflavonoid

A **bioflavonoid** is a pigment within plants and fruits that acts as an antioxidant to protect the body against damage from free radicals and excess oxygen. In the body, bioflavonoids enhance the beneficial activities of vitamin C, and they are often included in vitamin C supplements. Originally called vitamin P, these vitamin C "helper" substances include citrin, hesperidin, catechin, rutin, and quercetin. When taken with vitamin C, bioflavonoids increase the absorption of vitamin C in the liver, kidneys, and adrenal glands. As antioxidants, they also protect vitamin C from destruction by free radicals.

Calorie

A **calorie** is a measure of the energy-producing potential contained in food. In practical terms, the number of calories in a particular food tells you how much fuel you're getting from eating it.

Diabetes Mellitus

Diabetes mellitus is a degenerative illness that centers around the hormone insulin and the pancreas. In type 1 diabetes, the pancreas is unable to manufacture insulin. This accounts for a very low percentage of people who have diabetes. In type 2 diabetes, the pancreas produces insulin, but the body's cells don't respond to it and can't absorb glucose from food. As blood glucose levels continue to rise, the pancreas releases more insulin to deal with the excess blood sugar. The result is both a state of low blood sugar and too much insulin (hyperinsulinism).

Endocrine Glands

The **endocrine glands**, including the testicles, ovaries, pancreas, adrenals, thyroid, parathyroid, and pituitary, are central to the regulation and normalization of all the body's complex, interconnected systems, from metabolism and heat production to spermatogenesis and uterine preparations for pregnancy.

Environmental Estrogens

Environmental estrogens are foreign compounds and/or chemical toxins that mimic the effects of estrogen in the body. Environmental estrogens, also called xenobiotics or xenoestrogens, are present primarily in man-made chemicals ("greenhouse gases," herbicides, and pesticides such as DDT) and industrial by-products (from manufacture of plastics and paper, as well as from the incineration of hazardous wastes).

Essential Fatty Acids

Essential fatty acids (EFAs) are unsaturated fats required in the diet. Omega-3 and omega-6 fatty acids are the two principal types. Omega-3 fatty acids are found in flaxseed, canola, pumpkin, walnut, and soy oils. Fish oils, especially from salmon, cod, and mackerel, also contain important omega-3 fatty acids. Omega-6 fatty acids are found in most plant and vegetable oils, including safflower, corn, peanut, and sesame, as well as evening primrose, black currant, and borage.

Free Radicals

Free radicals are a major molecular cause of damage to healthy cells. A free radical is an unstable molecule with an unpaired electron that steals electrons from other molecules, producing harmful effects, such as membrane destruction and changes in the cell nucleus, which can lead to mutations. Free radicals form when molecules react with oxygen and are "oxidized." This occurs due to normal metabolic processes, as well as increased chemical, physical, or emotional stress. Environmental toxicity in food, air, water, and cigarette smoke increases the production of free radicals.

Glucagon

Glucagon is secreted by the pancreas and helps to unlock the body's fat stores to be burned as fuel. If too much insulin is present in the bloodstream, due to a steady diet of carbohydrates for example, glucagon is blocked and the body's fat stores aren't available as an energy source. As a result, the person may feel lethargic, and may crave carbohydrates as a result.

Glucose

Glucose, a type of sugar, is the main fuel used by the brain. After a meal is eaten, the pancreas produces insulin to enable sugars to be metabolized. If you are eating a lot of carbohydrates, your body will become accustomed to producing a lot of insulin and, over time, you may experience insulin resistance. The result is that your body may store the carbohydrates as fat rather than making them available as fuel that can be burned off by your body.

Hypoglycemia

Hypoglycemia, or low blood sugar (glucose), is a condition often associated with diabetes. Glucose is the primary source of fuel for the brain. In healthy people, the release of insulin acts to keep blood sugar levels fairly constant. When the pancreas produces too much insulin, however, blood glucose levels drop suddenly. Symptoms of hypoglycemia include anxiety, weakness, and sweating.

Immune System

The **immune system** guards the body against foreign, disease-producing substances. Its "workers" are various white blood cells including 1 trillion lymphocytes and 100 million trillion antibodies. Lymphocytes are found in high numbers in the lymph nodes, bone marrow, spleen, and thymus gland.

Immunoglobulin

An **immunoglobulin** is one of a class of five specially designed antibody proteins produced in the spleen, bone marrow, or lymph tissue and involved in the immune system's defense response to foreign substances. The main types of immunoglobulins, grouped according to their concentration in the blood, are IgG (80%), IgA (10% to 15%), IgM (5% to 10%), IgD (less than 0.1%), and IgE (less than 0.01%).

Lectins

Lectins are protein fragments of incompletely digested foods that bind with specific sugar receptors on the surface of all cells of the body. They tend to stick like Velcro to the lining of the gastrointestinal tract, where they irritate the tissues and can destroy cell membranes. Most dietary lectins come from the indigestible fractions of plant products, often deriving from beans, grains, soy, and wheat. Lectins can lead to food allergies and toxic reactions at the mucosal membranes in the intestines. In particular, soybean and wheat lectins can produce an increase in permeability in the cells they bind to, often leading to cell death. Further, lectins can cause atrophying of the intestinal villi (the fingerlike projections that afford the intestines their absorptive surface area).

Lipotropic Factors

Lipotropic factors are substances that naturally prevent excess fat from accumulating in the liver. They help cleanse the liver by promoting the flow of fat and bile into the gallbladder. They also stimulate the growth of phagocytes (the bacteria-eating cells in the liver).

Lymphatic System

The **lymphatic system** consists of lymph fluid and the structures (vessels, ducts, and nodes) involved in transporting it from tissues to the bloodstream. Lymph fluid occupies the space between the body's cells and contains plasma proteins, foreign particles, and cellular wastes. Lymph nodes are clusters of immune tissue that work as filters, or "inspection stations," for detecting and removing foreign and potentially harmful substances in the lymph fluid. While the body has hundreds of lymph nodes (more than 500), they are mostly clustered in the neck, armpits, chest, groin, and abdomen. The lymphatic system is the body's master drain, collecting and filtering the lymph fluid and conveying waste products and cellular debris to the bloodstream, ultimately allowing them to be cleared from the body.

Metabolism

Metabolism is the biological process by which energy is extracted from the foods consumed, producing carbon dioxide and water as by-products for elimination. There are two kinds of metabolism constantly underway in the cells: anabolic and catabolic. The anabolic function produces substances for cell growth and repair, while the catabolic function controls digestion, disassembling food into forms the body can use for energy.

Mitochondria

Mitochondria are organelles present in every cell of the body. They have a highly organized internal structure with many internal membranes. Enzymes responsible for converting proteins, carbohydrates, and fats into energy are located on these membranes.

Neurotransmitter

A **neurotransmitter** is a brain chemical with the specific function of enabling communications to happen between brain cells. Chief among the 100 identified to date are acetylcholine, gamma-aminobutyric acid (GABA), serotonin, dopamine, and norepinephrine.

Qi

Qi or chi (pronounced CHEE) is a Chinese word variously translated to mean "vital energy," "essence of life," and "living force." In Chinese medicine, the proper flow of qi along energy channels (meridians) within the body is crucial to a person's health and vitality. There are many types of qi, classified according to source, location, and function (such as activation, warming, defense, transformation, and containment). Within the body, qi and blood are closely linked, as each is considered to flow along with the other. Qi may be stagnant (nonmoving), deficient (partially absent), or excessive (inappropriately abundant) from a given organ system. Qi has two essential qualities: yang (active, fiery, moving, bright, energizing) and yin (passive, watery, stationary, dark, calming).

Thermogenesis

As with basal metabolism, the rate of **thermogenesis** will determine whether the body sheds or accumulates fat. *Thermogenesis* means, simply, to generate heat in the body during metabolism. The digestion of food, movement of the muscles, and other metabolic processes all produce heat as a by-product. In certain metabolic activities, however, heat is the primary product. This type of pure thermogenesis is one of the body's key weight-control mechanisms and serves as a kind of waste incinerator for excess calories. When this mechanism does not burn fat as it should, weight gain is sure to follow.

Thyroid Gland

The **thyroid gland**, one of the body's seven endocrine glands, is located in the throat area, and wraps around the windpipe right behind the Adam's apple. It is the body's metabolic thermostat, controlling body temperature, energy use, and, in children, the body's growth rate. The thyroid controls the rate at which organs function and the speed with which the body uses food. Hypothyroidism is a condition of low or underactive thyroid gland function that can produce one or more of as many as 47 symptoms, including fatigue, depression, lethargy, weakness, weight gain, and low body temperature. A resting body temperature below 97.8°F may indicate hypothyroidism.

Traditional Chinese Medicine

Traditional Chinese medicine (TCM), which originated over 5,000 years ago, is a comprehensive system of medical practice that heals the body according to the principles of nature and balance. A TCM physician considers the flow of vital life force energy (qi) in a patient through close examination of the person's pulse, tongue, body odor, voice tone and strength, and general demeanor, among other elements. Underlying imbalances and disharmony in the body are described in terminology analogous to the natural world (heat, cold, dryness, dampness, or wind).

Trans Fats

Although some **trans fats** occur naturally in minute quantities in certain foods, most of them are man-made, created by a process wherein vegetable oil is chemically and structurally altered by being combined with hydrogen to lengthen shelf life. This process transforms some of the fatty acids in the oil into trans-fatty acids (TFAs). Trans-fatty acid composition of commercially prepared hydrogenated fats varies from 8% to 70%, and until very recently, trans fats comprised about 60% of the fat found in processed foods. It is estimated that Americans consume over 600 million pounds of TFAs annually in the form of frying fats. TFAs can increase the risk of heart disease when consumed as at least 12% of the total fat intake. TFAs also reduce production of prostaglandins (hormones that act locally to control all cell-to-cell interactions) and interfere with fatty acid metabolism.

Resources

Aromatherapy

Amrita Aromatherapy, P.O. Box 2178, Fairfield, IA 52556; tel: 800-410-9651 or 5 15-472-9136; www.amrita.net.

National Association for Holistic Aromatherapy, P.O. Box 17622, Boulder, CO 80308-0622; tel: 303-258-3791; www.naha.com.

Bodywork

American Chiropractic Association, 1701 Clarendon Boulevard, Arlington, VA 22209; tel: 703-276-8800; www.amerchiro.org.

American Massage Therapy Association, 820 Davis Street, Suite 100, Evanston, IL 60201; tel: 312-761-2682; www.amtamassage.org.

International Institute of Reflexology, P.O. Box 12462, St. Petersburg, FL 33733; tel: 813-343-4811; www.reflexology-usa.net.

International Rolf Institute, P.O. Box 1868, Boulder, CO 80306; tel: 800-530-8875 or 303-449-5903; www.rolf.org.

Cognitive Therapy

American Institute for Cognitive Therapy, 136 E. 57th Street, Suite 1101, New York, NY 10022; tel: 212-308-2440; fax 212-308-9847; www.cognitivetherapynyc.com.

University of Pennsylvania Center for Cognitive Therapy, 3600 Market Street, 8th Floor, Philadelphia, PA 19104; tel: 215-898-4100; fax: 215-898-1865; www. uphs.upenn.edu/psycct/.

Exercise

American Association of Taoist Studies, 445 Richmond Park West, Suite 603-B, Richmond Heights, OH 44143; tel: 800-646-5731, ext. 4619, or 216-646-9129. Information on tai chi and qigong.

American Foundation of Traditional Chinese Medicine, 505 Beach Street, San Francisco, CA 94133; tel: 415-776-0502.

Chinese Healing Arts Center, 266 Smith Avenue, Kingston, NY 12401; tel: 845-338-6045; fax: 845-338-5438; www.qihealer.com. Offers an instructional video-cassette (*The Swimming Dragon: Ancient Chinese Exercise for Rapid Weight Loss*) and book (*The Swimming Dragon*) on the swimming dragon exercise.

International Association of Yoga Therapists, P.O. Box 1386, Lower Lake, CA 95457; tel: 707-928-9898; www.iayt.org.

President's Council on Physical Fitness and Sports, 200 Independence Avenue SW, Room 738-H, Washington, DC 20201; tel: 202-690-9000; fax: 202-690-5211; www.fitness.gov. Excellent fitness tips.

Titus Kahoutek, BS, and Jasson Zurilgen, Certified Personal Trainers/ C.H.E.K. Practitioners, Heroics Exercise Systems, 5102 239th Street, Mount Lake Terrace, WA 98043, tel: 206-714-6483; www.urbanmonkeys.com.

Flower Essences

Aum Himalaya Sanjeevini Essences,15 E Jaybharat Society, 3rd Road, Khar (West), Mumbai 400052, India; tel: (00-91-22) 26486819;

fax: (00-91-22) 26050975; email: infoaumhimalaya.com; www.aumhimalaya.com. Offers electromagnetic field deflectingdevices and flower and gemstone essence remedies.

Flower Essence Society, P.O. Box 459, Nevada City, CA 95959; tel: 800-548-0075 or 916-265-9163; fax: 916-265-6467; www.flowersociety.org.

Perelandra, P.O. Box 3603, Warrenton, VA 20188; tel: 800-960-8806; fax: 540-937-3360; email: email@perelandra-ltd.com; www.perelandra-ltd.com.

Full-Spectrum Lighting

Seventh Generation, 1 Mill Street, Box A-26, Burlington, VT 05401-1530; tel: 800-456-1191 or 802-658-3773; fax: 802-658-1771; www.seventhgeneration.com.

Verilux, 9 Viaduct Road, Stamford, CT 06907; tel: 800-786-6850 or 203-921-2430; fax: 203-921-2427; www.ergolight.com.

Guided Imagery

Academy for Guided Imagery, P.O. Box 2070, Mill Valley, CA 94942; tel: 800-726-2070 or 415-389-9325; fax: 415-389-9342; www.healthy.net/agi.

Herbs and Nutritional Supplements

Lin Sister Herb Shop, 4 Bowery Street, New York, NY 10013; tel: 212-962-5417; email: linsisterherb@aol.com. Sells traditional Chinese medicine herbs and formulas.

Metagenics, 971 Calle Negocio, San Clemente, CA 92673; tel: 800-692-9400; fax: 714-366-0818; www.metagenics.com. (Available to professionals only.)

Nature's Answer, 75 Commerce Drive, Hauppauge, NY 11788; tel: 800-439-2324 or 631-231-7492; fax: 631-231-8391; www.naturesanswer.com. Holistically balanced herbal and nutritional products since 1972.

NutriCology/Allergy Research Group, P.O. Box 55907, Hayward, CA 94544; tel: 510-487-8526 or 800-782-4274; fax: 510-487-8682; www.nutricology.com.

Pure Encapsulations, 490 Boston Post Road, Sudbury, MA 01776; tel: 800-753-2277 or 508-443-1999; fax: 888-783-2277; www.purecaps.com.

Vitamin Shoppe, 2101 91st Street, North Bergen, NJ 07047; tel: 800-223-1216; fax: 800-852-7153; www.vitaminshoppe.com. Has locations across the United States.

Hypnotherapy

American Institute of Hypnotherapy, 1805 East Garry Avenue, Suite 100, Santa Ana, CA 92606; tel: 800-634-8766 or 949-261-6400.

American Society of Clinical Hypnosis, 2200 East Devon Avenue, Suite 291, Des Plaines, IL 60018; tel: 708-297-3317; www.asch.net.

Laboratories

American College for Advancement in Medicine, 23121 Verdugo Drive, Suite 204, Laguna Hills, CA 92653; tel: 800-532-3688 or 714-583-7666; www.acam.org. Contact this organization to find a physician who performs the EDTA lead versenate 24-hour urine collection test.

Analytical Research Laboratories, 840 Research Parkway, Suite 546, Oklahoma City, OK 73104; tel: 800-393-1595 or 405-271-1144; fax: 405-271-1174; www.arlok.com. Hair mineral analysis.

Diagnos-Techs, 6620 South 192nd Place, J-104, Kent, WA 98032; tel: 800-878-3787 or 425-251-0596; fax: 425-251-0637; www.diagnostechs.com. Offers Adrenal Stress Index test.

Genox Corporation, 1414 Key Highway, Baltimore, MD 21230; tel: 410-347-7616 (office); tel: 410-347-7637 (lab); fax: 410-347-7617; www.genox.com. Oxidative stress profile.

Great Smokies Diagnostic Laboratory (Genove Diagnostics), 63 Zillicoa Street, Asheville, NC 28801; tel: 704-253-0621 or 800-522-4762; fax: 704-252-9303; www.gsdl.com. Offers comprehensive digestive stool analysis, functional liver detoxification profile, and oxidative stress profile.

Immuno Laboratories, 1620 West Oakland Park Boulevard, Fort Lauderdale, FL 33311; tel: 800-231-9197 or 954-486-4500; fax: 954-739-8583; www. immunolabs.com. Offers the IgG ELISA test.

International Iridology Practitioners Association, P.O. Box 339, Pinehurst, TX 77362; tel: 888-682-2208; http://iridologyassn.org. Provides referrals to iridologists.

Lita Lee, Ph.D., P.O. Box 516, Lowell, OR 97452; tel: 541-431-1099; www. litalee.com. Offers the Loomis urinalysis; click on the Loomis Test Kit link.

Meridian Valley Laboratory, 24030 132nd Avenue SE, Kent, WA 98042; tel: 800-234-6825 or 206-631-8922; http://meridianvalleylab.com.

Metametrix Medical Laboratory, 5000 Peachtree Boulevard, Suite 110, Norcross, GA 30071; tel: 800-221-4640 or 770-446-5483; fax: 770-441-2237; www. metametrix.com. Offers cell membrane lipid profile and toxic metal screening.

Optimal Wellness Center (Dr. Joseph Mercola), 1443 W. Schaumburg, Suite 250, Schaumburg, IL 60194; tel: 847-985-1777; www.mercola.com. Offers an email mini course in metabolic typing.

SpectraCell, 515 Post Oak Boulevard, Suite 830, Houston, TX 77027; tel: 800-227-5227 or 713-621-3101; www.spectracell.com. Offers functional intracellular analysis.

Light Therapy

College of Syntonic Optometry, 1200 Robeson Street, Fall River, MA 02720-5508; tel: 508-673-1251; www.syntonicphototherapy.com.

Society for Light Treatment and Biological Rhythms, 10200 West 44th Avenue, Suite 304, Wheat Ridge, CO 80033-2840; tel: 303-422-7905; fax: 303-422-8894; www.sltbr.org.

Natural Healthcare Professionals

Hyla Cass, MD, 1608 Michael Lane, Pacific Palisades, CA 90272; tel: 310-459-9866; fax: 310-564-0328; www.drcass.com; e-mail: hyla@drcass.com.

Susan Groh, MD, 2916 Frankel Boulevard, Merrick, NY 11566; tel: 516-867-5132; fax: 516-867-5519; www.grohwellhealingcenter.com.

Ronald Hoffman, MD, The Hoffman Center, 40 East 30th Street, New York, NY 10016; tel: 212-779-1744; www.drhoffman.com

Stephen Holt, MD, Natures Benefit Inc., 61 Stevens Avenue, Little Falls, NJ 07424; tel: 973-890-2378; fax: 973-890-8654; www.naturesbenefit.com.

Ellen Kamhi, Ph.D., RN, P.O. Box 525, Oyster Bay, NY 11771; tel: 800-829-0918; www.naturalnurse.com.

Eugene Zampieron, ND, 413 Grassy Hill Road, Woodbury, CT 06798; tel/fax: 203-263-2970; www.drznaturally.com.

Neuro-Linguistic Programming

NLP Comprehensive, 5695 Yukon Street, Arvada, CO 80002; tel: 800-233-1657 or 303-940-8888; fax 303-940-8889; www.nlpco.com.

NLP Seminars Group International, P.O. Box 424, Hopatcong, NJ 07843; tel: 201-770-1084; www.purenlp.com.

NLP University/Dynamic Learning Center, P.O. Box 1112, Ben Lomond, CA 95005; tel: 408-336-3457; fax: 408-336-5854; www.nlpu.com.

Organic and Nontoxic Products

American Water Council, tel: 866-278-2634; www.aquamd.com. Provides water testing services.

Consumer Health Research, P.O. Box 1884, Bandon, OR 97411; tel: 800-282-9274 or 609-645-1110; fax: 609-645-8881; www.vegiwash.com. Makers of VegiWash.

EarthSafe (a division of National Research and Chemical Company), 15600 New Century Drive, Gardena, CA 90248; tel: 310-515-1700; fax: 310-527-9963; www.earthsafe.net.

Environmental Detoxification Consultants, 413 Grassy Hill Road, Woodbury, CT 06798; tel/fax: 203-263-2970; www.drznaturally.com.

Northeast Organic Farmers Association, 411 Sheldon Road, Barre, MA 01005; tel: 978-355-2853; www.nofamass.org.

Organic Consumers Association, 6771 South Silver Hill Drive, Finland, MN 55603; tel: 218-353-7454; fax: 218-353-7652; www.organicconsumers.org.

Science Air Products USA, 809 San Antonio Road, Unit 7, Palo Alto, CA 94303; tel: 888-682-0273; www.freshairmachine.com.

Seventh Generation, 1 Mill Street, Box A-26, Burlington, VT 05401; tel: 800-456-1191 or 802-658-3773; fax: 802-658-1771; www.seventh generation.com. Offers environmentally friendly cleaning products.

Sprouts Farmers Market, 11811 N. Tatum Blvd., Suite 2400, Phoenix, AZ 85028; tel: 480-814-8016; fax: 480-814-8017; www.sprouts.com.

Walnut Acres Organic Farms, 4600 Sleepytime Road, Boulder, CO 80301; tel: 800-433-3998; www.walnutacres.com. Offers a wide selection of organically grown foods.

Whole Foods Market; www.wholefoods.com. Organic foods, healthy recipes, and more. Locations across the United States.

Support Groups

American Self-Help Group Clearinghouse, Saint Clare's Health Services, 25 Pocono Road, Denville, NJ 07834; tel: 973-326-6789; fax: 973-625-8848; http:// mentalhelp.net/selfhelp/.

National Self-Help Clearinghouse, 25 West 43rd Street, New York, NY 10036; tel: 212-817-1822; www.selfhelpweb.org.

Therapeutic Touch

Nurse Healers—Professional Associates International, 175 Fifth Avenue, Suite 2755, New York, NY 10010; tel: 212-886-3776; www.therapeutic-touch.org.

Workshops

Ellen Kamhi, Ph.D., RN, and Eugene Zampieron, ND, MH (AHG), conduct the EcoTours for Cures series of workshops internationally, focusing on the ethnobotany of wild edible and medicinal plants. For more information on any of the EcoTours for Cures workshops, call 800-829-0918 or visit www.naturalnurse.com.

Radio Shows

Herbally Yours, Wednesday, 12 noon EST on 90.3 FM (WHPC, in the New York area).

It's All About Health, Monday through Friday, 8 to 10 a.m. (listen online at www.newstalk1220.com).

Natural Alternatives, Friday 6 to 7 p.m. EST on 90.1 FM (listen online at www.wusb.org).

The Natural Nurse and Dr. Z, Monday 10 to 11 a.m. EST on Gary Null's Progressive Radio Network (listen online or check archives anytime at www.progressiveradionetwork.org).

Books by the Author

Cycles of Life: Herbs and Energy Techniques for the Stages of a Woman's Life

The Natural Guide to Great Sex

Arthritis: An Alternative Medicine Definitive Guide (with Eugene Zampieron, ND)

The Natural Medicine Chest (with Eugene Zampieron, ND)

Endnotes

Introduction: Dieting Is Not the Answer

1. D. E. Cummings et al., "Plasma ghrelin levels after diet-induced weight loss or gastric bypass surgery," *New England Journal of Medicine* 346, no. 21 (2002): 1623–30.

2. A. J. Caban et al., "Obesity in US workers: The National Health Interview Survey, 1986 to 2002," *American Journal of Public Health* 95, no. 9 (2005): 1614–22.

3. National Institutes of Health guidelines for obesity, 2005, available at www.nhlbi.nih.gov/guidelines/obesity/ob_home.htm.

4. S. Jay Olshansky et al., "A potential decline in life expectancy in the United States in the 21st century," *New England Journal of Medicine* 352, no. 11 (2005): 1138–45.

5. Health Scout, "Obesity causes society-wide cost burden," *Daily News Central: Health News,* June 27, 2005, available at http://health.dailynewscentral.com/content/view/1146/0.

6. D. M. Eddy et al., "Clinical outcomes and cost-effectiveness of strategies for managing people at high risk for diabetes," *Annals of Internal Medicine* 143, no. 4 (2005): 251–64.

7. A. V. Joshi et al., "Relationship between obesity and cardiovascular risk factors: Findings from a multi-state screening project in the United States," *Current Medical Research and Opinion* 21, no. 11 (2005): 1755–61.

8. T. B. Van Itallie, "Health implications of overweight and obesity in the United States," *Annals of Internal Medicine* 103, no. 6, part 2 (1985): 983–88.

9. K. M. Rexrode et al., "A prospective study of body mass index, weight change, and risk of stroke in women," *Journal of the American Medical Association* 277, no. 19 (1997): 1539–45.

10. A. Lukanova et al., "Body mass index and cancer: Results from the Northern Sweden Health and Disease Cohort," *International Journal of Cancer* 118, no. 2 (2006): 458–66; K. Rapp et al., "Obesity and incidence of cancer: A large cohort study of over 145,000 adults in Austria," *British Journal of Cancer*

93, no. 9 (2005): 1062–67; E. E. Calle et al., "Overweight, obesity, and mortality from cancer in a prospectively studied cohort of U.S. Adults," *New England Journal of Medicine* 348, no. 17 (2003): 1625–38.

11. T. M. Griffin and F. Guilak, "The role of mechanical loading in the onset and progression of osteoarthritis," *Exercise and Sport Sciences Reviews* 33, no. 4 (2005): 195–200.

12. A. C. Cannella and T. R. Mikuls, "Understanding treatments for gout," *American Journal of Managed Care* 11, suppl. 15 (2005): S451–58.

13. C. Younan et al., "Cardiovascular disease, vascular risk factors and the incidence of cataract and cataract surgery: The Blue Mountains Eye Study," *Opthalmic Epidemiology* 10, no. 4 (2003): 227–40.

14. K. Krahnstoever Davison et al., "Reexamining obesigenic families: Parents' obesity-related behaviors predict girls' change in BMI," *Obesity Research* 13, no. 11 (2005): 1980–90.

15. www.supersizeme.com. Film that follows the health of a man who eats McDonald's food for a month.

16. American Academy of Pediatrics Committee on Communications, "Children, adolescents, and advertising," *Pediatrics*, 95 (1995): 295–97.

17. National Institute of Diabetes and Digestive and Kidney Diseases, *Understanding Adult Obesity*, NIH Publication No. 94-3680 (Washington, DC: National Institutes of Health, 1998).

18. M. Fenton, "Battling America's epidemic of physical inactivity: Building more walkable, livable communities," *Journal of Nutrition Education and Behavior* 37, suppl. 2 (2005): S115–20.

19. Thomas N. Robinson, "Does television cause childhood obesity?" *Journal of the American Medical Assocation* 279, no. 12 (1998): 959–60; Ross E. Andersen et al., "Relationship of physical activity and television watching with body weight and level of fatness among children," *Journal of the American Medical Assocation* 279, no. 12 (1998): 938–42.

20. National Heart, Lung, and Blood Institute, Obesity Education Initiative, "Calculate Your Body Mass," available at www.nhlbisupport.com/bmi/bmicalc. htm.

21. C. J. Dobbelsteyn et al., "A comparative evaluation of waist circumference, waist-to-hip ratio and body mass index as indicators of cardiovascular risk factors: The Canadian Heart Health Surveys," *International Journal of Obesity and Related Metabolic Disorders* 25, no. 5 (2001): 652–61.

Chapter 1. Detoxification

1. Bill Wolverton, *How to Grow Fresh Air: 50 Houseplants That Purify Your Home or Office* (New York: Penguin, 1997).

2. William J. Rea, Chemical Sensitivity, vol. 4 (Boca Raton, FL: CRC Lewis, 1997), 2434.

3. Environmental Working Group, BodyBurden Study, available at www. ewg.org/issues/siteindex/issues.php?issueid=5004#report'%20or%20content_ type='project.'

4. D. P. Wyon, "The effects of indoor air quality on performance and productivity," *Indoor Air* 14, suppl. 7 (2004): 92–101.

5. B. Thriene et al., "Man-made mineral fiber boards in buildings: Health

risks caused by quality deficiencies," *Toxicology Letters* 88, nos. 1–3 (1996): 299–303.

6. R. J. Laumbach and H. M. Kipen, "Bioaerosols and sick building syndrome: Particles, inflammation, and allergy," *Current Opinion in Allergy and Clinical Immunology* 5, no. 2 (2005): 135–39.

7. B. McFadden, "Phenotypic variation in xenobiotic metabolism and adverse environmental response: Focus on sulfur-dependent detoxification pathways," *Toxicology* 111, nos. 1–3 (1996): 43–65; B. Crotty, "Ulcerative colitis and xenobiotic metabolism," *Lancet* 343, no. 8888 (1994): 35–38.

8. William Lee Cowden, "Is your shower toxic? Some pollution solutions," *Alternative Medicine* 29 (1999): 69; Joseph Mercola, comments on Mercola.com, available at www.mercola.com/2004/sep/4/heavy_metals_water.htm.

9. M. E. Crespo-Lopez et al., "Mercury and neurotoxicity," *Revista de Neurologia* 40, no. 7 (2005): 441; World Health Organization, Environmental Health Criteria for Inorganic Mercury (Geneva, Switzerland: World Health Organization, 1991), 118.

10. C. M. Galhardi et al., "Toxicity of copper intake: Lipid profile, oxidative stress and susceptibility to renal dysfunction," *Food and Chemical Toxicology* 42, no. 12 (2004): 2053–60.

11. H. Xu et al., "Exposure to trichloroethylene and its metabolites causes impairment of sperm fertilizing ability in mice," *Toxicological Sciences* 82, no. 2 (2004): 590–97.

12. D. Pizzetti et al., "Colonic hydrotherapy for obstructed defecation," *Colorectal Disease* 7, no. 1 (2005): 107–108.

13. Edmond Bordeaux Szekeley, *Essene Gospel of Peace* (London: International Biogenic Society, 1937), 16.

14. John Harvey Kellogg, "Should the colon be sacrificed or may it be reformed?" *Journal of the American Medical Association* 68, no. 26 (1917): 1957–59.

15. C. E. Ruhl and J. E. Everhart, "Coffee and caffeine consumption reduce the risk of elevated serum alanine aminotransferase activity in the United States," *Gastroenterology* 128, no. 1 (2005): 24-32; L. K. T. Lam et al., "Isolation and identification of kahweol palmitate and cafestol palmitate as active constituents of green coffee beans that enhance glutathione S-transferase activity in the mouse," *Cancer Research* 42, no. 4 (1982): 1193–98.

16. N. H. Shear et al., "Acetaminophen-induced toxicity to human epidermoid cell line A431 and hepatoblastoma cell line Hep G2, in vitro, is diminished by silymarin," *Skin Pharmacology* 8, no. 6 (1995): 279–91.

17. Kerry Bone, "Picrorrhiza: Important modulator of immune function," *Townsend Letter for Doctors and Patients* 1995: 88–94, available at www.herbalgram.org/herbclip/review.asp?i=41604.

18. Eugene Zampieron and Ellen Kamhi, *The Natural Medicine Chest* (New York: M. Evans, 1999), 65–67.

19. D. Chen et al., "Inhibition of human liver catechol-O-methyltransferase by tea catechins and their metabolites: Structure-activity relationship and molecular-modeling studies," *Biochemical Pharmacology* 69, no. 10 (2005): 1523–31.

20. W. Siems et al., "Anti-fibrosclerotic effects of shock wave therapy in lipedema and cellulite," *Biofactors* 24, nos. 1–4 (2005): 275–82.

21. A. Bhattacharya et al., "Body acceleration distribution and O2 uptake

in humans during running and jumping," *Journal of Applied Physiology* 49, no. 5 (1980): 881–87; Joan Bartlett et al., "Rebounding on a mini-trampoline: Implications for physical fitness and coronary risk factors," *Journal of Cardiopulmonary Rehabilitation* 10 (1990): 401–8.

22. N. Kap-Soon et al., "Protein biomarkers in the plasma of workers occupationally exposed to polycyclic aromatic hydrocarbons," *Proteomics* 4, no. 11 (2004): 3505–13.

23. D. W. Schnare et al., "Body burden reductions of PCBs, PBBs, and chlorinated pesticides in human subjects," *Ambio* 13 (1984): 5–6.

24. William J. Rea, *Chemical Sensitivity*, vol. 4 (Boca Raton, FL: CRC Lewis, 1997), 2463.

Chapter 2. Start Exercising

1. J. M. Jakicic and A. D. Otto, "Treatment and prevention of obesity: What is the role of exercise?" *Nutrition Review* 64, no. 2, part 2 (2006): S57–S61.

2. F. G. Toledo et al., "Changes induced by physical activity and weight loss in the morphology of inter-myofibrillar mitochondria in obese men and women," *Journal of Clinical Endocrinology and Metabolism* 91, no. 8 (2006): 3224–27.

3. J. Gonzalez-Alonso et al., "Erythrocytes and the regulation of human skeletal muscle blood flow and oxygen delivery: Role of erythrocyte count and oxygenation state of hemoglobin," *Journal of Physiology* 572, part 1 (Apr. 1, 2006): 295–305.

4. T. S. Altena et al., "Lipoprotein subfraction changes after continuous or intermittent exercise training," *Medicine and Science in Sports and Exercise* 38, no. 2 (2006): 367–72.

5. Kathryn Woolf-May et al., "Effects of an 18-week walking programme on cardiac function in previously sedentary or relatively inactive adults," *British Journal of Sports Medicine* 31, no. 1 (1997): 48–53.

6. The President's Council on Physical Fitness and Sports, "Fitness fundamentals: Guidelines for personal fitness programs," October 15, 2004, available via www.fitness.gov/exerciseweight.htm.

7. D. E. Warburton et al., "Prescribing exercise as preventive therapy," *Canadian Medical Association Journal* 174, no. 7 (2006): 961–74.

8. K. I. Gallagher et al., "Psychosocial factors related to physical activity and weight loss in overweight women," *Medicine and Science in Sports and Exercise* 38, no. 5 (2006): 971–80.

9. The President's Council on Physical Fitness and Sports, "Fitness fundamentals: Guidelines for personal fitness programs," October 15, 2004, available via www.fitness.gov/fitness.htm.

10. A. I. Zeni et al., "Energy expenditure with indoor exercise machines," *Journal of the American Medical Association* 275, no. 18 (1996): 1424–27.

11. A. Bhattacharya et al., "Body Acceleration Distribution and O_2 Uptake in Humans during Running and Jumping," *Journal of Applied Physiology* 49, no. 5 (1980): 881–87; Joan Bartlett et al., "Rebounding on a Mini-Trampoline: Implications for Physical Fitness and Coronary Risk Factors," *Journal of Cardiopulmonary Rehabilitation* 10 (1990): 401–8.

12. Steven L. Wolf et al., "Exploring the basis for tai chi chuan as a therapeutic exercise approach," *Archives of Physical Medicine and Rehabilitation* 78, no. 8 (1997): 886–92.

13. S. H. Yeh et al., "Regular tai chi chuan exercise enhances functional mobility and CD4CD25 regulatory T cells," *British Journal of Sports Medicine* 40, no. 3 (2006): 239–43.

14. Philip S. Lansky and Yu Shen, "The Swimming Dragon," *Health World* (July/August 1990): 47.

Chapter 3. Healthy Eating

1. D. Forman and B. E. Bulwer, "Cardiovascular disease: Optimal approaches to risk factor modification of diet and lifestyle," *Current Treatment Options in Cardiovascular Medicine* 8, no. 1 (2006): 47-57.

2. Robert Garrison, Jr., and Elizabeth Somer, *Nutrition Desk Reference* (New Canaan, CT: Keats, 1995), 27.

3. H. Trowell et al., *Dietary Fibre, Fibre-Depleted Foods and Disease* (New York: Academic Press, 1985).

4. N. M. Delzenne and P. D. Cani, "A place for dietary fibre in the management of the metabolic syndrome," *Current Opinion in Clinical Nutrition and Metabolic Care* 8, no. 6 (2005): 636–40; M. H. Davidson et al., "The hypocholesterolemic effects of beta-glucan in oatmeal and oat bran: A dose-controlled study," *Journal of the American Medical Association* 265, no. 14 (1991): 1833–39; J. W. Anderson and C. A. Bryant. "Dietary fiber: Diabetes and obesity," *American Journal of Gastroenterology* 81, no. 10 (1986), 898–906.

5. American Cancer Society, "Controlling portion sizes," available at www.cancer.org/docroot/PED/content/PED_3_2x_Portion_Control.asp.

6. Y. Schutz et al., "Failure of dietary fat to promote fat oxidation: A factor favoring the development of obesity," *American Journal of Clinical Nutrition* 50, no. 2 (1989), 307–14.

7. J. P. Flatt. "Body weight, fat storage, and alcohol metabolism," *Nutrition Reviews* 50, no. 9 (1992): 267–70.

8. C. M. Chen et al., "Consumption of purple sweet potato leaves modulates human immune response: T-lymphocyte functions, lytic activity of natural killer cell and antibody production," *World Journal of Gastroenterology* 11, no. 37 (2005): 5777–81; A. C. Ross, "Vitamin A status: Relationship to immunity and the antibody response," *Proceedings of the Society for Experimental Biology and Medicine* 200, no. 3 (1992): 303–20; G. Dennert, "Retinoids and the immune system: Immunostimulation by vitamin A" in M. B. Sporn et al., eds. *The Retinoids* (Orlando, FL: Academic Press, 1984), 373–90; B. E. Cohen et al., "Reversal of postoperative immunosuppression in man by vitamin A," *Surgery, Gynecology, and Obstetrics* 149, no. 5 (1979): 658–62.

9. B. Watzl et al., "A 4-wk intervention with high intake of carotenoid-rich vegetables and fruit reduces plasma C-reactive protein in healthy, nonsmoking men," *American Journal of Clinical Nutrition* 82, no. 5 (2005): 1052–58.

10. D. Canoy et al., "Plasma ascorbic acid concentrations and fat distribution in 19,068 British men and women in the European Prospective Investigation into Cancer and Nutrition Norfolk cohort study," *American Journal of Clinical Nutrition* 82, no. 6 (2005): 1203–9.

11. Dean Ornish, *Stress, Diet and Your Heart* (New York: Holt, Rinehart, and Winston, 1983).

12. American Dietetic Association, "Vegetarian diets," *ADA Reports: Journal of the American Dietetic Association* 88, no. 3 (1988): 351–55.

13. J. Sabate, "The contribution of vegetarian diets to human health," *Forum of Nutrition* 56 (2003): 218–20.

14. H. Breiteneder and E. N. Mills, "Molecular properties of food allergens," *Journal of Allergy and Clinical Immunology* 115, no. 1 (2005): 14–23.

15. David S. Ludwig et al., "Dietary fiber, weight gain, and cardiovascular disease risk factors in young adults," *Journal of the American Medical Association* 282, no. 16 (1999): 1539–46.

16. R. L. Walford et al., "The calorically restricted low-fat nutrient-dense diet in Biosphere 2 significantly lowers blood glucose, total leukocyte count, cholesterol, and blood pressure in humans," *Proceedings of the National Academy of Sciences* 89, no. 23 (1992): 11533–37.

17. B. V. Howard et al., "Low-fat dietary pattern and weight change over 7 years: The Women's Health Initiative Dietary Modification Trial," *Journal of the American Medical Association* 295, no. 1 (2006): 39–49.

18. X. Zhao et al., "Modification of lymphocyte DNA damage by carotenoid supplementation in postmenopausal women," *American Journal of Clinical Nutrition* 83, no. 1 (2006): 163–69; A. L. Ray et al., "Low serum selenium and total carotenoids predict mortality among older women living in the community: The Women's Health and Aging Studies," *Journal of Nutrition* 136, no. 1 (2006): 172–76; B. Cartmel et al., "A randomized trial of an intervention to increase fruit and vegetable intake in curatively treated patients with early-stage head and neck cancer," *Cancer Epidemiology Biomarkers and Prevention* 14, no. 12 (2005): 2848–54.

19. Walter C. Willett, M.D., et al. Letter to David Kessler, M.D., Commissioner, U.S. Food and Drug Administration (November 23, 1995).

20. J. S. Vander Wal et al., "Short-term effect of eggs on satiety in overweight and obese subjects," *Journal of the American College of Nutrition* 24, no. 6 (2005): 510–15.

21. K. Meksawan et al., "Effect of low and high fat diets on nutrient intakes and selected cardiovascular risk factors in sedentary men and women," *Journal of the American College of Nutrition* 23, no. 2 (2004): 131–40.

22. J. E. Upritchard et al., "Modern fat technology: What is the potential for heart health?" *Proceedings of the Nutrition Society* 64, no. 3 (2005): 379–86.

23. E. Giovannucci, "Diet, body weight, and colorectal cancer: A summary of the epidemiologic evidence," *Journal of Women's Health* 12, no. 2 (2003): 173–82.

24. G. Nagel and J. Linseisen, "Dietary intake of fatty acids, antioxidants and selected food groups and asthma in adults," *European Journal of Clinical Nutrition* 59, no. 1 (2005): 8–15.

25. K. Murakami et al., "Effect of dietary factors on incidence of type 2 diabetes: A systematic review of cohort studies," *Journal of Nutritional Science and Vitaminology* 51, no. 4 (2005): 292–310.

26. S. Stender and J. Dyerberg, "Influence of trans fatty acids on health," *Annals of Nutrition and Metabolism* 48, no. 2 (2004): 61–66.

27. Center for Science the Public Interest http://www.cspinet.org/olestra/history.html.

28. C. Zhang et al., "Activation of JNK and xanthine oxidase by TNF-alpha impairs nitric oxide-mediated dilation of coronary arterioles," *Journal of Molecular and Cellular Cardiology* 40, no. 2 (2006): 247–57.

29. William Campbell Douglass, *The Milk Book: How Science Is Destroying Nature's Nearly Perfect Food* (Dunwoody, GA: Second Opinion Publishing, 1993), 103–10.

30. B. Hennig, "Dietary fat and macronutrients: Relationships to artherosclerosis," *Journal of Optimal Nutrition* 1, no. 1 (1992): 21–23.

31. J. L. Quiles et al., "Dietary fat type (virgin olive vs. sunflower oils) affects age-related changes in DNA double-strand-breaks, antioxidant capacity and blood lipids in rats," *Experimental Gerontology* 39, no. 8 (2004): 1189–98.

32. I. A. Prior et al., "Cholesterol, coconuts, and diet on Polynesian atolls: A natural experiment: The Pukapuka and Tokelau island studies," *American Journal of Clinical Nutrition* 34, no. 8 (1981): 1552–61.

33. K. G. Nevin and T. Rajamohan, "Beneficial effects of virgin coconut oil on lipid parameters and in vitro LDL oxidation," *Clinical Biochemistry* 37, no. 9 (2004): 830–35.

34. K. M. Hargrave et al., "Dietary coconut oil increases conjugated linoleic acid-induced body fat loss in mice independent of essential fatty acid deficiency," *Biochimica et Biophysica Acta* 1737, no. 1 (2005): 52-60.

35. M. P. Portillo et al., "Energy restriction with high-fat diet enriched with coconut oil gives higher UCP1 and lower white fat in rats," *International Journal of Obesity and Related Metabolic Disorders* 22, no. 10 (1998): 974–79.

36. J. Han et al., "Medium-chain oil reduces fat mass and down-regulates expression of adipogenic genes in rats," *Obesity Research* 11, no. 6 (2003): 734–44.

37. M. Kasai et al., "Comparison of diet-induced thermogenesis of foods containing medium- versus long-chain triacylglycerols," *Journal of Nutritional Science and Vitaminology* 48, no. 6 (2002): 536–40.

38. M. P. St-Onge and P. J. Jones, "Physiological effects of medium-chain triglycerides: Potential agents in the prevention of obesity," *Journal of Nutrition* 132, no. 3 (2002): 329–32; M. P. St-Onge et al., "Medium-chain triglycerides increase energy expenditure and decrease adiposity in overweight men," *Obesity Research* 11, no. 3 (2003): 395–402.

39. S. Bartolotta et al., "Effect of fatty acids on arenavirus replication: Inhibition of virus production by lauric acid," *Archives of Virology* 146, no. 4 (2001): 777–90; C. E. Isaacs, et al., "Inactivation of enveloped viruses in human bodily fluids by purified lipids," *Annals of the New York Academy of Sciences* 724 (June 6, 1994): 457–64; J. J. Kabara, "Antimicrobial agents derived from fatty acids," *Journal of the American Oil Chemists Society* 61 (1984): 397–403.

Chapter 4. Heal Your Emotional Appetite

1. E. M. Webber, "Psychological characteristics of bingeing and nonbingeing obese women," *Journal of Psychology* 128, no. 3 (1994): 339–51.

2. T. A. Wadden et al., "Comparison of psychosocial status in treatment-seeking women with class III vs. class I–II obesity," *Obesity* 14, suppl. 3 (2006): 90S–98S.

3. K. Raikkonen et al., "Anger, hostility, and visceral adipose tissue in healthy postmenopausal women," *Metabolism* 48, no. 9 (1999): 1146–51; T. P. Carmody et al., "Hostility, dieting, and nutrition attitudes in overweight and weight-cycling men and women," *International Journal of Eating Disorders* 26, no. 1 (1999): 37–42; A. J. Hill et al., "Food craving, dietary restraint, and mood," *Appetite* 17, no. 3 (1991): 187–97.

4. American Psychological Association, "Mind/body health: Did you know?" (2004), available at www.apahelpcenter.org/articles/article.php?id=103.

5. S. C. Segerstrom and G. E. Miller, "Psychological stress and the human immune system: A meta-analytic study of 30 years of inquiry, *Psychological Bulletin* 130, no. 4 (2004): 601–30.

6. D. Boey et al., "Peptide YY ablation in mice leads to the development of hyperinsulinaemia and obesity," *Diabetologia* 49, no. 6 (2006): 1360–70.

7. M. Moorhouse et al., "Carbohydrate craving by alcohol-dependent men during sobriety: Relationship to nutrition and serotonergic function," *Alcohol Clinical and Experimental Research* 24, no. 5 (2000): 635–43.

8. A. C. Need et al., "Obesity is associated with genetic variants that alter dopamine availability," *Annals of Human Genetics* 70, part 3 (2006): 293–303.

9. K. Masuo et al., "Rebound weight gain as associated with high plasma norepinephrine levels that are mediated through polymorphisms in the beta 2-adrenoceptor," *American Journal of Hypertension* 18, no. 11 (2005): 1508–16.

10. Shad Helmsetter, *What to Say When You Talk to Yourself* (Scottsdale, AZ: Grindle Press/Audio, 1986).

11. C. M. Grilo and R. M. Masheb, "A randomized controlled comparison of guided self-help cognitive behavioral therapy and behavioral weight loss for binge eating disorder," *Behavior Research and Therapy* 43, no. 11 (2005): 1509–25.

12. J. Achterberg, "Ritual: The foundation for transpersonal medicine," *Re-vision* 14, no. 3 (1992): 158–64.

13. J. Stradling et al., "Controlled trial of hypnotherapy for weight loss in patients with obstructive sleep apnoea," *International Journal of Obesity and Related Metabolic Disorders* 22, no. 3 (1998): 278–81.

14. Christina Northrup, *Women's Health: A Special Supplement to Health Wisdom for Women* (January 1996), 15.

15. R. W. Lam et al., "The Can-SAD Study: A randomized controlled trial of the effectiveness of light therapy and fluoxetine in patients with winter seasonal affective disorder," *American Journal of Psychiatry* 163, no. 5 (2006): 805–12.

16. R. A. Chalmers et al., eds., *Scientific Research on Maharishi's Transcendental Meditation and TM-Sidih Program: Collected Papers*, vols. 2–4 (Vlodrop, Netherlands: Maharishi Vedic University Press, 1989).

17. R. K. Wallace et al., "Physiological effects of Transcendental Meditation," *Science* 167, no. 926 (1970): 1751–54; M. C. Dillbeck et al., "Physiological differences between TM and rest," *American Physiologist* 42 (1987): 879–81.

18. R. W. Cranson et al., "Transcendental Meditation and improved performance on intelligence-related measures: A longitudinal study," *Personality and Individual Differences* 12, no. 10 (1991): 1105–16.

19. D. H. Shapiro and R. N. Walsh, *Meditation: Classic and Contemporary Perspectives* (New York: Aldine, 1984).

20. M. T. Cabyoglu et al., "The treatment of obesity by acupuncture," *Inter-*

national Jounal of Neuroscience 116, no. 2 (2006): 165–75.

21. Z. Movaffaghi et al., "Effects of therapeutic touch on blood hemoglobin and hematocrit level," *Journal of Holistic Nursing* 24, no. 1 (2006): 41–48.

22. Patricia Kaminski and Richard Katz, *Flower Essence Repertory* (Nevada City, CA: The Flower Essence Society, 1994), 118–19.

23. Ibid.

Chapter 5. Strengthen Your Sugar Controls

1. J. James and D. Kerr, "Prevention of childhood obesity by reducing soft drinks," *International Journal of Obesity* 29, suppl. 2 (2005): S54–S57.

2. E. Braunwald et al., eds., *Harrison's Principles of Internal Medicine*, 15th ed. (New York : McGraw-Hill, 2001), 2138–43.

3. N. Barzilai, "Disorders of carbohydrate metabolism," in M. H. Beers and R. Berkow, eds., *The Merck Manual of Diagnosis and Therapy* (Rahway, NJ: Merck Research Laboratories, 1999).

4. D. L. Kasper et al., *Harrison's Principles of Internal Medicine*, 16th ed. (New York: McGraw-Hill Professional, 2005).

5. A. Astrup et al., "Failure to increase lipid oxidation in response to increasing dietary fat content in formerly obese women," *American Journal of Physiology* 266, no. 4, part 1 (1994): E592–99.

6. S. Lee et al., "Waist circumference is an independent predictor of insulin resistance in black and white youths," *Journal of Pediatrics* 148, no. 2 (2006): 188–94.

7. Scott M. Grundy, "Third Report of the National Cholesterol Education Program Expert Panel on Detection, Evaluation, and Treatment of High Blood Cholesterol in Adults (ATP III)," press conference remarks, available at www.nhlbi.nih.gov/guidelines/cholesterol/grundy.htm.

8. C. Lorenzo et al., "Trend in the prevalence of the metabolic syndrome and its impact on cardiovascular disease incidence: The San Antonio Heart Study," *Diabetes* 29, no. 3 (2006): 625–30; P. Kohli and P. Greenland, "Role of the metabolic syndrome in risk assessment for coronary heart disease," *Journal of the American Medical Association* 295, no. 7 (2006): 819–21.

9. A. Macchia et al., "A clinically practicable diagnostic score for metabolic syndrome improves its predictivity of diabetes mellitus," *American Heart Journal* 151, no. 3 (2006): 754.e7–754.e17.

10. P. Pasanisi et al., "Metabolic syndrome as a prognostic factor for breast cancer recurrences," *International Journal of Cancer* 119, no. 1 (2006): 236–38.

11. A. S. Gonzalez et al., "Metabolic syndrome, insulin resistance and the inflammation markers C-reactive protein and ferritin," *European Journal of Clinical Nutrition* 60, no. 6 (2006): 802–9.

12. Mayo Clinic, "Metabolic syndrome," available at www.mayoclinic.com/health/metabolic%20syndrome/DS00522/DSECTION=6.

13. I. Lemieux et al., "Elevated C-reactive protein: Another component of the atherothrombotic profile of abdominal obesity," *Arteriosclerosis, Thrombosis, and Vascular Biology* 21, no. 6 (2001): 961–67.

14. K. N. Englyst and H. N. Englyst, "Carbohydrate bioavailability," *British Journal of Nutrition* 94, no. 1 (2005): 1–11.

15. V. J. Vieira et al., "Elevated atopy in healthy obese women," *American*

Journal of Clinical Nutrition 82, no. 3 (2005): 504–9.

16. K. Bhat et al., "Perceived food and drug allergies in functional and organic gastrointestinal disorders," *Alimentary Pharmacology and Therapeutics* 16, no. 5 (2002): 969–73.

17. American Diabetes Association, "How to tell if you have pre-diabetes," available at www.diabetes.org/pre-diabetes/pre-diabetes-symptoms.jsp.

18. S. K. Raatz et al., "Reduced glycemic index and glycemic load diets do not increase the effects of energy restriction on weight loss and insulin sensitivity in obese men and women," *Journal of Nutrition* 135, no. 10 (2005): 2387–91; E. J. Mayer-Davis et al., "Towards understanding of glycaemic index and glycaemic load in habitual diet: Associations with measures of glycaemia in the Insulin Resistance Atherosclerosis Study," *British Journal of Nutrition* 95, no. 2 (2006): 397–405

19. W. C. Knowler et al., "Reduction in the incidence of type 2 diabetes with lifestyle intervention or metformin," *New England Journal of Medicine* 346, no. 6 (2002): 393–403.

20. M. K. Song et al., "Raw vegetable food containing high cyclo (his-pro) improved insulin sensitivity and body weight control," *Metabolism* 54, no. 11 (2005): 1480–89.

21. T. Tsuda et al., "Microarray profiling of gene expression in human adipocytes in response to anthocyanins," *Biochemical Pharmacology* 71, no. 8 (2006): 1184–97.

22. T. L. Davidson and S. E. Swithers, "A Pavlovian approach to the problem of obesity," *International Journal of Obesity and Related Metabolic Disorders* 28, no. 7 (2004): 933–35.

23. W. Bell et al., "Carcinogenicity of saccharin in laboratory animals and humans: Letter to Dr. Harry Conacher of Health Canada," *International Journal of Occupational and Environmental Health* 8, no. 4 (2002): 387–93.

24. See FDA list of Aspartame Adverse Reactions: http://www.sweetpoison.com/articles/0706/aspartame_symptoms_submit.html. Also http://www.sweetpoison.com/aspartame-side-effects.html.

25. FDA document IA #45-06, revised February 2, 1996, attachment revised October 27, 2005, available at www.fda.gov/ora/fiars/ora_import_ia4506.html.

26. Julian Whitaker, "The nefarious FDA strikes again," *Free American* April, 1999, available at www.dorway.com/jwstevia.txt.

27. S. Gregersen et al., "Antihyperglycemic effects of stevioside in type 2 diabetic subjects," *Metabolism* 53, no. 1 (2004): 73–76.

28. T. H. Chen et al., "Mechanism of the hypoglycemic effect of stevioside, a glycoside of *Stevia rebaudiana*," *Planta Medica* 71, no. 2 (2005): 108–13.

29. J. C. Chang et al., "Increase of insulin sensitivity by stevioside in fructose-rich chow-fed rats," *Hormone and Metabolic Research* 37, no. 10 (2005): 610–16.

30. C. Boonkaewwan et al., "Anti-inflammatory and immunomodulatory activities of stevioside and its metabolite steviol on THP-1 cells," *Journal of Agricultural Food Chemistry* 54, no. 3 (2006): 785–89.

31. W. Hassinger et al., "The effects of equal caloric amounts of xylitol, sucrose and starch on insulin requirements and blood glucose levels in insulin-dependent diabetics," *Diabetologia* 21, no. 1 (1981): 37–40.

32. K. A. Ly et al., "Linear response of mutans streptococci to increas-

ing frequency of xylitol chewing gum use: A randomized controlled trial [ISRCTN43479664]," *BMC Oral Health* 6 (2006): 6.

33. T. Tapiainen et al., "Ultrastructure of Streptococcus pneumoniae after exposure to xylitol," *Journal of Antimicrobial Chemotherapy* 54, no. 1 (2004): 225–28.

34. Xylitol. Code of Federal Regulations, Title 21, Volume 3. U.S. Government Printing Office, 2003: 21CFR172.395.

35. E. K. Dunayer, "Hypoglycemia following canine ingestion of xylitol-containing gum," *Veterinary and Human Toxicology* 46, no. 2 (2004): 87–88.

36. "A scientific review: The role of chromium in insulin resistance," *Diabetes Education* 2004 suppl.: 2–14.

37. W. Mertz, "Chromium in human nutrition: A review," *Journal of Nutrition* 123, no. 4 (1993): 626-633; R. A. Anderson, "Chromium, glucose intolerance and diabetes," *Journal of the American College of Nutrition* 17, no. 6 (1998): 548–55.

38. J. Racek, "Chromium as an essential element," *Casopis Lekaru Ceskych* 142, no. 6 (2003): 335–39; R. S. Lucidi et al., "Effect of chromium supplementation on insulin resistance and ovarian and menstrual cyclicity in women with polycystic ovary syndrome," *Fertility and Sterility* 84, no. 6 (2005): 1755–57.

39. H. Wang et al., "Cellular chromium enhances activation of insulin receptor kinase," *Biochemistry* 44, no. 22 (2005): 8167–75.

40. S. K. Jain et al., "Trivalent chromium inhibits protein glycosylation and lipid peroxidation in high glucose-treated erythrocytes," *Antioxidants and Redox Signaling* 8, nos. 1–2 (2006): 238–241.

41. M. Z. Mehdi et al., "Insulin signal mimicry as a mechanism for the insulin-like effects of vanadium," *Cell Biochemistry and Biophysiology* 44, no. 1 (2006): 73–81.

42. K. A. Jelveh et al., "Inhibition of cyclic AMP dependent protein kinase by vanadyl sulfate," *Journal of Biological Inorganic Chemistry* 11, no. 3 (2006): 379–88.

43. K. M. Wasan et al., "Differences in plasma homocysteine levels between Zucker fatty and Zucker diabetic fatty rats following 3 weeks oral administration of organic vanadium compounds," *Journal of Trace Elements in Medicine and Biology* 19, no. 4 (2006): 251–58.

44. G. Boden et al., "Effects of vanadyl sulfate on carbohydrate and lipid metabolism in patients with non-insulin-dependent diabetes mellitus," *Metabolism* 45, no. 9 (1996): 1130–35.

45. V. Kagan et al., "Antioxidant action of thioctic acid and dihydrolipoic acid," *Free Radical Biology and Medicine* 9S (1990): 15.

46. A. E. Midaoui and J. de Champlain, "Effects of glucose and insulin on the development of oxidative stress and hypertension in animal models of type 1 and type 2 diabetes," *Journal of Hypertension* 23, no. 3 (2005): 581–88.

47. S. Jacob et al., "The antioxidant alpha-lipoic acid enhances insulin-stimulated glucose metabolism in insulin-resistant rat skeletal muscle," *Diabetes* 45, no. 8 (1996): 1024–29.

48. W. J. Lee et al., "Alpha-lipoic acid increases insulin sensitivity by activating AMPK in skeletal muscle," *Biochemical and Biophysical Research Communications* 332, no. 3 (2005): 885–91.

49. S. Sola et al., "Irbesartan and lipoic acid improve endothelial function

and reduce markers of inflammation in the metabolic syndrome: Results of the Irbesartan and Lipoic Acid in Endothelial Dysfunction (ISLAND) study," *Circulation* 111, no. 3 (2005): 343–48.

50. J. Zempleni, "Lipoic acid reduces the activities of biotin-dependent carboxylases in rat liver," *Journal of Nutrition* 127, no. 9 (1997): 1776–81.

51. K. S. Mhasker and J. F. Caius, "A study of Indian medicinal plants. II. *Gymnema sylvestre* R.Br.," *Indian Journal of Medical Research Memoirs* 16 (1930): 2–75.

52. I. Kimura, "Medical benefits of using natural compounds and their derivatives having multiple pharmacological actions," *Yakugaku Zasshi* [Journal of the Pharmaceutical Society of Japan] 126, no. 3 (2006): 133–43.

53. E. R. Shanmugasundaram et al., "Possible regeneration of the islets of Langerhans in streptozotocin diabetic rats given *Gymnema sylvestre* leaf extracts," *Journal of Ethnopharmacology* 30, no. 3 (1990): 265–79.

54. S. Gholap and A. Kar, "Effects of *Inula racemosa* root and *Gymnema sylvestre* leaf extracts in the regulation of corticosteroid induced diabetes mellitus: Involvement of thyroid hormones," *Pharmazie* 58, no. 6 (2003): 413–15.

55. T. Nakagawa et al., "A causal role for uric acid in fructose-induced metabolic syndrome," *American Journal of Physiology: Renal Physiology* 290, no. 3 (2006): F625–31.

56. B. Levi and M. J. Werman, "Long-term fructose consumption accelerates glycation and several age-related variables in male rats," *Journal of Nutrition* 128, no. 9 (1998): 1442–49.

57. J. P. Bantle et al., "Effects of dietary fructose on plasma lipids in healthy subjects," *American Journal of Clinical Nutrition* 72, no. 5 (2000): 1128–34.

58. P. J. Havel, "Dietary fructose: Implications for dysregulation of energy homeostasis and lipid/carbohydrate metabolism," *Nutrition Reviews* 63, no. 5 (2005): 133–57.

59. D. B. Milne and F. H. Nielsen, "The interaction between dietary fructose and magnesium adversely affects macromineral homeostasis in men," *Journal of the American College of Nutrition* 19, no. 1 (2000): 31–37.

60. A. R. Gaby, "Adverse effects of dietary fructose," *Alternative Medicine Review* 10, no. 4 (2005): 294–306.

61. H. G. Preuss et al., "Effects of a natural extract of (-)-hydroxycitric acid (HCA-SX) and a combination of HCA-SX plus niacin-bound chromium and *Gymnema sylvestre* extract on weight loss," *Diabetes, Obesity and Metabolism* 6, no. 3 (2004): 171–80.

62. R. K. Satdive et al., "Antimicrobial activity of *Gymnema sylvestre* leaf extract," *Fitoterapia* 74, nos. 7–8 (2003): 699–701.

63. B. Khan B et al., "Hypogylcemic activity of aqueous extract of some indigenous plants," *Pakistan Journal of Pharmaceutical Sciences* 18, no. 1 (2005): 62–64.

64. B. A. Reyes et al., "Anti-diabetic potentials of *Momordica charantia* and *Andrographis paniculata* and their effects on estrous cyclicity of alloxan-induced diabetic rats," *Journal of Ethnopharmacology* 105, nos. 1–2 (2006): 196–200.

65. L. L. Chan et al., "Reduced adiposity in bitter melon (*Momordica charantia*)-fed rats is associated with increased lipid oxidative enzyme activities and uncoupling protein expression," *Journal of Nutrition* 135, no. 11 (2005): 2517–23.

66. A. Tongia et al., "Phytochemical determination and extraction of

Momordica charantia fruit and its hypoglycemic potentiation of oral hypoglycemic drugs in diabetes mellitus (NIDDM)," *Indian Journal of Physiology and Pharmacology* 48, no. 2 (2004): 241–44.

67. C. C. Jimenez, "Diabetes and exercise: The role of the athletic trainer,"
Journal of Athletic Training 32, no. 4 (1997): 339–43.

Chapter 6. Overcome a Sluggish Thyroid

1. G. J. Canaris et al., "The Colorado Thyroid Disease Prevalence Study,"
Archives of Internal Medicine 160, no. 4 (2000): 526–34.

2. M. Imaizumi et al., "Radiation dose-response relationships for thyroid
nodules and autoimmune thyroid diseases in Hiroshima and Nagasaki atomic
bomb survivors 55–58 years after radiation exposure," *Journal of the American
Medical Association* 295, no. 9 (2006): 1011–22.

3. I. V. Tereshchenko et al., "Trace elements and endemic goiter" [in Rus-
sian], *Klinicheskaia Meditsina* 82, no. 1 (2004): 62–68.

4. M. Yaman, "The improvement of sensitivity in lead and cadmium deter-
minations using flame atomic absorption spectrometry," *Annals of Biochemistry*
339, no. 1 (2005): 1–8.

5. L. Takser et al., "Thyroid hormones in pregnancy in relation to environmental exposure to organochlorine compounds and mercury," *Environmental
Health Perspectives* 113, no. 8 (2005): 1039–45.

6. O. E. Paynter et al., "Goitrogens and thyroid follicular cell neoplasia:
Evidence for a threshold process," *Regulatory Toxicology and Pharmacology* 8, no.
1 (1988): 102–19.

7. M. Messina and G. Redmond, "Effects of soy protein and soybean isofla-
vones on thyroid function in healthy adults and hypothyroid patients: A review
of the relevant literature," *Thyroid* 16, no. 3 (2006): 249–58.

8. M. A. Michalaki et al., "Thyroid function in humans with morbid obesity," *Thyroid* 16, no. 1 (2006): 73–78.

9. R. Bunevicius et al., "Effects of thyroxine as compared with thyroxine
plus triiodothyronine in patients with hypothyroidism," *New England Journal of
Medicine* 340, no. 6 (1999): 424–29.

10. U. C. Goswami and S. Choudhury, "The status of retinoids in women
suffering from hyper- and hypothyroidism: Interrelationship between vitamin
A, beta-carotene and thyroid hormones," *International Journal for Vitamin and
Nutrition Research* 69, no. 2 (1999): 132–35; D. Aktuna et al., "Beta-carotene,
vitamin A and carrier proteins in thyroid diseases," *Acta Medica Austriaca* 20,
nos. 1–2 (1993): 17–20.

11. S. J. Zhao et al., "Experimental study on effects of iodine deficiency and
excess on thyroid autoimmunity," *Chinese Journal of Preventive Medicine* 40, no. 1
(2006): 18–20.

12. A. J. Seal et al., "Excess dietary iodine intake in long-term African refu-
gees," *Public Health Nutrition* 9, no. 1 (2006): 35–39.

13. S. A. Evans et al., "Regulation of metabolic rate and substrate utilization
by zinc deficiency," *Metabolism* 53, no. 6 (2004): 727–32.

14. C. Coudray et al., "Introduction to the ZENITH study and summary
of baseline results," *European Journal of Clinical Nutrition* 59, suppl. 2 (2005):
S5–S7.

15. C. Feillet-Coudray et al., "Long-term moderate zinc supplementation increases exchangeable zinc pool masses in late-middle-aged men: The ZENITH Study," *American Journal of Clinical Nutrition* 82, no. 1 (2005): 103–10.

16. S. A. Evans et al., "Regulation of metabolic rate and substrate utilization by zinc deficiency," *Metabolism* 53, no. 6 (2004): 727–32.

17. B. Contempre et al., "Effect of selenium supplementation in hypothyroid subjects of an iodine and selenium deficient area: The possible danger of indiscriminate supplementation of iodine-deficient subjects with selenium," *Journal of Clinical Endocrinology and Metabolism*, 73, no. 1 (1991): 213–15.

18. C. S. Hotz et al., "Dietary iodine and selenium interact to affect thyroid hormone metabolism of rats," *Journal of Nutrition* 127, no. 6 (1997): 1214–18.

19. M. H. Eftekhari et al., "The relationship between iron status and thyroid hormone concentration in iron-deficient adolescent Iranian girls," *Asia Pacific Journal of Clinical Nutrition* 15, no. 1 (2006): 50–55.

20. M. B. Zimmerman, "The influence of iron status on iodine utilization and thyroid function," *Annual Review of Nutrition* 26 (2006): 367–89.

21. C. M. Hansen, "Oral iron supplements," *American Pharmacy* NS34, no. 3 (1994): 66–71.

22. D. Casparis et al., "Effectiveness and tolerability of oral liquid ferrous gluconate in iron-deficiency anemia in pregnancy and in the immediate postpartum period: Comparison with other liquid or solid formulations containing bivalent or trivalent iron," [in Italian] *Minerva Ginecologica* 48, no. 11 (1996): 511–18.

23. Y. B. Tripathi et al., "Thyroid-stimulatory action of (Z)-guggulsterone: Mechanism of action," *Planta Medica* 54, no. 4 (1988): 271–77.

24. N. A. Tritos and E. G. Kokkotou, "The physiology and potential clinical applications of ghrelin, a novel peptide hormone," *Mayo Clinic Proceedings* 81, no. 5 (2006): 653–60.

25. M. Owecki and J. Sowinski, "Adiponectin and its role in the pathogenesis of obesity, diabetes mellitus and insulin resistance," [in Polish] *Polski Merkuriusz Lekarski* 20, no. 117 (2006): 355–57.

26. T. T. Antunes et al., "Thyroid-stimulating hormone stimulates interleukin-6 release from 3T3-L1 adipocytes through a cAMP-protein kinase A pathway," *Obesity Research* 13, no. 12 (2005): 2066–71; B. Saunier et al., "Cyclic AMP regulation of Gs protein: Thyrotropin and forskolin increase the quantity of stimulatory guanine nucleotide-binding proteins in cultured thyroid follicles," *Journal of Biological Chemistry* 265, no. 32 (1990): 19942–46; P. P. Roger et al., "Regulation of dog thyroid epithelial cell cycle by forskolin: An adenylate cyclase activator," *Experimental Cell Research* 172, no. 2 (1990): 282–92; B. Haye et al., "Chronic and acute effects of forskolin on isolated thyroid cell metabolism," *Molecular and Cellular Endocrinology* 43, no. 1 (1990): 41–50.

Chapter 7. Break Food Allergies and Addictions

1. P. Humbert et al., "Gluten intolerance and skin diseases," *European Journal of Dermatology* 16, no. 1 (2006): 4–11; P. J. Ciclitira et al., "The pathogenesis of coeliac disease," *Molecular Aspects of Medicine* 26, no. 6 (2005): 421–58; S. Jacob et al., "Gluten sensitivity and neuromyelitis optica: Two case reports,"

Journal of Neurology, Neurosurgery, and Psychiatry 76, no. 7 (2005): 1028–30.

2. G. J. Wang et al., "Similarity between obesity and drug addiction as assessed by neurofunctional imaging: A concept review," *Journal of Addictive Diseases* 23, no. 3 (2004): 39–53.

3. T. T. Macdonald and G. Monteleone, "Immunity, inflammation, and allergy in the gut," *Science* 307, no. 5717 (2005): 1920–25.

4. K. J. Simansky, "NIH symposium series: Ingestive mechanisms in obesity, substance abuse and mental disorders. *Physiology and Behavior* 86, nos. 1–2 (2005): 1–4.

5. M. Lessner, *Nutrition and Vitamin Therapy* (Berkeley, CA: Parker House, 1982).

6. M. T. Cabyoglu et al., "The treatment of obesity by acupuncture," *International Journal of Neuroscience* 116, no. 2 (2006): 165–75.

7. K. C. Otto, "Acupuncture and substance abuse: A synopsis, with indications for further research," *American Journal on Addictions* 12, no. 1 (2003): 43–51.

8. Roberta Wilson. *Aromatherapy for Vibrant Health and Beauty* (Garden City Park, NY: Avery Publishing, 1994), 99.

Chapter 8. Individualize Your Diet

1. Swami Sada Shiva Tirtha, *The Ayurveda Encyclopedia: Natural Secrets to Healing, Prevention, and Longevity* (Bayville, NY: Ayurveda Holistic Center Press, 1998), introduction to chapter 1.

2. United Blood Services, "Human blood types," available at www.united-bloodservices.org/humanbloodtypes.html.

3. W. E. Connor et al., "Benefits and hazards of dietary carbohydrate," *Current Atherosclerosis Reports* 7, no. 6 (2005): 428–34.

4. C. D. Gardner et al., "The effect of a plant-based diet on plasma lipids in hypercholesterolemic adults: A randomized trial," *Annals of Internal Medicine* 142, no. 9 (2005): 725–33.

5. E. J. Schaefer et al., "The effects of low-fat, high-carbohydrate diets on plasma lipoproteins, weight loss, and heart disease risk reduction," *Current Atherosclerosis Reports* 7, no. 6 (2005): 421-27.

6. C. Erlanson-Albertsson and J. Mei, "The effect of low carbohydrate on energy metabolism," *International Journal of Obesity* 29, suppl. 2 (2005): S26–30.

7. J. S. Volek and R. D. Feinman, "Carbohydrate restriction improves the features of metabolic syndrome. Metabolic syndrome may be defined by the response to carbohydrate restriction," *Nutrition and Metabolism* 16, no. 2 (2005): 31.

8. D. Giugliano and K. Esposito, "Mediterranean diet and cardiovascular health," *Annals of the New York Academy of Science* 1056 (2005): 253–60.

9. P. Kris-Etherton et al., "AHA science advisory: Lyon Diet Heart Study: Benefits of a Mediterranean-style, National Cholesterol Education Program/ American Heart Association Step I dietary pattern on cardiovascular disease," *Circulation* 103, no. 13 (2001): 1823–25.

10. G. Flynn and D. Colquhoun, "Successful long-term weight loss with a Mediterranean style diet in a primary care medical centre," *Asia Pacific Journal of Clinical Nutrition* 13, suppl. (2004): S139.

Chapter 9. Supplements for Weight Loss

1. L. Gillis and A. Gillis, "Nutrient inadequacy in obese and non-obese youth," *Canadian Journal of Dietary Practice and Research* 66, no. 4 (2005): 237–42.

2. S. J. Nielsen and B. M. Popkin, "Changes in beverage intake between 1977 and 2001," *American Journal of Preventive Medicine* 27, no. 3 (2004): 205–10.

3. Paul Bergner, *The Healing Power of Minerals: Special Nutrients and Trace Minerals* (Rocklin, CA: Prima, 1997), 68–75.

4. K. J. Rothman et al., "Teratogenicity of high vitamin A intake," *New England Journal of Medicine* 333, no. 21 (1995): 1369–73.

5. "Don't overlook niacin for treating cholesterol problems," *Harvard Heart Letter* 14, no. 8 (2004): 4–5.

6. R. B. Norris, "'Flush-free niacin': Dietary supplement may be 'benefit-free,'" *Preventive Cardiology* 9, no. 1 (2006): 64–65.

7. M. R. Werbach, *Nutritional Influences on Illness* (Tarzana, CA: Third Line Press, 1993).

8. C. T. Wittwer et al., "Mild pantothenate deficiency in rats elevates serum triglyceride and free fatty acid levels," *Journal of Nutrition* 120, no. 7 (1990): 719–25.

9. L. H. Leung, "Pantothenic acid as a weight-reducing agent: Fasting without hunger, weakness and ketosis," *Medical Hypotheses* 44, no. 5 (1995): 403–05.

10. V. Teplan et al., "Obesity and hyperhomocysteinaemia after kidney transplantation," *Nephrology, Dialysis, Transplantation* 18, suppl. 5 (2003): v71–73.

11. M. Cohen and A. Bendich. "Safety of pyridoxine: A review of human and animal studies," *Toxicology Letters* 34, no. 2–3 (1986): 129–39.

12. Stephen Langer and James F. Scheer, *Solved: The Riddle of Weight Loss* (Rochester, VT: Healing Arts Press, 1989), 67.

13. D. Canoy D et al., "Plasma ascorbic acid concentrations and fat distribution in 19,068 British men and women in the European Prospective Investigation into Cancer and Nutrition Norfolk cohort study," *American Journal of Clinical Nutrition* 82, no. 6 (2005): 1203–9.

14. Frank Murray, "Advanced new form of vitamin C: Ester C," *Better Nutrition for Today's Living* (January 1993).

15. M. Levine et al., "Vitamin C pharmacokinetics in healthy volunteers: Evidence for a recommended dietary allowance," *Proceedings of the National Academy of Sciences* 93, no. 8 (1996): 3704–9.

16. Tamas Decsi et al., "Obese kids can lack antioxidants," *Journal of Pediatrics* 130 (1997), 653–55.

17. B. Eaton and D. A. Nelson, "Calcium in evolutionary perspective," *American Journal of Clinical Nutrition* 54, suppl. 1 (1991): 281S–87S.

18. M. B. Zemel et al., "Calcium and dairy acceleration of weight and fat loss during energy restriction in obese adults," *Obesity Research* 12, no. 4. (2004): 582–90.

19. S. A. Shapses et al., "Effect of calcium supplementation on weight and fat loss in women," *Journal of Clinical Endocrinology and Metabolism* 89, no. 2 (2004): 632–37.

20. M. B. Zemel, "The role of dairy foods in weight management," *Journal of the American College of Nutrition* 24, suppl. 6 (2005): 537S–46S.

21. Betty Kamen, *The Chromium Connection* (Novato, CA: Nutrition Encounter, 1992), 118.

22. G. R. Kaats et al., "A randomized, double-masked, placebo-controlled study of the effects of chromium picolinate supplementation on body composition: A replication and extension of a previous study," *Current Therapeutic Research* 59 (1998): 379–88.

23. B. L. Creech et al., "Effect of dietary trace mineral concentration and source (inorganic vs. chelated) on performance, mineral status, and fecal mineral excretion in pigs from weaning through finishing," *Journal of Animal Science* 82, no. 7 (2004): 2140–47.

24. Michael A. Schmidt and Jeffrey Bland, "Thyroid gland as sentinel: Interface between internal and external environment," *Alternative Therapies* 3, no. 1 (1997): 78–81.

25. J. Beard et al., "Changes in iron status during weight-loss with very-low-energy diets," *American Journal of Clinical Nutrition* 66, no. 1 (1997): 104–10.

26. J. T. Salonen et al., "High stored iron levels are associated with excess risk of myocardial infarction in eastern Finnish men," *Circulation* 86, no. 3 (1992): 803–11.

27. L. H. Duntas et al., "Kinetics and effects of selenomethionine in patients with autoimmune thyroiditis," *Journal of Endocrinological Investigation* 25, suppl. to no. 7 (2002): 21.

28. C. Chen et al., "The roles of serum selenium and selenoproteins on mercury toxicity in environmental and occupational exposure," *Environmental Health Perspectives* 114, no. 2 (2006): 297–301.

29. U.S. Centers for Disease Control, "Selenium intoxication," *Morbidity and Mortality Weekly Report* 33 (1984): 157.

30. J. R. Hunt, "Bioavailability of iron, zinc, and other trace minerals from vegetarian diets," *American Journal of Clinical Nutrition* 78, suppl. 3 (2003): 633S–39S.

31. M. Al-Qunaibit et al., "The effect of solvents on metal ion adsorption by the alga *Chlorella vulgaris*," *Chemosphere* 60, no. 3 (2005): 412–18.

32. J. Simpore et al., "Nutrition rehabilitation of undernourished children utilizing Spiruline and Misola," *Nutrition Journal* 5 (2006): 3.

33. L. K. Han et al., "Isolation of pancreatic lipase activity-inhibitory component of *Spirulina platensis* and it reduce postprandial triacylglycerolemia," [in Japanese] *Yakugaku Zasshi* [Journal of the Pharmaceutical Society of Japan] 126, no. 1 (2006): 43–49.

34. K. Jeyaprakash and P. Chinnaswamy, "Effect of spirulina and Liv-52 on cadmium induced toxicity in albino rats," *Indian Journal of Experimental Biology* 43, no. 9 (2005): 773–81.

35. A. D. Liese et al., "Dietary glycemic index and glycemic load, carbohydrate and fiber intake, and measures of insulin sensitivity, secretion, and adiposity in the Insulin Resistance Atherosclerosis Study," *Diabetes Care* 28, no. 12 (2005): 2832–38.

36. N. C. Howarth et al., "Dietary fiber and weight regulation," *Nutrition Review* 59, no. 5 (2001): 129–39.

37. K. I. Inokuma et al., "Indispensable role of mitochondrial uncoupling protein 1(UCP1) for anti-obesity effect of 3-adrenergic stimulation," *American Journal of Physiology, Endocrinology, and Metabolism* 290, no. 5 (2005): E1014–E1021.

38. A. S. Avram et al., "Subcutaneous fat in normal and diseased states: 2. Anatomy and physiology of white and brown adipose tissue," *Journal of the American Academy of Dermatology* 53, no. 4 (2005): 671–83.

39. Laura Austgen, "Brown adipose tissue," *Hypertexts for Biomedical Sciences* August 8, 2002, available at http://arbl.cvmbs.colostate.edu/hbooks/pathphys/misc_topics/brownfat.html.

40. A. M. Valverde and M. Benito, "The brown adipose cell: A unique model for understanding the molecular mechanism of insulin resistance," *Mini Reviews in Medical Chemistry* 5, no. 3 (2005): 269–78.

41. J. Himms-Hagen, "Exercise in a pill: Feasibility of energy expenditure targets," *Current Drug Targets: CNS and Neurological Disorders* 3, no. 5 (2004): 389–409.

42. M. Yoshioka et al., "Combined effects of red pepper and caffeine consumption on 24 h energy balance in subjects given free access to foods," *British Journal of Nutrition* 85, no. 2 (2001): 203–11; M. Yoshioka et al., "Effects of red pepper on appetite and energy intake," *British Journal of Nutrition* 82, no. 2 (1999): 115–23.

43. S. Renault et al., "CAY-1, a novel antifungal compound from cayenne pepper," *Medical Mycology* 41, no. 1 (2003): 75–81.

44. C. S. Coffey et al., "A randomized double-blind placebo-controlled clinical trial of a product containing ephedrine, caffeine, and other ingredients from herbal sources for treatment of overweight and obesity in the absence of lifestyle treatment," *International Journal of Obesity and Related Metabolic Disorders* 28, no. 11 (2004): 1411–19.

45. C. N. Boozer et al., "Herbal ephedra/caffeine for weight loss: A 6-month randomized safety and efficacy trial," *International Journal of Obesity and Related Metabolic Disorders* 26, no. 5 (2002): 593–604.

46. F. Charatan, "Ephedra supplement may have contributed to sportsman's death," *British Medical Journal* 326, no. 7487 (2003): 464.

47. S. Haaz et al., "*Citrus aurantium* and synephrine alkaloids in the treatment of overweight and obesity: An update," *Obesity Review* 7, no. 1 (2006): 79–88.

48. L. T. Bui et al., "Blood pressure and heart rate effects following a single dose of bitter orange," *Annals of Pharmacotherapy* 40, no. 1 (2006): 53–57.

49. Y. Oi et al., "Garlic supplementation enhances norepinephrine secretion, growth of brown adipose tissue, and triglyceride catabolism in rats," *Journal of Nutritional Biochemistry* 6, no. 5 (1995): 250–255.

50. A. Elkayam et al., "The effects of allicin on weight in fructose-induced hyperinsulinemic, hyperlipidemic, hypertensive rats," *American Journal of Hypertension* 16, no. 12 (2003): 1053–56.

51. S. H. Kim et al., "Effects of *Panax ginseng* extract on exercise-induced oxidative stress," *Journal of Sports Medicine and Physical Fitness* 45, no. 2, (2005): 178–82.

52. J. H. Kim et al., "Effect of crude saponin of Korean red ginseng on high-fat diet-induced obesity in the rat," *Journal of Pharmacological Sciences* 97, no. 1 (2005): 124–31.

53. L. Dey et al., "Anti-hyperglycemic effects of ginseng: Comparison between root and berry," *Phytomedicine* 10, nos. 6–7 (2003): 600–5.

54. M. S. Westerterp-Plantenga et al., "Body weight loss and weight maintenance in relation to habitual caffeine intake and green tea supplementation," *Obesity Research* 13, no. 7 (2005): 1195–1204.

55. A. G. Dulloo et al., "Efficacy of a green tea extract rich in catechin polyphenols and caffeine in increasing 24-h energy expenditure and fat oxidation in humans," *American Journal of Clinical Nutrition* 70 (1999): 1040–45.

56. C. Juhel et al., "Green tea extract (AR25) inhibits lipolysis of triglycerides in gastric and duodenal medium in vitro," *Journal of Nutritional Biochemistry* 11, no. 1 (2000): 45–51.

57. J. Lin et al., "Green tea polyphenol epigallocatechin gallate inhibits adipogenesis and induces apoptosis in 3T3-L1 adipocytes," *Obesity Research* 13, no. 6 (2005): 982–90.

58. Y. Lu et al., "Fluoride content in tea and its relationship with tea quality," "Journal of Agricultural and Food Chemistry," 52, no. 14 (2004): 4472–76.

59. D. B. MacLean and L. G. Luo, "Increased ATP content/production in the hypothalamus may be a signal for energy-sensing of satiety: Studies of the anorectic mechanism of a plant steroidal glycoside," *Brain Research* 1020, nos. 1–2 (2004): 1–11.

60. M. S. Kim et al., "Anti-adipogenic effects of Garcinia extract on the lipid droplet accumulation and the expression of transcription factor," *Biofactors* 22, nos. 1–4 (2004): 193–96.

61. D. W. Foster, "The role of the carnitine system in human metabolism," *Annals of the New York Academy of Sciences* 1033 (Nov. 2004): 1–16.

62. C. Brandsch and K. Eder, "Effect of L-carnitine on weight loss and body composition of rats fed a hypocaloric diet," *Annals of Nutrition and Metabolism* 46, no. 5 (2002): 205–10; R. G. Villani et al., "L-carnitine supplementation combined with aerobic training does not promote weight loss in moderately obese women," *International Journal of Sports Nutrition and Exercise Metabolism* 10, no. 2 (2000): 199–207.

63. D. S. Sachan et al., "Decreasing oxidative stress with choline and carnitine in women," *Journal of the American College of Nutrition* 24, no. 3 (2005): 172–76.

64. H. Karlicand and A. Lohninger. "Supplementation of L-carnitine in athletes: Does it make sense?" *Nutrition* 20, nos. 7–8 (2004): 709–715.

65. E. Thom et al., "Conjugated linoleic acid reduces body fat in healthy exercising humans," *Journal of Internal Medicine Research* 29, no. 5 (2001): 392–96; J. M. Gaullier et al., "Conjugated linoleic acid supplementation for 1 y reduces body fat mass in healthy overweight humans," *American Journal of Clinical Nutrition* 79, no. 6 (2004): 1118–25.

66. V. Mougios et al., "Effect of supplementation with conjugated linoleic acid on human serum lipids and body fat," *Journal of Nutritional Biochemistry* 12, no. 10 (2001): 585–94; K. L. Zambell et al., "Conjugated linoleic acid supplementation in humans: Effects on body composition and energy expenditure," *Lipids* 35, no. 7 (2000): 777–82.

67. F. Moloney et al., "Conjugated linoleic acid supplementation, insulin sensitivity, and lipoprotein metabolism in patients with type 2 diabetes mellitus," *American Journal of Clinical Nutrition* 80, no. 4 (2004): 887–95.

68. J. M. Arbones-Mainar et al., "Trans-10, cis-12- and cis-9, trans-11-conju-

gated linoleic acid isomers selectively modify HDL-apolipoprotein composition in apolipoprotein E knockout mice," *Journal of Nutrition* 136, no. 2 (2006): 353–59.

69. D. S. Kalman et al., "A randomized, double-blind, placebo-controlled study of 3-acetyl-7-oxo-dehydroepiandrosterone in healthy overweight adults," *Current Therapeutic Research* 61 (2000): 435–42.

70. J. Keithley and B. Swanson, "Glucomannan and obesity: A critical review," *Alternative Therapies in Health and Medicine* 11, no. 6 (2005): 30–34.

71. V. Vuksan et al., "Konjac-mannan (glucomannan) improves glycemia and other associated risk factors for coronary heart disease in type 2 diabetes: A randomized controlled metabolic trial," *Diabetes Care* 22, no. 6 (1999): 913–19.

72. R. T. Stanko et al., "Pyruvate supplementation of a low-cholesterol, low-fat diet: Effects on plasma lipid concentration and body composition in hyperlipidemic patients," *American Journal of Clinical Nutrition* 59, no. 2 (1994): 423–27; D. Kalman et al., "The effects of pyruvate supplementation on body composition in overweight individuals," *Nutrition* 15, no. 5 (1999): 337–40.

73. P. K. Koh-Banerjee et al., "Effects of calcium pyruvate supplementation during training on body composition, exercise capacity, and metabolic responses to exercise," *Nutrition* 21, no. 3 (2005): 312–19.

74. P. Koh et al., "Effects of pyruvate supplementation during training on hematologic and metabolic profiles," *Medicine and Science in Sports and Exercise* 30 (1998): S62.

75. M. Dufer et al., "Methyl pyruvate stimulates pancreatic beta-cells by a direct effect on KATP channels, and not as a mitochondrial substrate," *Biochemical Journal* 368, part 3 (2002): 817–25.

Index

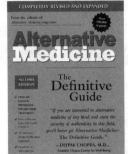
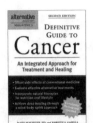

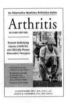
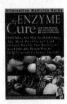
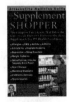
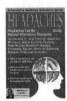

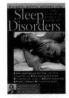

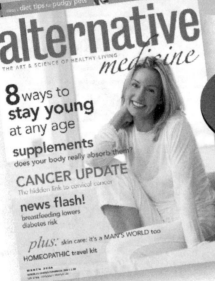